Tarnished Gold

The Sickness of Evidence-Based Medicine

Steve Hickey PhD

and

Hilary Roberts PhD

Consider two physicians, A and B:

A is a conventional physician, he diagnoses ailments on the basis of what he has learned in school, what he has read about and his experience in treating patients.

B is not a conventional physician. He is 'objective' [using evidence-based medicine]. His [clinically proven] diagnosis is entirely 'by the book' - things he has learned in school that are universally accepted. He tries as hard as he can to make his judgements free of any bias that might be brought about by his own experience in treating patients.

As a lawyer, I might prefer defending B's decisions in court, but as a patient, I would prefer A's intelligently biased diagnosis and treatment.

Ray Solomonoff

Copyright Steve Hickey and Hilary Roberts (2011). All rights reserved. The authors assert their moral rights to the book and its content. All trademarks are acknowledged.

Preface

Medicine is a science of uncertainty and an art of probability.

Sir William Osler

Our aim in this book is to present an argument that is accessible to a general reader. The ideas presented are subtle and might have been expressed more precisely using mathematics. Nevertheless, we decided to write the book in a relatively simple style, without recourse to equations or mathematical treatment.

We have tried to present sophisticated concepts in the areas of mathematics, theoretical computer science, and decision science, without resorting to confusing nomenclature or jargon. We hope readers will find they have followed the complex ideas without too much effort. A word of warning: some of our examples, though amusing, are fiendishly difficult to understand. This is deliberate, so we ask the reader not to worry! The point we are making is that since even leading mathematicians have misunderstood superficially simple experiments, the massive complexity of evidence-based medicine (EBM) is self-defeating. We have included a summary of important points at the end of each chapter.

We ask mathematically and statistically expert readers to bear with the simplifications. Parts of the text are novel and involve a high degree of sophistication. Keep with the text, for we hope that you will realise the profound implications. One of our reviewers confirmed our analysis of the probability problems was correct but warned us to expect many emails on the topic. However, we can simply state that if your interpretation of, say, the Monte Hall problem differs from ours, you have joined numerous mathematicians and scientists in indirectly making our point. Even simple probability problems are hard to understand and this has profound implications for the mega-studies of evidence-based medicine.

This book covers a broad range of topics, from a collection of sciences. While medicine is a central theme, we necessarily cover aspects of decision science and the scientific method. We hope medical readers will tolerate the seemingly irrelevant puzzles, descriptions of simplicity, and the information content of a sentence; be patient, we will eventually relate these theoretical concepts to practical medicine. In addition to the background theory, some sections deal with the current practice of evidence-based medicine. EBM as presently implemented is not what is claimed in the hype that surrounds it.

On occasion, we use the word *belief* to express an appreciation of the evidence. Belief, in this context, does not imply irrationally holding a point of view in the absence of supporting data. Similarly, we criticize the use of the word *best*, as in "best evidence", as often being meaningless or worse. Best means optimal and refers to a specific criterion. Nevertheless, in evidence-based medicine, its use is misleading. For simplicity, we have tried to use the word only where the meaning is clear.

Throughout the text, we have scattered quotations for fun and illumination. Partly, they have been included as an invitation to think more deeply about the issues. Sometimes they are there to break up sophisticated arguments and give the reader a rest. Some of the quotations are from J.E.H. Shaw's *Some Quotable Quotes for Statistics*. Similarly, we have broken chapters into short sections, so the book can be read in segments. If you do not understand a section, don't worry—just read over it lightly and then continue. If in doubt, you can always return and study it in detail. The overall picture will emerge, as it does not depend on the detail.

Often, we return to demonstrate a point using a different approach. The foundations of EBM break the scientific rules of several disciplines. It is reassuring to know that the limitations of EBM can be illustrated in several different ways. We hope readers will realise that the apparent repetition is part of the story.

We may have been somewhat *laissez-faire* with our definitions of random, chance, probability, and similar technical terms. The meaning should be clear from the context. Similarly, we use the terms meta-analysis and systematic review interchangeably, as is often the case in normal discussion. Meta-analysis is a statistical technique often employed to combine data from various studies in a systematic review of the literature. This book describes how even the simplest experiment is profoundly difficult to analyse with EBM's standard "frequentist" statistics. We suggest the use of Bayesian statistics, decision trees, and heuristics (rules of thumb) to overcome this and other confusions. In particular, we describe a simple and inexpensive clinical trial that could be performed by a family doctor, yet is at least as powerful as EBM's mega-trials.

We would like to think that supporters and promoters of EBM will read the book with an open mind. We are fully aware of Upton Sinclair's comment "It is difficult to get a man to understand something, when his salary depends upon his not understanding it." Anyone practicing the current selective evidence-based medicine owes it to their patients to consider its limitations and to substitute a rational approach.

Supporters of evidence-based medicine may consider trying to attack this book and discredit our analysis. We would welcome such attempts; if we are wrong, we would rather know it! We assert that EBM suffers from the accumulation of a series of independent problems, any one of which is sufficient to classify it as a *cargo-cult science*. As readers progress through the text, we trust it will become increasingly clear that EBM is junk science and there is little, if any, prospect of a rational defence of its methods.

As scientists, we have taken the viewpoint of the patient. EBM has developed from organised medicine. Doctors are experts in the field and are able to present their own case for or against EBM. We take the perspective of expert patients, dissatisfied with the approach and progress of so-called evidence-based medicine. Although some of the arguments in this book are theoretical, many are practical and pragmatic. The problems with EBM have real consequences for patients and, at some point, we are all patients.

EBM harms patients and suppresses medical progress. Sometimes, there are duties that people need to carry out; for the authors, writing this book was such a responsibility.

Acknowledgements

> The important thing in science is not so much to obtain new facts as to discover new ways of thinking about them.
>
> Sir William Bragg

This book arose following SH's use of examples from evidence-based medicine to illustrate his lectures on artificial intelligence, cybernetics, and decision making. Many of the pitfalls of decision science were exemplified by the current practice of so-called evidence-based medicine. During this time, Dr Len Noriega helped with background research and discussion of the central points. Students of Artificial Intelligence and Decision Science at Staffordshire University provided feedback in seminars, during which we discussed and clarified many of the issues presented in this book. Professors Hongnian Yu and Bernadette Sharp also provided help and encouragement with aspects of the underlying research.

Andrew Hickey conducted the literature search on inappropriate sampling in the meta-analyses published by the Cochrane Foundation and the Journal of the American Medical Association. He also carried out background checking of the book and proofreading, for which we are most grateful.

The authors would like to thank Dr Gert Schuitemaker and Elsedien de Groot for discussion and assistance in developing the thesis. Thanks to their support, we were also helped by discussion with delegates of the 2008 Anholt meeting on Orthomolecular Medicine. Dr Damien Downing, President of the British Society for Ecological Medicine, provided us with helpful background information, commented on an early version of the book and agreed to provide a short introduction. Stephanie Morgan, Elizabeth Hickey, and Chris Hickey kindly checked the manuscript and the calculations.

Dr Abram Hoffer discussed with us his thoughts concerning the abuse of the scientific method in medicine and the restriction of information by the establishment. Dr Hoffer gave his time in developing his ideas on the limitations of randomized placebo controlled trials; the fact that Hoffer was a pioneer of these clinical trials allowed him a broad perspective of the change in scientific methods over the last 50 years. Our work and discussions with Dr Robert F. Cathcart III and Dr Thomas Levy also stimulated our interest in the lack of rationality in modern statistical medicine.

Dr Olga Gregson and Professor Terry Looker have also given consistent encouragement and the benefit of their knowledge. Over the years, Michael Roberts, retired surgeon, has helped by sharing his viewpoint in detailed discussions and interpretation of medical data. Bill Sardi has generously provided us with insights into the use and abuse of EBM in modern healthcare. We would also like to thank Owen Fonorow, Andrew Saul and Drs Bo Jonsson, John Ely, Carolyn Dean, Erik Paterson, Ralph Campbell, Michael Ellis, Ian Brighthope, and Todd Penberthy.

In the UK, our friends in the British Society for Ecological Medicine have pioneered the use of rational treatment based on a patient's individuality. In Japan, Atsuo Yanagisawa and his colleagues have demonstrated how an individual approach to medicine can function in a technological society. Internationally, Drs Michael Gonzalez, Jorge Miranda-Massari, Jim Jackson, and Ron Hunninghake have been consistent in supporting a more rational approach to medicine. We reserve particular thanks to Karen Davies and Professor David Hukins who inspired us to take an uncompromising rational view as young scientists.

This book depends upon the work of numerous others who we should acknowledge; many are referenced in the text. While we are critical of the core ideas of EBM, there is no implication of disparagement of any particular individual or organisation; everyone is entitled to an opinion and for scientists an individual viewpoint is essential. The diagram of systematic reviews and clinical guidelines is modified, after a US Institute of Medicine image.

Foreword

> Scientific behaviour can be classified as appropriately under cybernetics as under logic.
>
> Sir Peter Medawar

Patient-Based Medicine

Very large trials, statistics, systematic reviews, meta-analyses; evidence-based medicine (EBM) has taken medical science to a new level of clarity—or has it? At last, here are the insights you need to form your own judgement.

Of course I'm biased—I know Hickey and Roberts personally, admire their work, and they are very nice about me in their preface. Now you know that, you can take it into account when you read what I say. What a pity you can't do the same with medical research, or indeed with your doctor's advice. You may think you can, because they tell us that EBM can now provide us with certainty about the effects of treatments, tests, and risk factors on our health. But EBM is about populations, not individuals, so it's useful for governments seeking to regulate us, and for companies seeking to market drugs; it's almost useless in the consulting room, for the doctor and patient trying to decide on the best treatment. People are not widgets, all reacting identically, we are complex and individual, and we need and deserve fully personal care—not guidelines that remove the thinking from medicine.

Read this book to discover some startling facts about EBM, and gain valuable tools in reading and interpreting research. As a doctor or therapist, it will even enable you to do your own small-scale research with direct benefit for your patients. You only need a very large trial to demonstrate a very small effect. This of course is why they do them.

Comparing treatment to a placebo? Unethical, say Hickey and Roberts, and unnecessary; if the treatment were any good they would compare it to the current best treatment. But systematic reviews get rid of all the bias in the research, surely? In fact, they offer an opportunity to introduce new bias; they are another chance to get the result you want from the data.

Read this book and you will see medical research in a new light—a clearer, far more revealing light.

> Dr Damien Downing MB BS MSP, President of the British Society for Ecological Medicine and Former editor of the Journal for Nutritional and Environmental Medicine, Sept 2011.

A Patient's View

The median isn't the message.

Stephen Jay Gould

In late November 2010, I visited my GP as I was suffering from a chest infection. With little meaningful dialogue and without averting his gaze from a computer screen on which my medical history was summarised, he wrote a prescription for an antibiotic. No doubt the drug I was given was "on average" the appropriate one for a member of a population with these symptoms and of my height, weight, age, and star sign. I returned a week later having completed the course of treatment, with no improvement in my condition. This time, the GP looked away from his computer screen and examined my chest with a stethoscope. He wrote another prescription for slightly stronger antibiotics, after a minimal dialogue. Perhaps my hair colour and shoe size had been ignored in assessing the appropriate "on average" drug in the first place! He also gave me a form to get an x-ray at the local hospital. The x-ray revealed that I needed even stronger antibiotics. This third prescription had an effect and a week later I returned to work, having been absent for three weeks.

Had a more individualistic approach to diagnosis been taken at my first visit, it is likely that I would have received appropriate treatment at an earlier stage and been off work for a much shorter period. If my experience is extrapolated across the general population, how great a cost to the economy results from inappropriate treatment? This is in addition to the costs and waste of the unrepeatable and statistically unfathomable clinical trials advocated by "evidence"-based medicine practitioners.

As individual human beings, we are all complex cybernetic systems and are supposed to be autonomous. When confronted with more serious complaints than chest infections, there is an increasing expectation on the part of medical professionals that we take an active role in making decisions about our own treatment. Despite this, the obfuscation of evidence-based medicine makes it impossible for the layman (or in some cases the experienced statistician) to make an informed choice.

This book makes an important case for scientific scepticism and the rehabilitation of cybernetics. With great clarity and economy of expression, the authors summarise two of the more important maxims or dicta of cybernetics: "there is no safety in numbers" and "data is not information." This is achieved in fewer pages than most statistics textbooks usually manage, and with infinitely more transparency than any meta-analysis. It is far too important to ignore.

>	Len Noriega BA MSc PhD LLB MBCS, Staffordshire University, England, Sept, 2011.

Contents

Evidence-based Medicine	13
Populations Are Not People	23
Prove It!	47
Beating the Odds	70
Understanding Results	89
What Is Evidence?	106
The Search for Simplicity	118
Science is Induction	137
Doctoring Evidence	152
Authority	181
Powerfully Deceptive Trials	205
Beyond Right and Wrong	225
Meta-analysis as Pseudoscience	244
Predictable Irrationality	261
Simply Brilliant Heuristics	280
Worshiping a Cult	302
Glossary	315
Index	321

Let us suppose that an ichthyologist is exploring the life of the ocean. He casts a net into the water and brings up a fishy assortment. Surveying his catch, he proceeds in the usual manner of a scientist to systematise what it reveals. He arrives at two generalisations:

(1) No sea-creature is less than two inches long.

(2) All sea-creatures have gills.

These are both true of his catch, and he assumes tentatively that they will remain true however often he repeats it.

In applying this analogy, the catch stands for the body of knowledge which constitutes physical science, and the net for the sensory and intellectual equipment which we use in obtaining it. The casting of the net corresponds to observation; for knowledge which has not been or could not be obtained by observation is not admitted into physical science.

An onlooker may object that the first generalisation is wrong. 'There are plenty of sea-creatures under two inches long, only your net is not adapted to catch them.' The ichthyologist dismisses this objection contemptuously.

'Anything uncatchable by my net is *ipso facto* outside the scope of ichthyologic knowledge.' In short, 'what my net can't catch isn't fish.'

Sir Arthur Eddington[1]

Evidence-based Medicine

> Any intelligent fool can make things bigger and more complex... It takes a touch of genius—and a lot of courage—to move in the opposite direction.
>
> E.F. Schumacher

The phrase "evidence-based medicine" is a wonderful slogan—surely, no reasonable person could object to the idea of medicine based on evidence? This book presents a different view: that medicine should be rational and based on science. Although these approaches to medical science may sound similar, they are mutually exclusive. Our aim is to demonstrate that evidence-based medicine (EBM) is both irrational and unscientific. The explanation involves some fascinating ideas, drawn from mathematics, science, and computing.

Criticism of EBM may be disconcerting to anyone who has taken its claims at face value. Nevertheless, the issue is too important to ignore, as the "evidence-based" culture affects the health of millions. For this reason, we hope you will consider our analysis before making up your mind—you may be surprised by what you read.

Historically, evidence-based medicine grew out of a social studies discipline called clinical epidemiology.[2] The name evidence-based medicine, or EBM, was introduced in about 1991.[3] Such a fantastic slogan could not go to waste and, a year later, the Journal of the American Medical Association (JAMA) launched EBM as a new initiative.[4] Supporters of evidence-based medicine declared it as a new paradigm and a major scientific advance.[5] They claimed the ideal way of making decisions about patients involved selective use of the best evidence from large-scale studies, using techniques derived from social science and statistics.

In 2001, the New York Times Magazine described evidence-based medicine as one of the most influential ideas of the year.[6]

Since then, EBM has been on its way to replacing traditional medicine, which depended on understanding physiology and disease processes. In this new brand of medicine, basic science and clinical experience—previously the bedrock of clinical practice—were relegated to the lower divisions of medical evidence.[5]

The phenomenon of evidence-based medicine expanded rapidly and supporters claimed it as a major advance. An expert panel of the British Medical Journal described it as one of the greatest milestones in medicine since the forerunner of the BMJ was first published, in 1840.[7,8] Nevertheless, it has become apparent that EBM cannot answer many medical problems.[9] With time and experience, EBM has become somewhat less pretentious and a little more practical.[5]

Evidence-based medicine enjoys considerable support from corporate medicine, governments, and the medical establishment. It is of particular use to such organisations, as its statistical approach provides a legal framework that aids the management and governance of medicine. Furthermore, EBM supports the medical industries in offering a structure for the development and introduction of new drugs and treatments.

This book is a direct counter to this dominant ideology. In developing the challenge, we need to state our case clearly and unambiguously. We will often write the term "evidence-based" in quotes, to avoid falling into EBM's marketing trap. We hope to provide a fair appraisal, while specifying a series of fundamental errors.

One aim of this book is to consider whether or not EBM allows patients and doctors to make decisions in a way that provides a near-optimal result for each individual. In seeking a rational approach, it will be necessary to challenge EBM's widely accepted claims of providing "scientific proof" and "gold standard" methods. At first sight, our critiques may appear alarming to readers who support evidence-based medicine; we hope you will approach the issues with an open mind. We are not trying to convert you but merely to deliver sophisticated information in a simple, direct, and understandable way. We hope our readers will put preconceived notions to one side, view statements critically, and think for themselves.

The story of how and why EBM might be flawed is at the heart of this book. We describe a series of problems, each of which raises fundamental issues. An overriding question is whether or not EBM is the method of choice for treating a specific patient.

In particular, we are concerned with the viewpoint of patients who take the time and effort to consider what they need from their medical treatment. We are all patients at some point and, when ill, want to be cured or at least to receive effective treatment. We will demonstrate that "evidence-based" medicine is of little benefit to an individual patient and, when considered rationally, is likely to be rejected by both doctors and patients. We hope that our book may help patients to defend themselves against the overwhelming authority of the medical establishment and its associated industries.

What's in a name?

By adopting the title "evidence-based" medicine, one group of doctors and statisticians sought to appropriate the scientific high ground. Their particular claim of being evidence-based seems to imply that other forms of medicine rest on the shifting sands of prejudice and intuition.

Superficially, the term evidence-based medicine gives the impression of a solid scientific discipline. Nevertheless, there is something odd about this name. If we were to speak of "evidence-based physics", it would sound absurd: physics is a rigorous discipline, based on direct observation and measurement. The phrase "evidence-based physics" amounts to a tautology, as in a "round circle". Similarly, medicine should be a practical discipline, based on scientific observation and experiment. There is only one valid form of medicine, which *must* be based on science. Anything else is not medicine, it is quackery.

What is EBM?

According to a widely quoted definition:

> Evidence based medicine is the conscientious, explicit, and judicious use of current best evidence in making decisions about the care of individual patients.[10]

Before we get round to what EBM is all about, a couple of terms in this definition merit examination. The word *evidence* suggests the information or data that are used to corroborate an idea. Police use the expression during their investigations, as do lawyers, in reference to the testimony given in a court. Indeed, the phrase "evidence-based" medicine sounds legalistic, compared to "data-based" or "science-based" medicine. This is not an accident, since the origins of EBM lie in the legal system, rather than in science. It will become clear that EBM's evidence does not mean scientific information or data, but refers to legal justification.

A second word in the definition leaps out at someone trained in scientific methods, though it is so common the non-scientist may overlook it; that word is *best*. However laudable the aim of basing medical science on the "best evidence" may sound, it is irrational. Used in this manner, *best* is an ill-defined word, since we do not know what criteria determine whether one bit of evidence is better than another. University science students are frequently taken to task for lack of specificity in describing something as "best", so they learn to avoid the word. We will show that in the context of scientific medicine, there is no such thing as best evidence, there is only information.

As we shall see, when making decisions, *all* information is potentially useful and, until you know the answer, it is prudent not to pre-select which evidence you think will be "best". We should point out that in decision science and game theory, the word best is used in determining strategy, or selecting between options. Here "best" is shorthand for choosing an optimal strategy. Having stated the problem, we can reclaim the word; an ideal approach will select the most useful outcome or diagnosis.

EBM: bad for your health

There are currently numerous criticisms of EBM. Dr Des Spence, a general practitioner in Glasgow, Scotland, reported some of these at a recent conference and listed them in the British Medical Journal.[11] His criticisms are well established, and are included here:

Epidemiological Changes

EBM is based on epidemiology, the study of disease in populations or groups. However, the illnesses a population suffers from change with time. Thus, EBM is always out of date. With its cumbersome large-scale trials, EBM is forever fighting the last war, while its adversary moves on.

Commissioning Bias

Unless the research is done, there is no evidence. The hugely expensive scale of EBM trials means that drug companies have a near-monopoly on research. This means that treatment is dominant, whereas prevention is side-lined. Only potentially profitable treatments—mainly those that can be patented—are pursued. Another often-used term for this trend is patentability bias.

Rules of Evidence

EBM creates a reductionist, rule-based approach to medicine. Doctors are often unwilling to go against the "evidence". The freedom of doctors to treat their patients is inevitably compromised.

Inadequate Data

Even when clinical trials are performed, the data is incomplete. Trials are not properly registered and the drug companies often own and control the results. Corporate medicine publishes results that help profits and suppress any negative findings. The literature is biased towards new drug treatments.

Medicalization

New diseases are being invented to provide new markets for drugs. By extending existing ideas of chronic disease, more drugs can be sold. The result is an increasingly medicated population.

Statistical Tricks

Statistics are used to manipulate results. Many doctors are not highly trained in statistics so are vulnerable to being deliberately misled by disreputable analysis. In Dr Spence's words, reports are presented in a way that "is just cheating".

Study Design

The design of clinical trials and related studies is biased by design. Results from high-risk groups are used to market drugs to low-risk groups.

These are potentially important issues, though they are not the primary focus of this book. Proponents of EBM might counter that no-one was claiming EBM was perfect and there remain some questions that are currently being addressed. Faced with Dr Spence's list, they could claim that EBM is better than the alternatives. It may be frustrating to Dr Spence and others, but supporters of EBM can claim to be hard-headed scientists, bringing a new rigorous approach; they consider themselves the sceptics of medicine. As this book shows, this defence of EBM is both incorrect and misleading.

Science and EBM

Science works by testing ideas using experiments and direct observation, which form the basis of the scientific method. Medicine is a technical discipline; it gains credibility because it has a scientific base. Many doctors we know are proud to assert that their subject is scientific; some older and wiser practitioners are also happy to claim it as an art. Medicine is an interdisciplinary technology, which can encompass both art and science.

Unfortunately, in modern medicine, basic experimental science (the sort conducted in a laboratory) is being downgraded and overruled. The best-known illustration of this new form of medicine concerns the link between smoking and lung cancer, along with subsequent efforts by medical authorities and politicians to modify smokers' habits. Another example relates to cholesterol and heart disease; we shall say more about these later. The originators of "evidence-based" medicine intended their new approach to introduce rigor and certainty. However, critics suggest it generates a form of cookbook medicine,[12] according to which doctors are supposed to adhere rigidly to official best practice. From this point of view, EBM erodes the autonomy of the physician and restricts patient choice.

In EBM, as we shall explain, some forms of data rate more highly than others. Over the centuries, the success of science has depended on observation and measurement. Repeated experiments lead to the collection of reproducible data. These help generate theories against which information can be judged. Repeatable experiments are particularly convincing, since other scientists can check to see if they get the same results. In science, we *trust but verify*. In this context, statistics acts as a supporting technology, for use when clear and repeatable measurement is impractical.

EBM, with its emphasis on statistical methods, seems locked into a form of physics envy. In physics, the aim is to describe natural events and generate theoretical models of the underlying mechanisms. From Archimedes through to quantum mechanics, its advances have depended on mathematics. This approach has been highly successful and has helped produce our current civilization. There is little doubt that medicine should strive for the sort of scientific and mathematical sophistication that was historically so successful in physics and other basic sciences. Such methods support the art of the practicing doctor. Unfortunately, as we show, EBM lacks this rigour and does not help patients.

Proponents claim that "evidence-based" medical investigation is relevant to the health of individuals. We will demonstrate that this idea is incorrect—it is not generally possible to use group statistics to predict the response of an individual patient. EBM has little to offer the doctor treating a patient, beyond suggestions about what might be expected with an *average* patient. An old Northern English saying tells us *"There's nowt so queer as folk."* Nowadays, such a phrase may be misunderstood, but it has nothing to do with sexuality. Rather, it reflects what Sir Robert Megarry, a senior judge who took the side of the individual in his rulings and writings, has called the "infinite charm and variety of human nature". In other words, we all have our idiosyncrasies—biochemical as well as psychological—and finding an average person is highly improbable.

Scientists avoid selecting evidence, it is a sign of bias. While concentrating on the statistics of large groups, however, proponents of EBM claim to consider all the relevant clinical evidence. This avoids the criticism that EBM is highly selective, by claiming that clinical observations and basic experimental results may be taken into account. In practise, however, we have found that EBM excludes important medical data.[13]

Patients need doctors, not statistics

Effective medical science could be straightforward. Later in the book, we describe an inexpensive clinical trial that a family doctor might perform. Our simple experiment is more robust than a large-scale EBM trial. Applying the principles of science leads us back to a more traditional form of medicine, based on heuristics (problem-solving rules of thumb), direct observation, and experimental testing. According to this approach, the critical authority in scientific medicine rests in the decision-making skills of each doctor-patient partnership.

Doctors and patients should take back the power in medical decision-making from EBM's statisticians and meta-analysts. Using a traditional medical approach, a typical examination may involve a doctor asking the patient questions, taking measurements (e.g. blood pressure), and getting test results. An experienced doctor can arrive at a diagnosis with surprisingly little information. Often, only a few questions may be needed to find the appropriate treatment.

Simplicity

Decision scientists have discovered that most practical systems have a limited complexity; as a rule, just a few parameters can describe most of them. By contrast, the explanations of disease produced within the framework of EBM are extremely complicated. EBM relies on numerous risk factors and complex multifactorial explanations, which are confusing for doctor and patient alike. Multiple risk factors are a tacit admission of ignorance; indeed, most doctors must have overheard the jest that describing something as multifactorial is just a more impressive way of saying "we don't know what causes this disease."

A fundamental principle of decision science is that too many risk factors produce information overload. This overload obscures the solution.[14,15] When doctors increase the number of risk-factors they use to investigate a problem, it becomes harder for them to find a real solution. This may sound counter-intuitive: it implies that as you increase the number of factors, your ability to solve a problem goes down. The explanation is that each new factor introduces an element of noise, and, eventually, the accumulated clatter hides the solution. We need a certain amount of information to solve a problem and no more than this. Adding excessive information does not help: it simply introduces error. We demonstrate that the multiple risk factors in EBM generate confusion rather than explanation.[16,17]

The word "evidence" in EBM, if it means anything at all, must be interpreted in terms of information. This information should reduce the amount of uncertainty in diagnosis and treatment. However, the skill of the individual doctor is essential. With only 20 questions, a doctor could theoretically diagnose over a million diseases. Doctors undertake years of training, learning key knowledge, accumulated over centuries of research and practice, in order to be able to ask the right questions. As poet and philosopher, Solomon Ibn Gabirol, put it: "A wise man's question contains half the answer."[18]

Decisions, decisions

The aim of science is to get the simplest explanation for complex phenomena.[19] This book explains some basic requirements for good decision making. It comes as a shock to many students of the decision sciences to realize that simple methods can be more useful and accurate than those produced by the most advanced and complex technologies. Simple rules, or heuristics, can match the amount of information necessary to address the problem. They are also intuitive and easy to use. In treating patients, decisions guided by simple rules offer doctors their most powerful approach.

EBM arose from legal, political, and commercial needs. Such requirements are inconsistent with scientific investigation. Unfortunately, this emphasis on social science has the consequence that scientists using traditional methods may be ignored and their results not accepted as evidence in a court case.

In this book, we will outline the limitations of current "evidence-based" medicine. In brief, EBM does not conform to the scientific method. It wastes resources and fails to advance medicine. Surprisingly, its statistical methods break basic rules of probability. The techniques used are incompatible with cybernetics, game theory, pattern recognition, and decision science. In short, we show that EBM increases uncertainty, confuses doctors, and ultimately kills patients. However, we don't ask you to take our word for this—rather, we hope readers will consider the evidence presented here critically and come to their own conclusions.

Main Points

- The name "evidence-based" medicine is a marketing ploy.
- EBM claims its authority from science, so it should obey the rules of science.
- Decision science and cybernetics show EBM is irrational.
- EBM is authoritarian and legalistic; it is cookbook medicine.
- EBM is dangerous to patients' health and wellbeing.

> All science is intelligent inference.
> Stephen Jay Gould

Populations Are Not People

> The average human has one breast and one testicle.
> Des McHale

Doctors may not realise the sophistication of the diagnoses and decisions they make on a daily basis when dealing with their patients. A doctor's judgement can be more balanced and effective than the most advanced offerings of "evidence-based" medicine. Rational doctors should avoid practising medicine based on large-scale trials and statistical theory.

A medical decision

Suppose someone asks you to donate one of your kidneys or part of your liver, for a transplant. Several issues influence your response. Firstly, your answer may depend on who the recipient will be. To take an extreme example, most people would be more predisposed to donate to a loved relative than to a serial killer. The anticipated benefit is also relevant: a young spouse or a child, who potentially has decades of productive and happy life ahead, seems more worthy than someone on death row, whose life expectancy is short.

Additional questions include asking why the transplant is necessary. Donating a lobe of your liver to an unreformed alcoholic would not seem wise, as he might continue drinking after the operation. You would probably want to be reassured that the recipient would be responsible and not destroy your life-giving gift. Also, you might factor in how closely your tissues match: unless the beneficiary is your identical twin, rejection is an important consideration. The recipient might need to be on anti-rejection medication for life, so, as a possible donor, you may want to make sure you were the most suitable candidate in terms of tissue typing.

In addition, you would probably want to consider the risks of exposing yourself to surgery or hospital infections. Moreover, loss of the organ could cause you future health problems. Donating a kidney would leave you dependent on just one, for the rest of your life. A motor vehicle accident, or similar, could damage your remaining kidney, leaving you in need of a transplant.

Organ donation is a typical medical decision. Your choice depends on the responses to numerous questions. Those questions relate to you as an individual and to the particular circumstances in which you find yourself. It is relatively rare for statistical information to be centrally important. It might be comforting to be told that, statistically, there are few complications in the proposed transplant surgery. Perhaps, on average, people have a 2% chance (one in fifty) of a serious problem—some people may find this reassuring.

Most of these statistics provide some indication of risk. However, they do not apply directly to you, personally. For example, suppose you know you are highly sensitive to a range of anaesthetic agents. In this case, standard surgery could be fatal, and a nonstandard form of pain relief would be needed. If you had this sensitivity but did not know it, you could be at unusually high risk, despite what the statistics suggest.

As a rational person, you might decide to donate or decline based on the information provided. The methods used to make decisions like this are the subject of the decision sciences. Decision science deals rationally with the process of arriving at a particular choice. Each decision depends primarily on the particular circumstances of the situation, rather than on group statistics.

The ecological fallacy

EBM is based on a statistical blunder: the assumption that a population value (such as the average risk of a complication during kidney surgery) can be applied to one specific individual. This is known as the *ecological fallacy*.[20] To take a simple example from physics, helium gas can be described in terms of temperature, volume, and pressure. The gas is a collection of a vast number of atoms and knowing its average temperature does not provide information about a particular helium atom.

Similarly, just because most people in Japan have black hair, it does not imply that the person sitting opposite you on a Tokyo train must have black hair. The seat could be occupied by a pink or blue coiffed Harajuku girl, a young man who has streaked his hair brown, a visiting Scandinavian blonde, an elderly person with grey hair, or even a bald person. The *average* hair colour in Tokyo might be black, but you will see many other colours on a trip around the city.

According to the ecological fallacy, it is fundamentally incorrect to apply the results of large-scale trials to individual patients. The problems associated with the application of clinical trial data to individuals are notorious—think of the tragedies associated with thalidomide or, more recently, with Vioxx. Despite this, the EBM myth is that individual patients should be treated according to a gold standard of population statistics.

Professor Trisha Greenhalgh wrote a book called *How To Read A Paper: The Basics of Evidence-Based Medicine*.[21] Greenhalgh's how-to book was aimed at introducing medical professionals to the new approach. The book begins with Greenhalgh seemingly enthralled that mathematics was being applied to medicine. In a later edition, she gives a definition of what EBM means to her:

> Evidence based medicine is the use of mathematical estimates of the risks of benefit and harm, derived from high quality research on population samples to inform clinical decision-making in the diagnosis, investigation or management of individual patients.

In a form of doublethink, the book quotes the ecological fallacy, but does not clarify its implications. Greenhalgh explains that "Evidence based clinical decision making involves the somewhat counterintuitive practice of assessing the current problem in the light of the aggregated results of hundreds or thousands of comparable cases in a distant population sample." The reason this process is, as she says, counterintuitive, is that decision science does not work in this way. You cannot apply a probability you get from a population to a specific individual and expect it to be accurate or useful.

Greenhalgh is aware of this problem but seems to miss the obvious contradiction, explaining that "the 'truths' established by the empirical observation of populations in randomised trials and cohort studies cannot be mechanistically applied to individual patients."[22] In other words, EBM does not work for any particular patient. Here, the term 'mechanistically' suggests that it might be possible for a human to interpret the EBM results, as a subjective guide to a patient's treatment. We agree. But we add that the patient's individual biology and circumstances dominate. So the

EBM population studies merely provide a vague context for human decision making.

Greenhalgh suggests that EBM is appropriate for questions of the form "If a 34 year old man presents with left sided chest pain, what is the probability that there is a serious heart problem, and if there is, will it show up on a resting ECG?" An ECG or electrocardiogram is a recording of the electrical activity of the heart. There does not appear to be a valid way of getting an answer to this and related problems using the group statistics of EBM. As we shall see, the young man needs to be treated as an individual; he requires a personal assessment.

Finally, Greenhalgh suggests that we can use Bayesian statistics to guide our decision making, based on EBM data.[22] Here she is suggesting avoiding the ecological fallacy by incorporating a more effective statistical method. In contrast to the complexity of standard techniques, Bayesian statistics are based on a single idea and can be described by a solitary equation. Essentially, it explains how to update a belief in terms of new evidence.

Reverend Bayes' belief system

Scientists can thank a theologian for explaining how we should use evidence. The Reverend Thomas Bayes was an eighteenth century British mathematician, who derived a special case of the theorem that bears his name. The decision trees we will use to evaluate mammography and other tests are constructed according to Bayes' ideas. Bayes' theorem is a simple method of interpreting the data from a clinical trial, experiment, or screening test.

An experiment is not conducted in isolation. At the start of a clinical trial we already know something about the problem and have a belief system. This knowledge is sometimes described as a *prior probability*, because it exists before we conduct the experiment. Thus, a mammogram checking for breast cancer is accepted on the understanding that the woman concerned is at some risk of the disease. The results of the test combine with our previous knowledge to improve our assessment; such evidence is the *belief system*. The use of the term belief is somewhat unfortunate; however, in this context, it means a rational interpretation of the data, rather than an act of faith.

Bayes' theorem is concerned with the chance of a result occurring, given our current beliefs. The results of experiments help update our beliefs, in the hope that they become a more accurate reflection of reality. There would be no point in performing a clinical trial if we were not going to use the results to increase our knowledge. Once we have done the test, our new belief combines the new result with our earlier knowledge.

When we use a medical experiment or clinical trial to increase our knowledge about a disease, we are performing a Bayesian process. Whatever approach a doctor uses to understand the data, if the method is accurate, it approximates to Bayes. As a result, our current scientific belief system is constantly updated. Clinical trials and other medical evidence provide information that adds to our knowledge and informs our way of thinking.

Good for the average patient?

At the beginning of this chapter, we quoted a humorous statement by Des McHale, who said "the average human has one breast and one testicle." Taking an average of the entire human population, we arrive at the strange half-man-half-woman suggested by the quote. National Geographic has described the typical human: a 28 year-old, right-handed, Han Chinese man, with a cell phone, an income of less than $12,000 a year, who does not have a bank account.[23] In the unlikely chance that this describes the reader, the average person changes with time and will be Indian in less than 20 years. It is evident that few, if any, people can truly be described as average.

Supporters of EBM may argue that if we use average results then, on average, we will all benefit. This argument is seductive, but things are not so straightforward. Suppose clinical trials show that, on average, 10 mg of a drug lowers blood pressure. The average member of a population is then found to have high blood pressure. So, if we give everyone, say, 10 mg of the drug, they should benefit, as the average blood pressure would be lower and the population as a whole would be healthier.

This is where the ecological fallacy kicks in. A relatively small number of people have extremely high blood pressure, but they increase the average (mean) value. Most people in our hypothetical population may have normal blood pressure. Some have low blood pressure and, for them, the drug is harmful—if they take it, they might die. Thus, indiscriminate application of the average dose will be dangerous to some. Only those with elevated blood pressure will benefit and the required dose depends on their individual circumstances. A rational physician would prescribe the drug only to patients with confirmed high blood pressure and would adjust the dose proportionately.

A doctor needs to treat every patient as a person with a unique problem. Moreover, that is what patients expect. A doctor practicing purely according to statistical expectations will inevitably harm patients. If the doctor wrongly assumes a chest pain is gastritis, rather than a coronary event, this may lead to the patient being discharged. Such mistakes can happen. The statistics might indicate that a heart attack is unlikely; gastritis is common, and the doctor might be too busy to check. At the other extreme, a doctor might run every available test and this might still lead to a wrong diagnosis, as the doctor suffers from information overload.

One of the first lessons in decision theory is how to avoid the ecological fallacy. This means not attempting to make predictions about an individual using data averaged from populations. The result of such attempts is inaccuracy. Our attempts to find a justification for EBM falter because it depends on applying the ecological fallacy. We know of no way of avoiding this limitation with group statistics. However, using pattern recognition or pattern matching in the diagnosis and treatment of disease avoids the ecological fallacy.

Pattern recognition

> The only possible conclusion the social sciences can draw is: some do, some don't.
>
> Ernest Rutherford

Collecting information from populations of people provides valuable data for governments and social scientists. For example, knowing the expected number of heart attacks in a city can be a guide to the number of cardiac beds the local hospitals need. Similarly, the government may use statistical results from clinical trials to recommend medicines that are likely to be cost effective. In the past, population studies helped show that cigarette smoking causes lung cancer and other illnesses; such information may help in regulating tobacco. Moreover, helping people become aware of the harmful effects of tobacco can allow them to make an informed *individual* choice on whether or not to smoke.

Despite these uses, statistics and social medicine are of little benefit to a particular individual: let's call him Uncle Charlie. We have all heard of someone's Uncle Charlie, he is 97 years-old, he smokes, drinks alcohol, eats poorly, and does not exercise. He has not suffered heart disease, arthritis, lung cancer, or any of the other expected illnesses. Indeed, he has never been in hospital in his life and does not believe in doctors. The statistical results apparently did not apply to Charlie, who is "nearly a hundred and still going strong!" Most people are aware that they need to be treated as an individual, but do not have the background knowledge to express this opinion adequately—so they tell us about Uncle Charlie.

Standard statistics indicate that, on average, people would be well advised not to smoke tobacco. This is not the whole story, scientists have shown that everyone who smokes even a single cigarette will suffer some injury. This knowledge comes directly from animal and laboratory experiments, not from clinical trials or epidemiology. Basic science demonstrates that everyone who smokes will suffer damage. Smoking introduces chemicals that direct measurement and observations in pharmacology, biochemistry, and biophysics have shown to be toxic.

Every puff of every cigarette harms the smoker; nevertheless, individual responses to this stress can vary. What medical statistics cannot say, with any accuracy, is whether their results apply to you, personally. It merely states that, on average, you increase your risk of illness by smoking. However, it is possible that, like Uncle Charlie, you have an unusual combination of features, perhaps antioxidants or detoxifying enzymes, that protects you from the effects of tobacco. If you fit this rare pattern, your life expectancy could exceed 100 years, even if you smoke.

The example of Uncle Charlie highlights the difference between standard population statistics and another form of decision-making, known as pattern recognition. Pattern recognition applies to individuals. Each person has an associated pattern of attributes, such as gender, eye colour, ethnicity, height, weight, and so on. Any person with this set of features has a particular propensity to illness or good health. Conventional statistics tells you the average and the spread of any of these values in a group or sample. Pattern recognition makes predictions for a particular patient, depending on the attributes they possess.

Until recently, computers were not powerful enough to carry out pattern recognition of any sophistication. Over the last thirty years, however, pattern recognition has come to surround us and, although we may not have noticed it, has become intimately involved in our lives. Pattern recognition applications started with military requirements, for example, to separate enemy submarines, aircraft, or missiles from friendly ones. Gradually, commercial systems have been developed for DNA profiling, fingerprint recognition, speech recognition, face recognition, reading postal codes on envelopes, automatically checking bank notes, and searching for explosives or contraband in airports. One of the authors (SH) has designed such systems for analysing medical and other images, stock market prediction, print inspection, reading car number plates, and so on. In these and numerous other applications, the aim is to recognize and classify individual items.

Medical pattern recognition

Pattern recognition is not new to medicine. In traditional methods of diagnosis, a doctor collects or elicits signs and symptoms from the patient; these are matched to different diseases, using the doctor's knowledge and experience. An experienced doctor will recognize the features of most common diseases quickly, having seen them many times before. During this process, the doctor is using pattern recognition.

Throughout medical training, doctors gain practical experience and expertise. This is another way of saying that they learn to recognize patterns. An excellent doctor may diagnose a condition with little information, seeking out just the relevant facts to make an accurate diagnosis. With practice, they can do this quickly, almost without realizing it. Malcolm Gladwell describes such rapid cognition in his book, *Blink*.[24] To take another example, chess grandmasters do not spend much time calculating moves but have learned to recognize whole positions on the board. They select moves that seem sensible and might be expected to give them some advantage. In diagnosing and treating their patients, expert doctors use similar methods.

Common diseases can normally be determined, with reasonable accuracy, from a short list of symptoms. In other cases, clinical or laboratory tests may be needed. However, doctors do not need the results of many questions to diagnose an illness. To see why, consider an electronic toy, called 20Q, which can appear to have almost magical mind-reading abilities.

The 20Q toy asks you to think of a word and then asks up to 20 questions, hence the name of the device. You are asked to respond "yes" or "no" and, in some variants, you can also respond "sometimes" or "unknown". Each question is designed to narrow the range of possible words. The device might ask if it is an animal and, if the answer is "yes", it might ask is it a mammal, and so on. These toys can guess most words accurately. In a few cases, you may be able choose a word that is not in the device's database, but that is a limitation of the toy, not the method of analysis. To many, this toy appears to have an almost magical mind-reading ability.

So, given relatively few questions, we can see that it is possible to find any word in the English language. Each yes/no question provides one bit of information. Asking 20 questions splits the list of possible words into over a million different categories. A large English dictionary contains about 500,000 words[25,26,27] and an additional half a million new words wait to be added.[28] Thus, in theory, the device could predict any word in a dictionary and many technical words that are not yet included. A typical educated person might know 20,000 words[29] and may use about 2,000 of them over a period of a week. So, even a badly programmed series of 20 questions can deal with the words most people might choose.

Similarly, an expert doctor does not need many questions to distinguish between a large number of disease possibilities. One question, with a yes or no answer, separates the possible diseases into two groups. A second question may split the symptoms into 4 groups. A third question renders 8 possible disease groups. Amazingly, just twenty questions are enough to split the list of possible diseases into 1,048,576 groups. That means twenty simple "yes or no" questions would be sufficient to specify a patient's particular disease from over a million possibilities.

When a doctor examines patients, he notes their gender, age, and other characteristics, asks about symptoms, and matches them to known diseases. While they are training, junior doctors memorize lists of symptoms, linked to illnesses. Later the lists are left behind, as the skill becomes automatic. During this process, the doctor formulates a diagnosis that is specific to each particular patient, in the current environment. In pattern recognition terms, the aim of the questions is to allow the doctor to determine the patient's set of attributes and then match them to a particular disease.

Population statistics are of limited help in reaching a diagnosis. For example, breast cancer is statistically rare in males, compared to females. Despite this, a man with breast cancer does not want his condition to be missed, just because it is less common. The patient expects the doctor to have specific diagnostic expertise and to apply this knowledge accurately, to help him regain his health.

Everyday miracles

> You should never bet against anything in science at odds of more than about 10-12 to 1.
>
> Ernest Rutherford

An adage commonly used by physicians, especially when teaching their juniors, is that "common things happen commonly."[30] This nonetheless allows for the possibility of rare or miraculous events, although the statement suggests that symptoms should be interpreted using the most likely explanation. Junior doctors may not have seen enough cases to know whether complaints are unusual or commonplace. They have yet to learn, through experience and from senior doctors.

Statements about common things happening frequently demonstrate one of the ways doctors learn to diagnose patients: they use heuristics as a guide. We all use heuristics to help us solve problems, even without realizing it. A common rule of thumb, for both doctors and laypeople, is that a person with a runny nose, cough, sore throat and a slight temperature probably has a common cold. Later, we will see that such simple heuristics, applied judiciously by the family doctor, can be at least as accurate as the most powerful statistical methods!

Few people will be surprised to hear that common things occur frequently. However, a more paradoxical idea is that unusual events also happen often. The chance of a particular person winning the lottery is highly unlikely but, as regular players will tell you, someone wins it almost every week. As they say, "Someone's got to win!" Unfortunately, that does not make it any more likely that the "someone" will be you. John Littlewood, a leading Cambridge mathematician, defined a miracle as an event with odds of a million to one against. Littlewood's law states that such a miracle can be expected to happen to a person about once a month.[31] Thus, Littlewood calculated that a person should expect to experience a strange occurrence relatively frequently.

Genetics, physiology, and environmental influences are all enormously complicated. Occasionally, Littlewood's miracles lead to breakthroughs, the classic example being Fleming's discovery of penicillin. Scientists are searching and hoping for the genius to be able to recognize such serendipitous miracles when they arise. As Nobel Prize winner Albert Szent-Györgyi put it, "discovery consists of seeing what everybody has seen, and thinking what nobody has thought."

Medical miracles are surprisingly common. Over the course of a year, a doctor might rationally expect to come across numerous rare symptoms and conditions. However, Littlewood's miracles and other unusual events are not covered by medical statistics.[32] Indeed, a patient that was truly average would be extremely unusual, easily rare enough to be considered one of Littlewood's miracles. Each individual has enough unusual biochemical parameters to be considered a statistical outlier.

Extraordinary claims

I don't see the logic of rejecting data just because they seem incredible.

Sir Fred Hoyle

In economics, Nassim Taleb explained the implications of unusual stock market events, which he famously described as "black swans". For centuries, people used the phrase *black swan* to describe the impossible, just as we might say "as rare as hen's teeth." Long ago, people thought all swans were white. Sampling swans from around the world, they covered most of the land mass of the globe. After a long period of history, no black swans were found. A practitioner of EBM might say this provides "proof" that all swans are white, and after such an extensive search, this might well sound plausible and rigorous.

Suppose then, that someone found black swans in Australia—where they do indeed occur—which the scientists had missed.[33] If people were convinced that *all* swans were white, this could affect how they received the new information. If you produced a specimen of a black swan, you might be accused of fraud, or asked how you had coloured its feathers. To a person working from a restricted evidence base, it could seem more plausible that your black swan was fake than the accepted idea was false. While the default position of many scientists is scepticism, we all need to be constantly aware of how little we know. Unfortunately, most standard statistical methods are not designed to cope with "black swans".

Taleb realized that many economic theories and stock market trading algorithms are based on linear statistics. However, the financial markets, just like medicine and many other aspects of life, are not linear. The world does not always obey the rules of EBM-style statistics: it is often complex, dynamic, and non-linear. Conventional statistics do not work well in this context; unusual events not only happen, they are to be expected.

Picking up pennies in front of a steamroller

In our discussions with supporters of EBM, the main defence of its methods has been that on average it provides consistent small benefits. Thus, "The drug may only help one patient in a hundred, but that one patient makes it all worthwhile." This interpretation is misguided, as the potential costs can greatly outweigh the benefits. Nassim Taleb has described a concept that applies to a system of financial returns that produces frequent small profits, punctuated by occasional catastrophic losses; this idea is known as the Taleb distribution. It is highly relevant to the practise of medicine.

Let us consider the case of Alice, who is health conscious and takes care to eat well and exercise regularly. She wants to stay healthy for as long as possible. Of course, she realises that eventually her life will end. But Alice wants to live a long active life, in good health. Her main concerns are "black swan" events that might drastically shorten her existence, such as a motor accident or heart attack. Her doctor provides check-ups and treatment according to EBM, giving Alice a little reassurance that she is taking precautions. The doctor provides painkillers to overcome an occasional stress headache and anti-inflammatories for her tennis elbow. The pills seem to reduce her symptoms, with acceptable side effects.

Apparently, Alice's doctor is providing multiple small benefits to her and his other patients. However, the idea that she is gaining an overall benefit is an illusion. EBM's statistics do not describe the outliers. Any particular drug or treatment, for example, has the potential for serious side effects, despite being tested in large-scale trials. It is assumed that side effects will be rare, but this is not necessarily true. Problems are often missed, partly because the statistical methods are limited and assume that a drug's response is well behaved. Despite this hope, the statistics often obscure serious side effects.

In this case, Alice gained 10 years of relief from her occasional tension headaches, only to find that the drug ultimately caused terminal liver failure. The liver damage was chronic, taking almost a decade to emerge; it was not apparent in the drug's clinical trials. History suggests that medical harm is not easily constrained. Anyone taking a new drug is at risk of potentially devastating side effects.

EBM is one of a number of activities that provide apparently stable and steady small benefits, but which can hide nasty events. Often it is not possible to predict these problems in advance or to use standard statistics to lower the risk. A classic description comes from the field of finance. Nobel Prize winning economist, Milton Friedman, described the "peso-problem". It was possible to borrow dollars at low rates of interest from US banks and invest at high interest in the Mexican peso. The returns were consistent and seemingly guaranteed—until the peso was allowed to float against the dollar. At that point, a peso investor, having gained, say, $10,000 profit a year, might find he had lost $2,000,000 and was wiped out. Unknown to our investor, the difference in interest rates reflected the market's expectation that the peso might be devalued.

Typically, a person has a relatively consistent low risk of severe illness but is subject to occasional catastrophic breakdowns. A person's health follows a Taleb distribution.[34] While it can be stable for long periods, it is always at risk of sudden unexpected illness or injury. The negative events will ultimately prevail, as everyone dies eventually. A heart attack is analogous to a stock market crash, in that it is a non-linear event, the timing of which is unpredictable.

Another example of a Taleb distribution is the driving behaviour known as tailgating. A motorist in a fast lane drives too close to the car ahead, in the hope of cutting a few extra seconds off his journey. If several drivers do the same thing, it only takes one near the front to brake a little too severely to cause a pile-up. The benefit is not worth the risk—the impatient drivers, their passengers, or other nearby drivers could by killed for the sake of a second or two. In placing their faith in statistical averages, EBM doctors act rather like these foolhardy motorists. Each decision may benefit a few people in some small way, but, given enough time, a calamitous event is almost certain.[35]

Doctors using what appear to be statistically-sensible treatments may expect to provide their patients with many small gains. However, these minor benefits, if they exist, can come with a large risk. Taleb has described the process as equivalent to picking up pennies in front of an advancing steamroller: the benefits are small but if you trip and fail to get up, you get flattened. A Taleb distribution can give steady returns for a time, but eventual ruin is almost certain.[36]

The characteristics of such a distribution are similar to those in the practise of medicine and include the following:

- High probability of extreme adverse events, such as the death of patients.
- Existence of hidden or unobserved events, such as side-effects, drug interactions, or superior "unproven" treatments.
- Unknown outcomes, as knowledge is limited, risks undetermined, and accurate expectations are difficult to compute.
- Belief in the management of risks, an unfounded belief in the ability of statistics to manage unknown risks, particularly as applied to individuals.

To avoid these problems, EBM should be replaced by robust methods, directed at supporting individual patients. The methods needed incorporate the following features:

- The patient avoids major risk. Each patient's risk needs to be considered separately, with little regard to population statistics.

- Methods should embrace uncertainty. Medical outcomes are tentative and remain so; rational doctors and patients have to accept this.
- Consider different options and their consequences. Compare both risks and benefits of any treatment options.
- Provision of information. It is important for doctors to focus on open sharing of information, including levels of uncertainty.
- Scenario analysis. Patients should be enabled to compare the likely outcomes of all available options, including the associated risks.
- Shared risk and responsibility. The ultimate risk, responsibility, and choice lie with the individual patient. Doctors have an obligation to assist with provision of information and decision-making.
- Freedom from bureaucratic interference. Governmental or organisational rules should not arbitrarily determine a patient's life or death.

Over time, doctors should expect most of their patients to encounter the occasional black swan event. It could be an unusual automobile accident, a rare cancer, or a tropical disease somehow contracted while on holiday in Alaska! Unfortunately, some people have difficulty with the thought that highly unusual events do sometimes occur.

The astronomer Carl Sagan famously said, "extraordinary claims require extraordinary evidence." His implication was that a highly unlikely claim demands powerful supporting evidence. Sagan was describing the interpretation of paranormal observations, near to the limits of scientific inference. This quotation is a variation on the suggestion that exceptional claims require exceptional evidence,[37] which reaches at least as far back as David Hume in the 18th Century. Hume said that "no testimony is sufficient to establish a miracle, unless the testimony be of such a kind that its falsehood would be more miraculous than the fact which it endeavours to establish."

However, the idea that an unusual report requires exceptional evidence is misguided: all data are important. A scientist should not ignore an observation, no matter how unlikely it appears. Apparently wild claims can easily be included, using Bayesian statistics. The importance of the claim is simply weighted by the likelihood that it is correct, given the other information we have. If a claim is unusual and does not agree with other findings, its importance is in proportion to the strength of the data. Any claim that is repeatable and can be tested easily with a simple low-cost experiment is particularly acceptable. This would mean that no matter how extraordinary a scientific claim is, we can test it, rather than just flatly denying it.

Ashby's law of requisite variety

William Ross Ashby was a psychiatrist who studied in Edinburgh and Cambridge, before taking a job at St. Bartholomew's Hospital in London. He became interested in how the brain worked and spent time wondering how a brain could evolve and function. Through this work, he discovered a simple law that governs all medical decisions, decision science, and computer applications. Ashby made an outstanding breakthrough in what was then a new discipline: *cybernetics*.

Cybernetics is the field of science concerned with control and communication in systems; it applies to both living organisms and machines. Ross Ashby's contribution was to discover a fundamental principle about how all systems work. This was his *law of requisite variety*, sometimes called *the first law of cybernetics*.[38] The link to EBM is immediate, since Ashby's law uses the word variety as another term for information—or what in EBM terms would be called evidence.

Ashby's law of requisite variety is, perhaps, the single most powerful statement concerning control, communication, or analysis of any system. His law is quite general in scope. It does not depend on external data for its validity: Ashby proved it using only logic and information theory. Put simply, the law implies that a complicated problem requires an equally complicated solution. We will expand it later to a Goldilocks principle, which means that the amount of information needed to control a system must be neither too little, nor too much, but—like Goldilocks' porridge—"just right".

In terms of information, Ashby's law is equivalent to Newton's third law of motion, often summarized as "every action has an equal and opposite reaction." This means that any applied force is balanced by an opposing force (reaction). In solving a problem,

Ashby's says there must be a similar balance: the person or computer providing a solution has to contain the same amount of relevant information (variety) as the problem itself. In other words, the solution to a complex problem will be more complicated than that to a straightforward problem.

The idea that an intricate problem is harder to solve than an easy one sounds like a banal statement. Nevertheless, Ashby's law is subtle, and understanding it is vital for understanding effective decisions. Ashby's law implies that, in order to reach an accurate diagnosis, a doctor needs sufficient knowledge of the individual patient, the environment, and the possible diseases. Of course, Ashby's law is not normally stated in this way, but in slightly obscure phrases, such as "variety absorbs variety."[39]

Another way of describing Ashby's law would be to say that if a doctor does not have enough knowledge, he will not be able to cure the disease. When stated in this way, it still sounds obvious, but so do many of the most powerful results in science. Ashby's law may appear simple but, as will become apparent, its implications are devastating. For example, trying to control the practice of a doctor using statistical rules breaks Ashby's law, as such rules restrict the amount of variety that a doctor can apply to diagnosis and treatment.

To solve a problem, you need sufficient ability, expertise, and knowledge. When a patient, such as Alice, is sick, she goes to a doctor to find out what is wrong. She does not go to a lawyer or an engineer, as it is highly unlikely that they will have sufficient medical expertise or knowledge. Alice is an individual, with unique characteristics, such as weight, genes, activities, and so on. Ashby's law means that all these must be taken into account when coming to a diagnosis and prescribing treatment.

Effective treatment of a patient like Alice depends on the skills and *variety* of the consulting doctor. The long medical training provides doctors with sufficient variety to help numerous different patients. We have spoken to many doctors, and have yet to come across one who supports the idea that results from statistical medicine should overrule a physician's expertise.

Game theory

Another branch of decision science, called *game theory*, is an effective way of addressing many aspects of human activity, whether military, economic, or medical. Its aim is to find the optimal strategy in a given situation. Despite the name, game theory is far from trivial. From its early origins in the fields of card games and economics, it developed further through use in cold war military analysis, and has frequently been applied to matters of life and death. Game theory is now incorporated into modern military strategy and progress in the field has been rapid.

Unfortunately, early game theory tended to be imbued with an almost sociopathic degree of rationalization. Theorists assumed that people would act only for their own limited benefit. The popular book and movie, *A Beautiful Mind*, about influential game theorist John Nash, illustrates this well. Nash suffered from paranoid schizophrenia, which may have influenced his thinking. Nash's genius in game theory was rewarded with a Nobel Prize. In rather an overstatement, his work has been described as affecting more disciplines than the theories of Newton or Einstein.[40]

Game theory applies to any situation that involves strategic interaction, such as social relationships. Much of medical practice can be described in this way. In a medical context, game theory provides a way for patients to ensure that they get the most effective treatment or disease prevention, with the lowest risk.

To take a simple example, suppose our patient, Alice, goes to her doctor, suffering from an infection. The treatment of choice is penicillin; best practice suggests this drug, as do government guidelines, cost, and the findings of multiple "evidence-based" studies. Despite all these factors pointing to a beneficial use of penicillin, it would be wrong to prescribe the treatment without considering Alice as an individual.

The doctor knows that Alice is unique; in this example, he remembers that she is allergic to penicillin and thus could go into acute shock and might even die. So her physician is likely to ignore part of the "evidence-base" and switch to an alternative, such as tetracycline. However, at this time, Alice is pregnant, so tetracycline should also be avoided because it may impair the development of her baby's bones. With this in mind, the doctor reconsiders the prescription. This process continues until the doctor has matched the treatment to the patient, the disease, and the current clinical conditions.

The doctor uses his skill and knowledge to battle Alice's infection, treating it as a unique event. He knows that a simple-minded approach will not work in every case. A bacterium has made the first move by invading Alice and causing symptoms. The doctor responds with an antibiotic. However, perhaps the bacterium has come up against this antibiotic before and has adapted, becoming resistant to the drug. The doctor needs to think again and find an alternative antibiotic. The process continues until an appropriate and effective treatment is found (or Alice's own immune system wins out) and hopefully Alice recovers. By analogy, the doctor is engaged in a game of chess against the illness.

> You have to learn the rules of the game.
> And then you have to play better than anyone else.
>
> Albert Einstein

Games can be surprisingly complex. Chess is played with simple rules, on a small board, with a limited number of pieces. Yet, despite its apparent simplicity, humans take years to master the game. A highly intelligent person might require a decade or more of intensive study to become a grandmaster. Modern computers can play the game at an advanced level, but it took a supercomputer to beat a world champion, Gary Kasparov—at the second attempt. The computer won a close match, after some between-game modifications to its program. Notably, the computer, known as Deep Blue, did not wait around for the requested rematch.

At the start of a game of chess, there are only 20 possible moves for the white pieces. Similarly, there are 20 possible responses for the black pieces. However, the number of different possible games is astronomically large. To understand how large such numbers can become, we can recall the well-known story of the King's prize. A King wished to reward a subject who had done a great and brave deed. The subject asked merely for a grain of rice on the first square of a chessboard, 2 grains on the second square, 4 on the third, 8 on the fourth, and so on. The amount doubled on each of the subsequent squares. The King thought this was too small a prize, and asked the subject to reconsider, but the man insisted this was all he wanted. In fact, his request was less modest than the King had realised. The sequence, 1, 2, 4, 8, 16, and so on, increases so rapidly that the value of rice on the 64 squares of the chessboard exceeded the worth of the entire kingdom. Even nowadays, it would be more than the rice production of the whole world for a century.

This sort of increase is described as exponential. The number of possible moves in a game of chess increases in a similar exponential way, which is why even the fastest supercomputers are currently unable to work out all the moves. The variety or information content in the game is astronomically large. As a result, it is typically not possible to work out the best current move. It is also not known if there is a winning strategy.

A simpler game, checkers (also called draughts), has a lower variety and all the moves can be calculated.[41,42] The standard game of checkers, using English rules, is probably the most complex game ever completely solved. It has over 500,000,000,000 possible moves and took a team of scientists almost 20 years to compute the solution, using dozens of computers. It is possible to build a computer program that is unbeatable at checkers. Played perfectly, a game of checkers will always end in a draw (like Tic-tac-toe, or, as it is called in England, noughts and crosses). There is no winning strategy, the only way you can win a game of checkers is if your opponent makes a mistake.

Medical problems are even more complex than such games and generally require a high level of human expertise. To provide the best possible treatment for a patient, the doctor has to solve a profoundly complicated problem. It is certainly not possible to provide a perfect solution to every doctor-patient game; it may be that the solution is not computable. Some decision problems have such staggering complexity that they are beyond an exact solution. The aim in such cases is to find an approximate solution or heuristic, which will give a satisfactory outcome. Most successful doctors would be happy if they could get their patients well again, regardless of whether or not the method was theoretically optimal.

Medical problems are too complex for doctors to be able to follow a list of instructions—they need to apply judgement. Current practice and guidelines may be helpful but, in practice, the problems faced by an individual doctor are too specific to allow a solution using standard statistical methods.

Individual medicine

Modern genetics is creating a new approach to personalized medicine. Pharmaceutical companies have embarked on an initiative to provide drugs tailored to a patient's individual genetic makeup. Excluding identical twins, triplets, and so on, every person on the planet is genetically unique. In addition to having distinctive genetics, we each have a characteristic anatomy, physiology, and biochemistry, which arose from the interactions between our genes and our environment. For example, one identical twin may be epileptic, while the other is not, which suggests that epilepsy can be a result of something more than genetics.

The aim of this initiative in medicine is to determine a person's genetic and biochemical profile, and then select the drugs that are most appropriate for each patient. This development of conventional medicine is an application of pattern recognition, which takes into account our biochemical individuality.

Personalised medicine is not a new idea, however. Surprisingly, the oft-derided alternative or complementary forms of medicine have led the way. For decades, practitioners of nutritional, ecological, and orthomolecular medicine have embraced the uniqueness of the individual. Roger Williams' excellent book, *Biochemical Individuality*, first published in 1956, demonstrates the incredible variability of human beings.[43] His approach may be summarized in his statement: "Statistical humans are of little interest." Biochemical individuality implies that direct application of statistical predictions must fail. To demonstrate this restriction, we return once again to Ross Ashby. Working with Roger Conant, Ashby came up with an extension to his first law, which further limits the applicability of statistical medicine.[44]

This extension is the *good regulator theorem*, which says that every good regulator must be a model of the regulated system. Daniel Scholten gives a practical example: every good key must be a model of the lock it opens.[45] Unless the key fits, it will not open the lock. Even picking a lock requires the locksmith or burglar to match the internal shape with his hairpin or other tools. The lock-and-key is an apt illustration for medicine, which uses similar analogies. The active site of an enzyme is a model of the substrate molecule. The receptor for a drug is a model of the drug. The head of the femur is a model of the acetabulum, and so on.

Hopefully the word theorem will not mislead you into thinking that this is some esoteric academic idea of no practical significance—this is basic information science and applies to any system. Applied to medicine, *a good regulator* could refer to an effective diagnosis and treatment. A *model of the regulated system* means the treatment is bespoke and customized to the idiosyncrasies of the patient.

Clearly, individual and customised treatment is not compatible with drawing "best evidence" from large-scale statistical trials. Statistics are aggregated from a population of unique individuals, but the process does not work in reverse because information is lost. For example, if we told you the height of each child in a class, you could calculate the average height for that class, by dividing the sum of all the heights by the number of children. Similarly, if Gemma is 4'10" and her best friend, Claire, is 5'10", you could calculate that their average height is 5'4". Clearly, clothes designed for their average height will not fit either of them! Calculating the average was easy. However, if we told you just the average value, it is not possible to work backwards to find the actual height of Gemma or Claire; that information is lost.

Population statistics do not discriminate between individuals. This is because when we calculate the statistics, we discard information. Statistics, such as the mean (a specific form of average) and standard deviation (a measure of the spread or variation), describe the population; they do not provide information about a particular person.

The variety in a group of individuals greatly exceeds that of the statistics used to describe them. This is a critical failure. Trying to apply group medical statistics to an individual patient not only results in the ecological fallacy and breaks Ashby's law, it does not provide an adequate model. The application of population statistics to a particular patient's medical problem does not provide a good solution, even in principle.

Normal Data

```
     -5  -4  -3  -2  -1   0   1   2   3   4   5
```
Standard Deviations

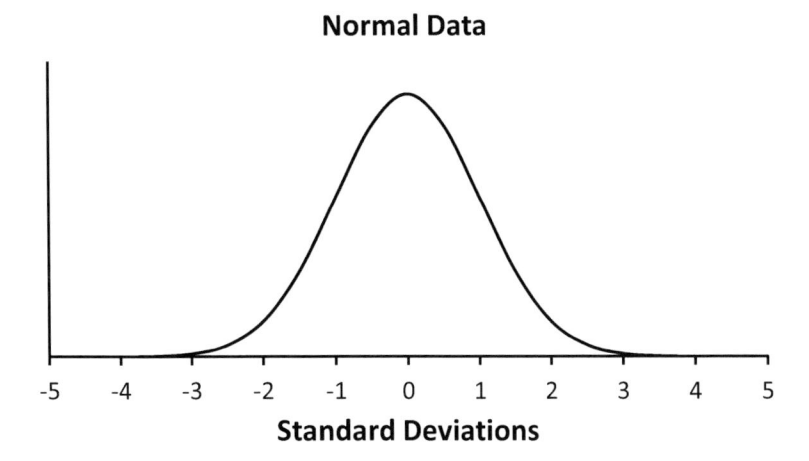

In this chart, the peak at zero is the mean, or average, value and the spread, or width, is measured in standard deviations

Scientific medicine

In this chapter, we have stressed the importance of biological individuality. This demands that diagnosis and treatment should be specific to the particular patient. We have seen why it is wrong to apply results from population statistics to an individual. The uniqueness of the patient overrides group statistics.

Because of its reliance on population averages and other aggregate statistics, blind use of "evidence-based" medicine is harmful. Modern decision science is specific to the individual and the situation. The decision sciences include several exciting sounding disciplines: decision theory, game theory, systems theory, chaos theory, complexity, heuristics, and pattern recognition, to name but a few. A typical family doctor will intuitively employ many of these advanced ideas in daily practice, though often without realizing it.

Contrary to the statistical notions of EBM, doctors' opinions, rules of thumb, and even gut feelings can be useful tools, helping the physician make a fast and accurate diagnosis. Doctors need to rediscover their instincts, rather than being made to feel inadequate for relying on age-old methods. A physician who uses individually-focused techniques can provide a more sophisticated diagnosis and treatment than the most "conclusive" edicts of "evidence-based" medicine.

Main Points

- Medicine is intelligent decision making.
- The science of decision making bears little relation to EBM.
- EBM can provide some degree of background information.
- EBM does not apply to individual patients (ecological fallacy).
- EBM does not provide enough information (Ashby's law).
- EBM does not provide a viable model (Ashby and Conant).
- The doctor-patient partnership is the primary decision making unit.
- Miracles should be expected—but don't bet on them.

Theory-free science makes about as much sense as value-free politics.
Stephen Jay Gould

Prove It!

> All scientific knowledge is uncertain.
>
> Richard Feynman

As a child in the school playground, you may recall having arguments that culminated in a demand to "prove it!" Children know the concept is powerful, so they often insist on proof as a last resort, when an argument is going against them. This ultimatum might turn a dispute, even when the evidence is stacked the other way. Their opponent's failure to "prove it" typically results in a stalemate, which is probably an acceptable result if the alternative is out-and-out defeat.

Of course, children are not stupid: they understand that proving something is difficult. An opponent is rarely able to produce the kind of definitive evidence that would end the argument. Asking another child to "prove it" is a way of dismissing him and his argument. He may be right, he may have a winning argument and data but, unless he provides overwhelming evidence, the demand for proof forces a draw.

Proponents of "evidence-based" medicine often make similar demands for scientific proof. A core feature of EBM is its requirement for scientific or clinical proof. Contradictory evidence is dismissed by saying "there is no proof", and unacceptable results are claimed to "need more proof." As in the playground, such demands can stifle objections.

Proof

It is important to realise that the concept of proof is not scientific, it is a feature of mathematics and logic. By definition, logical proof is absolute, so if a mathematical conjecture (equivalent to a guess or hypothesis) is proven, that means it is true. The proof consists of a series of logical deductive steps, which every mathematician accepts as being completely valid and forever true. Such proof is unconditionally correct, and not part of the scientific method.

A correct mathematical proof is, in some way, absolute. Tell a mathematician that you "need *more* proof" and he may well dismiss you as crazy. The only rebuttal to a proof is to show that it contains an error. You may have a better proof—one that is shorter, or more elegant and appealing—but, once a thing is proven, it is established as true.

The word proof gets its power from mathematics and logic: it provides a convincing demonstration that a mathematical statement is true, without debate or doubt. Once proof is established, it would be irrational to object. However, this definition provides the word with a powerful aura that can be exploited to shore up weak arguments.

Sometimes, arguments about unproven treatments are bizarre. One notably titled article by Dr Simon Wein was *Cancer, Unproven Therapies, and Magic*.[46] He claimed, "In order for unproven therapies to work, they need to remain unproven." Apparently, practitioners of unproven therapies do not want randomized controlled trials, as they need the treatment to be neither proven nor disproven. Wein suggests there is a requirement to avoid reality and the popularity of unproven treatments rests on the reassurance of magic. We prefer to consider that intelligent patients and their doctors are capable of rational decision making.

Beyond reasonable doubt?

In comparison with logical and mathematical proof, legal proof is tenuous: it merely requires the confirmation of a fact by evidence. To a lawyer, the idea of "proof" may be indistinguishable from that of "evidence". A driving license or a passport might be accepted as legal proof of identity, for example.

Nevertheless, the law does encompass a concept of proof that is similar to that found in mathematics; it is demonstrated in the phrase *proof beyond the shadow of a doubt*. This goes further than suggesting that not a single doubt is known, reported, or hinted at: it says that the possible doubt does not even cast a shadow. Not even the slightest hint of a hidden doubt remains to be uncovered.

Proof beyond the shadow of a doubt is not expected in a law court. In the real world, such a restriction would be impossible, as no-one would ever be convicted. The law uses a different standard for major crimes: *proof beyond a reasonable doubt.* According to Lord Denning, the most celebrated English judge of the 20th century: "Proof beyond reasonable doubt does not mean proof beyond a shadow of doubt. The law would fail to protect the community if it admitted fanciful possibilities to deflect the course of justice. If the evidence is so strong against a man as to leave only a remote possibility in his favour, which can be dismissed with the sentence 'of course it is possible but not in the least probable' the case is proved beyond reasonable doubt, but nothing short of that will suffice."[47]

"Proof beyond a reasonable doubt" implies that a jury may convict, even if they have doubts about the defendant's guilt. The jury is free to disregard doubts, provided they are unrealistic. This is the standard for many criminal systems. Beyond reasonable doubt is assumed to be a stringent criterion, but it simply means that a reasonable person would have no reasonable doubt of the defendant's guilt. This is a rather weak and variable measure; members of the Flat Earth Society might interpret "reasonable" quite differently to specialists in formal logic, for example.

One would hope that prisoners on death row would not be awaiting execution if there were doubt of their guilt. However, many innocent people are convicted or even executed. Despite this, once a person is convicted, we are supposed to accept that they really are guilty, as doubt or uncertainty at this point would make the legal system unworkable.

Turning "reasonable doubt" into numbers can destroy the illusion of certainty. Suppose someone is found guilty with a 95% probability, should that person be executed? Looked at the other way, if the person has a one in twenty chance of being innocent, does that justify a reprieve? Should we accept the likelihood of executing five innocents in every hundred? If this is too many, should those guilty of murder with, say, 99% probability be executed? In this case, we would only kill one innocent person in every hundred.

One of the first attempts to quantify the concept of "beyond reasonable doubt" measured it as equivalent to a perceived likelihood of guilt of between 70% and 74%.[48] If these figures are in any way reflective of true levels of guilt or innocence, then a large number of legal decisions must be wrong. Worryingly, if the figure holds true in death penalty cases, it suggests that about 1 in 4 executed prisoners were probably innocent. Not surprisingly, most law theorists hold that reasonable doubt cannot be quantified.

In the US, a lesser standard of evidence than "beyond reasonable doubt" may be used; this is known as the *clear and convincing* standard of proof. It is taken to mean that it is substantially more likely than not that the thing is, in fact, true. This standard is for child custody orders, involuntary commitment to a mental hospital, withdrawal of life support in comatose patients, and during disciplinary cases for professionals, such as attorneys or doctors.[49]

In civil cases, the concept of absence of reasonable doubt, with all its failings, is considered too restrictive. The typical criterion for civil cases is *proof on the balance of the evidence*. If your legal case for a billion dollars is just slightly more convincing than that of your opponent, you may win the lot.[49] Even the slightest smidgen of extra weight in support of your argument may be decisive. This form of legal "proof" potentially depends on the least possible evidence and takes us about as far from logical or mathematical proof as it is possible to get.

Being scientific

So far, we have seen that being reasonably sure that someone is guilty in a court of law does not require the same level of "proof" as that required in mathematics or computing. Legal proof is a social idea, subject to opinion, attitude, and bias. Most people would agree that a decision of the legal system is less powerful than a scientific fact. Thus, even when someone has been convicted "beyond reasonable doubt" of a most serious crime, the conviction can be overturned using scientific evidence.

DNA evidence has been used to demonstrate that convicted murderers were in fact innocent. For example, at Winchester Crown Court, England, in 1982, Sean Hodgson was convicted of raping and strangling Teresa de Simone.[50] In this case, the proof beyond reasonable doubt was based on a questionable confession and on evidence that his blood type matched samples found at the scene. Fortunately, Hodgson was not executed but jailed; he was released in 2009, after 27 years in captivity, because his DNA did not match samples found at the scene. On appeal, his conviction was considered "unsafe". Scientific evidence eventually corrected this miscarriage of justice, although not until ten years later than it might have. In 1998, the forensic science service told Hodgson's lawyers, wrongly, that the case exhibits had been destroyed, thus delaying rectification of this serious error.

Even DNA evidence does not provide certainty, although in the popular imagination it is probably equivalent to definitive proof. DNA analysis links a person to a tissue sample, such as blood. However, cross contamination can easily occur in the laboratory, rendering the DNA evidence invalid. There are other difficulties with the validity of DNA evidence but a recent development is particularly interesting. It is now known that, with access to standard laboratory equipment, a reasonably competent biologist could produce practically unlimited amounts of artificial DNA, to match a particular genetic profile.[51] This artificial DNA could be applied liberally to a crime scene, superficially establishing the guilt of the person whose DNA had been copied.

Unscientific proof

> In the empirical sciences, which alone can furnish us with information about the world we live in, proofs do not occur, if we mean by 'proof' an argument which establishes once and for ever the truth of a theory.
>
> Sir Karl Popper

Many people find it difficult to accept that the concept of "scientific proof" could itself be unscientific. However, all science is uncertain. The ultimate scientific criterion lies in the results of experiments that are designed to test whether an idea is false—a process known as *refutation* or *falsification*. The concept of proof is largely relegated to helping show that ideas are logically and mathematically consistent.

Science does not "prove it": demands for proof are contrary to the scientific method. Scientists aim to understand the world, in all its complexity. Nature is often unreasonable and is not constrained by human understanding or laws. Quantum mechanics, for example, is the most accurate and reliable model in physics, yet it defies common sense. Mathematical physicist Paul Dirac expressed this well, when he said "Pick a flower on Earth and you move the farthest star." Dirac was being precise, rather than poetic (or perhaps both precise and poetic). If you find Dirac's statement puzzling, you are not alone. The universe is strange and even our most accurate scientific knowledge is far from certain.

An example of something most people would consider proven might be gravity. In 1665, according to legend, Isaac Newton was taking afternoon tea in the shade of a fruit tree, when an apple fell on his head, prompting him to conceive his theory of gravitational attraction. Since then, countless apples have fallen to the ground, consistent with Newton's theory, providing an enormous body of supportive evidence. Despite this, in scientific terms, the matter is not fully settled.

While a physicist will probably accept that if you drop an apple it will fall, he might explain that some doubt remains. If you were to drop an apple in a tornado, for example, it may soar upwards into the air, at least initially. There are numerous reports of frogs falling in rainstorms, which suggest similar special atmospheric conditions. Even if we exclude such events, the physicist would still have some doubt. He might explain that quantum mechanics indicates a minute possibility that the apple will land on the surface of Mars, rather than on the earth. This probability is infinitesimally small and is unlikely to occur during the lifetime of the universe. However, in science, there is often residual doubt and uncertainty, even if it is of the kind that lawyers, such as Lord Denning, might refer to as "fanciful possibilities".

Scientists increase their understanding by building models, called theories. In science, even the most accepted theory can be disproved by experimental findings. Thus, if just one apple were to reproducibly fall upwards, for no apparent external reason, then gravity might have to be re-thought. People often consider physics the most rigorous of the sciences. While physicists use mathematical proof to demonstrate that their ideas are internally consistent and valid, a simple experiment can destroy the most elegant physical theory.

Science works by trial and error. A scientist designs and performs experiments, to check if current theories are valid. If the experiment agrees with the theory, little extra knowledge is obtained; we have simply shown that the theory explains our experimental results. An interesting result is one that contradicts the current theory or expectations. Scientists are always on the lookout for anomalies or unexpected events that do not agree with their current understanding. According to the eminent philosopher of science, Karl Popper, "statements or systems of statements, in order to be ranked as scientific, must be capable of conflicting with possible, or conceivable, observations."[52] In other words, the concept of scientific proof is an oxymoron.

The influential American biologist, Stephen Jay Gould, explained this well, when he said:

> Some beliefs may be subject to such instant, brutal and unambiguous rejection. For example: no left-coiling periwinkle has ever been found among millions of snails examined. If I happen to find one during my walk on Nobska beach tomorrow morning, a century of well nurtured negative evidence will collapse in an instant.

Legal proof adopted by EBM

The kind of proof that is claimed or, more frequently, demanded, by proponents of EBM is not determined according to a logical or mathematical gold standard. Perhaps surprisingly, lawyers rather than trained scientists determined the acceptability of the evidence base. Medicine's obsession with the idea of proof arose during attempts to legislate against tobacco. At this time, medical researchers were asked to "prove" to the law courts that smoking causes lung cancer and other diseases.

The campaign against tobacco began in 1950, when Richard Doll and Bradford Hill linked lung cancer with smoking.[53] Doll and Hill were not the first to recognize the link, though they reaped the credit. Before the Second World War, studies in Germany had demonstrated the connection, however these were largely ignored.[54] Doll achieved fame for his work on smoking and cancer. He became a Fellow of the Royal Society and was later knighted.

It soon became clear that tobacco companies would not stop marketing their products just because scientists said they were harmful. Unless the law forced the companies to comply, they would continue their activities—after all, it was their duty to maximize profits for their shareholders. Naturally, the tobacco companies challenged suggestions that their products were anything but healthy. As a result, medical experts were asked to provide sufficient evidence to establish the harm of smoking, for presentation in the law courts.

Demonstrating the harm of smoking to the courts was tough. Chemicals released from cigarettes promote cancer in experimental models,[55,56] though it can be difficult to cause the disease in healthy animals.[57,58] Nevertheless, if animals with spontaneous tumours are forced to smoke, they develop increased numbers of lung tumours.[59,60,61] However, lawyers argued that the results of animal experiments do not necessarily apply to humans.

Burning tobacco releases chemicals that cause genetic mutations, chromosome damage, irritation, and proliferation of cells, all of which are consistent with development of cancer.[62] The act of smoking delivers these carcinogens to the delicate tissues of the lung and into the blood. Despite this, lawyers did not accept *in vitro* (test tube) experiments, which showed that burning cigarettes produce numerous substances that cause mutations and cancerous changes in cells. What happens in a cell culture, they argued, could be quite different from what happens in a human lung.

In legal terms, the most acceptable evidence linking smoking and lung cancer came from epidemiology, which is the study of the health of populations. It estimated the risks of smoking, using statistics. While it took decades, eventually the medical profession relied on epidemiology to establish legally that tobacco causes cancer. As a result, medical theorists came to adopt the legally accepted idea of proof as their major criterion for evaluating research. This pragmatic tactic also provided doctors with a defensive position when it came to legal actions, which were a problem to clinical practice in an increasingly litigious society.

Realizing they were under attack, tobacco companies produced a solid and powerful defence of their deadly products. Like schoolchildren, they demanded that their medical adversaries should "prove it". At the same time, they used every opportunity to spread doubt. One quick and inexpensive tactic was to pay trusted experts to support the case for tobacco. The experts were well rewarded and companies used their opinions to mount effective media and legal campaigns.[63] Richard Doll himself became one of those medical experts, who formed close connections with industry,[64] and his later work appears ethically dubious. He defended asbestos, dioxin, lead in vehicle exhaust fumes, and ionizing radiation, while secretly being paid consultancy fees by the chemical and asbestos industries.[65,66] When these links became public, Doll's scientific reputation plummeted.

Acceptable evidence?

> Whoever undertakes to set himself up as a judge in the field of truth and knowledge is shipwrecked by the laughter of the gods.
>
> Albert Einstein

The legal conflict over what constitutes acceptable evidence in medical cases ultimately led to a US Supreme Court Ruling, which must rank as one of the silliest in scientific history. For comparison, there is a bizarre story that, in the 1897 *Indiana House Bill 246*, a physician attempted to redefine the constant Pi (π, 3.14159...). As children learn in school, this is the ratio of the circumference of a circle to its diameter. It is difficult to be sure of the proposed new value of Pi (perhaps about 3.2), since the Bill was contradictory. As one critic explained, "ignorance is consistently inconsistent."[67]

The idea that a government could consider a ruling to redefine Pi has become a metaphor for institutional arrogance. Pi is an irrational number: it cannot be expressed as the ratio between two integers, such as 22/7 (a common approximation), and the Indiana Bill was not passed.

Unfortunately, as recently as 1993, the Supreme Court made an equally ridiculous ruling on the legitimacy of scientific evidence, which has influenced the practice of medicine ever since. The parents of two children who were believed to have been harmed by drug toxicity asked the courts for help. Despite their lack of scientific training, the judges assumed the role of gatekeepers to scientific knowledge and validity.[68]

In *Daubert v Merrell Dow Pharmaceuticals*, the Supreme Court ruled that judges should consider whether the scientific evidence meets the following criteria, in order to determine whether it is admissible or credible:[69]

- The evidence is consistent with a testable technique or theory.
- The theory or technique has been peer reviewed and has widespread scientific acceptance.
- The technique should have a known error rate and standards.
- The underlying science should be generally acceptable.

These requirements seem superficially reasonable, but are misleading. Later, we will show that the court's demands—that evidence must be consistent, reliable, and accepted by the scientific community—are inconsistent with the scientific method. The insistence on being consistent with a testable theory is contrary to science, which rests on refutability. A primary criterion for evidence to be considered scientific is that it should be easily replicated, preferably using simple inexpensive experiments. We also need to be able to show it to be false. The Court did not properly include these crucial requirements for scientific belief.

The case concerned two children, Jason Daubert and Eric Schuller, who had been born with serious birth defects, which their parents attributed to a drug called Bendectin. The drug company, Merrell Dow, presented data from published studies of pregnant women who had taken the drug, apparently without harm. These studies had only indirect relevance to the children in the case—being equivalent to the early claim that all swans are white. Daubert's lawyers, however, introduced data from experimental and animal studies, which showed or suggested birth abnormalities when the drug was taken in pregnancy. This experimental work was supported by case studies, where birth defects had been reported in expectant mothers who had taken the drug. Daubert's lawyers also presented expert reanalysis of the defence's published studies.

The Supreme Court rejected the laboratory and animal studies, claiming these were irrelevant to side effects in humans. Case reports from human patients were also rejected as being an inappropriate form of evidence. It did not matter how many case reports the lawyers presented, they were not considered acceptable evidence. Expert testimony, pointing out errors and correcting the statistical analysis of published papers, was also ignored. In effect, the Supreme Court legislated that only epidemiological evidence mattered.[63] As Justice Blackmun concluded: "Given the vast body of epidemiological data concerning Bendectin, the court held, expert opinion which is not based on epidemiological evidence is not admissible to establish causation."

We could present a concise argument as to how and why the law is irrelevant to ruling on scientific facts. However, we will simply remind the reader of the story of King Canute the Great, former ruler of England and substantial parts of Western Europe. According to legend, King Canute went down to the seashore and, wanting to teach a lesson to his fawning subjects, ordered the tide to stop. Not surprisingly, this royal command was unsuccessful. The moral of this story is that it does not matter how important or powerful a human authority may be: it cannot override the laws of nature.

The judges were free to stipulate what evidence was required in a particular court case. However, they had no authority, right, or expertise for determining the relative importance of different kinds of scientific evidence. In this intention, they were repeating the error of the Catholic Church in trying to force Galileo to accept that the sun orbits the earth. Even though Galileo could be tortured or even killed for suggesting otherwise, the Catholic Church did not have authority over the solar system. We assume the judges in the *Daubert v Merrell Dow* case did not expect their pronouncements to extend to the wider practice of science.

Two of the judges (Chief Justice Rehnquist and Justice Stevens) dissented. In their words: "[This case deals] with definitions of scientific knowledge, scientific method, scientific validity, and peer review - in short, matters far afield from the expertise of judges." In addition, "the unusual subject matter should cause us to proceed with great caution in deciding more than we have to, because our reach can so easily exceed our grasp." The dissent continues, "I defer to no one in my confidence in federal judges; but I am at a loss to know what is meant when it is said that the scientific status of a theory depends on its 'falsifiability,' and I suspect some of them will be, too."

Perhaps the dissenting judges were anxious to avoid the *Daubert v Merrell Dow Pharmaceuticals* ruling ending as an anecdotal warning against authoritarian blunders, alongside the idea that the State of Indiana could specify the value of Pi. The judges were not qualified to rule on the scientific method. Unfortunately, their well-intentioned attempt to validate scientific evidence has since acted to protect companies from cases resulting from product liability, personal injury, and release of pollution.[70] Companies can use the ruling to prevent juries from hearing damaging evidence. Pharmaceutical companies can use it to defend their drugs against complaints. As a result, it has become difficult to stop products from causing harm, until they have injured enough people to fulfil the epidemiological requirements of legal proof.[63]

The supporters of EBM embraced the Supreme Court's Ruling on the relative importance of different kinds of scientific evidence. The Court's decision may have pleased epidemiologists and medical statisticians, as this ruling greatly increased their status. As a result, epidemiological evidence and large-scale clinical trials became the gold standard for legal proof in medicine. Statistical data became established as the official source of proof and was assumed to trump all other evidence.

The evidence hierarchy in practice

Let us put this into context. Imagine you are on a jury in a murder trial—Alice is accused of murdering Bob. The prosecution provides a series of respected professional witnesses, who have been trained in observation. The murder occurred at a medical conference and 10 scientists (of various disciplines), 5 engineers, and 21 physicians observed the shooting directly. Bob's body was found to have three bullet wounds, two in the head and one in the heart. All the witnesses say they clearly observed Alice shoot Bob in broad daylight. Two video recordings confirm these observations. The bullets matched the revolver found in Alice's hand. Alice had purchased the weapon. Chemical analysis suggested Alice had recently fired a gun. Furthermore, she admits the killing.

If you are a true believer in EBM, you should ignore all this anecdotal and physical evidence as unreliable, and pronounce Alice innocent! The defence is simple. Even multiple witnesses provide only anecdotal evidence, which is at the bottom of the EBM evidence hierarchy. The bullet wounds and video recordings are merely physical evidence. Similarly, the chemical analysis of the residue on Alice's hands is only a laboratory finding. Alice admitting the killing is just expert opinion. According to EBM, all this evidence is of low quality.

So now, we bring statistics to the rescue. Alice does not have the risk factors associated with a murderer. She is female, from a good family, is psychologically normal and well adjusted. There was no clear motive. Statistical probability and large-scale population studies have shown that such crimes have specific risk factors. Officially, these studies provide the best and only acceptable scientific evidence. The police should arrest Tom, a drug-abusing ethnic youth from the slums, with a criminal record of violence and gun crime, who was also present at the crime scene. The risk factors are all present, so we have "proof" and can convict him instead.

Obviously, this entire scenario is ridiculous, and is only intended to illustrate the silliness of the idea that population studies trump other forms of evidence.

Statistics are not proof!

The scientific method is a well-defined technique for increasing knowledge. Throughout history, however, authorities have attempted to override science and its methods. In every case, these attempts have ultimately failed.

To return to one of our examples, in 1632, Galileo Galilei published his *Dialogue Concerning the Two Chief World Systems*, whereupon the Inquisition charged him with heresy. It took a long time but eventually, between 1992 and 2008, Popes John Paul II and Benedict XVI recanted, acknowledging the contribution of Galileo to scientific understanding. In 2008, the Catholic Church even contemplated erecting a statue to the great man in the Vatican gardens, though these plans were quietly shelved in 2009. Similarly, we expect medicine ultimately to reject the misguided idea that statistics are more reliable than observation, measurement, and reasoning.

Zoologist and statistician, Lancelot Hodgben, illustrated the dominance of direct observation over statistical "proof".[71] In a modification of Hodgben's story, we will suppose that Alice is an artist and Bob, her husband, is an epidemiologist. Both are interested in the environment and nature so, for their holiday, they go on a botany course. During an exercise, a tutor asks them to sort a collection of leaves, originating from two different but related plants, according to species. They share the leaves out and move apart, to give themselves space. Alice puts red leaves in one pile and green in another and is soon finished.

"Done it!" Alice calls to Bob, who comes over to see her work. "That's not right" says Bob "You've got them all mixed up—come over here and look at mine." Alice looks at Bob's leaves: both piles contain a mixture of colours. Bob's sorting seems completely arbitrary. In response to Alice's objections, Bob decides that they should each test their sorting, to see if they can consistently reproduce the sorted piles. To Bob's surprise, Alice re-sorts her piles with 100% accuracy; the likelihood of her having done this by chance is infinitesimal. Bob sorts his leaves again and is similarly dependable. Statistics indicate that both their methods are perfectly reliable and equally valid.

While they are arguing about how to sort the leaves, the tutor overhears the resulting commotion. He gets his camera and takes three photos of the leaves: one with a red filter, one with a green filter, and a "black and white" or mono image. The problem becomes obvious: Bob suffers from red-green colour-blindness! Bob has sorted his leaves by shape and texture, which meant the colours got mixed together. Meanwhile, Alice had failed to notice the subtle differences in shading and texture, as her sorting was dominated by the overwhelming colour difference.

The moral of this story is that a person's viewpoint can skew their results, even though the results are repeatable and the statistics highly significant. Statistics have little bearing on the underlying reality and can be misleading, unless we consider alternate interpretations and data. The statistical "proof" valued by EBM merely suggests a level of consistency in performing a particular type of clinical trial. Likewise, the sorting methods of both Bob and Alice had similar levels of statistical significance. Nevertheless, Bob could not sort the leaves in the required manner, until he could use his tutor's camera filters to highlight the different colours.

Conflicting data is not a problem to a scientist: it may point the way to a new discovery. If a scientist is exceptionally fortunate, he will produce data that is both conflicting and reliable. The effort to understand and resolving such conflicts often leads to scientific innovations, just as Bob and Alice's conflicting data led their tutor to realise that Bob could not distinguish the colours of light reflected by the different leaves.

For many years, early physicists disputed the nature of light. Some followed Robert Hooke, claiming light was composed of waves. Others followed Isaac Newton and thought it was made of small particles, guided by waves. Strangely, if you design an experiment to show light is made of particles, you find the particles, but if you look for waves, you can find them also. There are anomalies in the experiments but, overall, either viewpoint is defensible. These and similar inconsistent results eventually led to the development of quantum mechanics, the most precise model of reality to be discovered so far. Strange as it may seem, light is simultaneously both a wave and a particle. As Nobel Prize winner, William Bragg, explained humorously, physicists use the wave theory on Mondays, Wednesdays, and Fridays, and the particle theory on Tuesdays, Thursdays, and Saturdays.

Before quantum theory, no-one thought that light might defy all common sense and have its own incomprehensible reality. The scientific world embraces fascinating observations, decisions, and fun; the universe is a more bizarre place than people can imagine.

Uncertainty before causation?

The scientist does not believe in effects without causes.

W Ross Ashby

Finding solutions to scientific problems is challenging. It requires hard work to collect and understand the relevant data, humility to discard long-held ideas or to change your frame of reference, and insight to recognise new ways of seeing things.

In this section, we are concerned with causality: the idea that an effect has a definite cause. We take causality as a given. A major limitation of EBM is that its method fails to identify direct causes of disease, though the claim that disease is multifactorial is often used as a get-out clause. Many problems, when solved, have a relatively simple solution.

A classic case of a "multifactorial disease" that was subsequently shown to have an underlying cause is peptic ulcers. Many possible risk factors were identified, including type A behaviour, hot drinks, stress, alcohol, smoking, spicy food, coffee, cola drinks, low dietary fibre, and so on. Doctors told patients they worried too much, were overworking, or were not eating properly. As recently as the 1980s, many doctors believed the illness was a psychosomatic disorder. One medical research paper, despite stating that psychosocial factors in ulcers had not been proven, claimed that "an unconscious conflict, by some yet unknown route, results in an increase in acid-pepsin secretion" and "some ulcer patients have a conflict over an exaggerated need for dependency and a desire to be a self-sufficient adult."[72] The paper's suggestion was that psychiatric intervention should be based on the individual's psychological profile and not just the existence of an ulcer. Fortunately, such imaginative ideas are gradually being replaced.

Stomach ulcers are typically a result of bacterial infection. Once this had been established, the relevance of the previously-assumed risk factors could be seen in context. Some people might be more prone to the infection, perhaps through poor eating or an immune system compromised by stress. In any illness, there will be numerous loose associations with the lifestyle of patients. These abundant associations do not mean the disease does not have a simple underlying cause. Most peptic ulcers (61% to 94%) are caused by infection with *Helicobacter pylori*.[73] Helicobacter is found in over 90% of cases, assuming the patient is not using aspirin or similar non-specific anti-inflammatory drugs that can damage the stomach. Many things can cause inflammation of the stomach or small intestine but, in most cases, a specific cause can be found for the individual patient and the disease explained. Nevertheless, despite the recent simple and direct explanations, modern medicine still describes peptic ulcer as a multifactorial disease.[73]

In the past, many infectious diseases were considered multifactorial in origin, including tuberculosis (TB). Factors that were blamed included bad smells, cold damp rooms, victims draining life from other family members, or masturbation. However, in 1905, Robert Koch won the Nobel Prize for showing that TB was caused by infection with the tubercle bacillus (*Mycobacterium tuberculosis*, and related organisms).

Koch's lecture on TB is considered one of the most important in medical history: his work showed the way for other scientists throughout the 20th century.[74] Not only did Koch demonstrate that TB was infectious and find the bacterial culprit, he developed rules, known as Koch's postulates, which show others how to associate a disease with an organism. According to Koch's postulates, the relevant organism:

- Must be found in all cases of the illness
- Must be isolated from the host and grown in a pure culture
- Must produce the infection after being cultured for several generations
- Should be recoverable from an experimentally infected host.

Koch's postulates are a minimum set of requirements for being reasonably sure that a particular organism causes the disease in question. However, they are difficult to achieve and some are starting to claim that they no longer apply. Ironically, the great new idea of modern "evidence-based" medicine appears to be a return to the idea of multifactorial illness, with numerous non-specific contributory factors.

What is a cause?

EBM has no cohesive theoretical structure. Ultimately, this may be a result of the philosophical notion of social construction.[75] According to this viewpoint, medicine, disease, and diagnosis are determined by social interpretation rather than underlying reality.[76] This approach suggests that with EBM, there are no real scientific facts, just socially constructed ideas and practical testing. This approach is useful for authoritarians who wish to control medicine. The alternative view is that the world is real and that science is describing reality. Science begins with the premise that direct observation and measurement are the fundamental building blocks of knowledge.

Practitioners of EBM often question the idea that a single organism or mechanism is directly responsible for the development of a disease. Their approach stresses disease susceptibility, co-factors, and multifactorial causation. This is a misunderstanding of the concept of causation. The presence of a causal factor is necessary for a specified event or illness to occur, although it may not be sufficient to produce it. For example, if a person has TB, he or she is infected with *Mycobacterium tuberculosis*, the bacterium that causes the disease. However, not all people who are infected with the bacterium develop the active form of the disease; their immune system is strong enough to prevent the bacteria from multiplying, so it remains inactive. Many people may be highly resistant to the bacteria: they have a dormant infection but no symptoms. However, all those who get active TB are infected with the bacteria that cause the disease.

Some supporters of EBM are starting to question the whole idea of causation. Researchers in epidemiology have claimed that there is little or no practical need to use the language of causation.[77] In one paper, researchers are encouraged to tell "a convincing story without resorting to metaphysical/unsupportable notions of cause." So, the authors assert that the statement "smoking two packs a day increases risk of lung cancer by 10 times" is preferable to saying that smoking causes lung cancer.

Let's take another example. A person executed by guillotine during the French revolution could have been the victim of an unfortunate pattern of circumstances. To tell a convincing story: he was in 18th century France, he had stayed in France even after being invited to England, and he was on the losing side. Furthermore, he insulted a local baker, who later accused him of counter-revolutionary activities. While attempting to escape, his horse went lame and he was caught. These might all be elements in the story of his death and each contributed a little to his ultimate demise. Despite this, the scientific cause of his death was not the risk of being in the wrong place at the wrong time, it was the removal of his head!

For most scientists, the statement that "smoking causes cancer" implies that some aspect of smoking produces a direct physical response, which leads to the illness. This is similar to the logical statement that A implies B. In classical physics, we might say that a force causes an object to move.

There are many direct cause-and-effect relationships in the physical sciences and the cause comes before the effect. To take a simple example, the light in a room does not come on before you throw the switch: setting the switch allows electricity to flow and thus the light comes on. However, this sequence of cause-first-effect-later may not always be apparent in the social sciences. We can demonstrate with a simple question: does the sale of Christmas trees cause Christmas?[78] Clearly, the answer is no—even if there were no Christmas trees sold one year, people would presumably still celebrate Christmas.

If you suggest that Christmas causes the sale of trees, the causality seems to be backwards: the cause (Christmas) comes after the sale of the trees (effect). Even if we go back to the first Christmas tree, or the first Yule log in pagan times, the tree or log did not cause the festival. We could assume that people remember previous years, so they predict Christmas will arrive on December 25th and buy a tree in anticipation. But regardless of how people learned to buy Christmas trees, it is clear that social and economic questions can have different characteristics to the linear cause-then-effect of classical physics.

Tarnished Gold

Genetics

Genetics is often associated with disease. In cases where there is heritable transmission, the existence of associated genes is to be expected. However, there are relatively few illnesses where a single gene is the cause. Such diseases, such as the devastating case of Huntington's chorea, are rare, and are usually easy to track in families. By contrast, cancer has numerous genetic disturbances, associated with many different genes. Cancer cells are variable: the genes that are active in one breast cancer cell may be absent from a second cell, even if they are next to each other in the same tumour! Despite this, the media frequently trumpet the discovery of a gene for a disease, such as cancer or schizophrenia. Such reports are overstated.

Whenever an association between a gene and illness is claimed, remember that a gene is merely a template—a blueprint for the production of a protein. Finding that a gene is related to an illness does not tell us what its linked protein does within the body. In addition, there are thousands of genes. This means that even in extremely large samples, researchers are likely to find many significant but irrelevant associations between genes and illnesses. Include a large number of genes and, by chance alone, you will find an apparent link.

When scientists claim to have found the gene for a disease, it does not mean they have a cure. Despite this, efforts to attract research funding or increase a newspaper's circulation may lead report writers to imply that this is just around the corner. Finding a gene means only that researchers have found a hint, which could potentially help suggest the nature of the disease in some patients and, perhaps, ultimately lead to an improved treatment. On the other hand, it is much more likely that the apparent link will be spurious and not result in a worthwhile therapy.

Statistical magic?

Part of the confusion about causation in EBM arises because its practitioners consider groups of people, rather than individuals. Some members of a group may have a specific disease and others might not. Taken at the level of the group, it can appear that cause and effect operate by way of chance.

In many common diseases, no single factor is both necessary and sufficient. In TB, as mentioned above, the infection is necessary but not sufficient. Similarly, if two people die from strokes, one may be found to be "occlusive" (caused by a blood clot from a vein in another part of the body) while the other is "haemorrhagic" (a result of an abnormal bleed in a blood vessel in the brain). Either of these causes was sufficient, but not necessary. A group of stroke patients is likely to contain a mixture of the different types.

Alice has a common cold. She gets one every year. As most people are aware, the common cold is a result of a viral infection. Alice is infected with a coronavirus. Relatively few colds (10-15%) are caused by coronaviruses. This virus became famous when a strain was found to cause the deadly SARS (Severe Acute Respiratory Syndrome). Alice was tested for various organisms and found to be infected with a coronavirus.

Like Alice, many people frequently get a common cold. Some people succumb to the condition far less often, perhaps once a decade or two. Frequently (in 30-50% of cases), people with colds are infected with a form of rhinovirus. Unfortunately, there are about 100 different serotypes of rhinovirus. If Alice becomes immune to one of these types of rhinovirus, there are many more waiting to infect her. About 200 or so recognised viruses can cause the common cold, such as adenovirus, enterovirus, and so on. When Alice gets a cold, she understands that a virus caused it, even though she does not know which species of virus is causing the problem.

In the city where Alice lives, let us say that on average each person gets one cold a year. Some people will suffer from an adenovirus, others from a coronavirus, and so on. A few people will suffer from multiple viral infections at the same time. While a typical individual's cold is caused by a specific viral infection, this is clearly not true for the population. In the population, each virus causes a proportion of the infections. So we might identify the viruses as risk factors: rhinovirus (probability 40%), coronavirus (10%), adenovirus (5%), and so on, where the percentage is the relative frequency of people with the associated colds. Rarely, a person may have common cold symptoms from a bacterial infection (perhaps 3%). For a given population, we might identify the various viruses and probabilities that caused a common cold.

The specific cause for each individual is converted into risk factors when considering the population.

Notice the difference between Alice as an individual and the population to which she belongs. Alice's cold has a specific cause—a particular form of coronavirus has caused her infection. However, only 10% of people with colds have this virus. In the population, the common cold has a number of risk factors (viruses), as multiple viruses are present and causing illness. At the population level, cause and effect apparently breaks down into risk factors and probabilities.

This lack of specific cause and effect when studying populations is a general issue. In different people, the same illness can have different causes. For example, a person might be born deaf, or have acquired deafness through being in a rock group, as a drug side effect, or as a result of an ear infection. For the individual patient this is not an issue, as in principle we can determine the cause. However, epidemiology, clinical trials, and social science deal with groups of people, so the underlying causation of the deafness is hidden. The result is that risk factors replace cause and effect.

Shaking trees do not cause the wind

Correlation does not imply causation is a phrase that is often taught to science students. It means that just because there is a statistical relationship between two factors, you can't say that one causes the other. For example, there is a correlation between the presence of firemen and fires, but firemen do not cause the fires! The suggestion that "correlation proves causation" is a logical fallacy. It is important to know the difference between a scientific model, with an underlying mechanism, and the kind of model we find in EBM, in which statistical relationships are perceived as driving events.[79]

We have some sympathy with the EBM researchers. EBM and epidemiology are built on group statistics. Clinical trials and population studies are pragmatic and do not directly involve mechanisms. EBM merely establishes that a treated group differs from an untreated group. A risk factor is associated with a disease. EBM tells us that, on average, a drug has a positive effect. It does not explain the molecular mechanisms involved. EBM exists in a world where direct mechanisms and causation are not relevant. An EBM researcher could have a successful career without ever commenting on a mechanism of action of a drug. It is quite consistent for EBM researchers to ignore causation.

Social medicine redefines what is meant by a cause. When everything else is held constant, the presence of an epidemiological "cause" changes the probability of an event, compared with when it is absent.[80] EBM also appears to accept causes that lack known mechanisms of action. With EBM, we are expected to accept a network or web of causation, formed by an interrelationship of variables.[81,82] While this redefinition of causation has the appearance of modern physics, systems, and complexity theory, it is simply muddled. The ultimate goal of science is to find an accurate model, or theory, with a logical chain of cause and effect.

Probabilistic causation has become more acceptable, because of quantum mechanics. Before quantum mechanics, physics was clearly deterministic, and physical events were described as having causes. One physical process causes another: heat causes ice to melt, for example. The increasing heat energy jiggles the ice molecules and their crystalline structure falls apart. With the advent of quantum mechanics, descriptions of what goes on with very small things, like atoms, became probabilistic. For example, you cannot accurately measure both the position and velocity of an electron. For large objects, like the movement and position of people, mice, or elephants, quantum mechanics is not relevant: normal cause and effect still apply. However, with quantum mechanics, we cannot apply strict causation directly to small particles or their interactions. It is necessary to work with probabilities and there is no way of getting around the uncertainty.

The uncertainty in medicine is of a different quality. People are complex systems with emergent behaviour. Logic, mathematics, and information theory are still relevant. EBM asks us to accept that the relationship between smoking and cancer requires a revision of the concept of cause and effect.[83] By accepting a legal definition of evidence, the EBM practitioners have to avoid hunting "the Holy Grail" of determinism[84] and, in doing so, they have given up real science.

Embracing uncertainty

The greatest enemy of knowledge is not ignorance,
it is the illusion of knowledge.

Stephen Hawking

There is an increasing tendency for medical authorities to require that a treatment be "proven". More strangely, when attending a medical conference, you may well hear phrases such as "more proof is required" or "it would be good to have more quality proof". This assumption of certainty in which EBM engages is a form of social proof.[85] Practitioners assume the behaviour and ideas of others dictate the correct thing to do. EBM is particularly prone to social proof, because people assume the experts are powerful, understand the process, and that accuracy is particularly important.[86] The collectivist organisation of "evidence-based" medicine makes it prone to this form of conformity.[87]

The notion of "scientific proof" is nonsense and should be expunged from discussions of medicine. Even the concept of such proof is destructive to scientific progress. A proven idea does not need to be subjected to scientific testing: it is already known to be true. Thus, the idea of scientific proof limits investigation, restricts scientific development, and is detrimental to patients.

Main Points

- There is no such thing as "scientific proof".
- EBM's "proof" protects corporate medicine, not patients.
- Clinical "proof" is for lawyers, not scientists.
- EBM arose out of the legal system, not science.
- Proof implies dogmatism, authority, and coercion.
- Science is free and embraces uncertainty.

If you thought that science was certain—well, that is just an error on your part.

Richard Feynman

Beating the Odds

> Games combining chance and skill give the best representation of human life, particularly of military affairs and of the practice of medicine, which necessarily depend partly on skill and partly on chance.... It would be desirable to have a complete study made of games, treated mathematically.
>
> Gottfried Wilhelm von Leibniz

In order to put EBM into context, we want to show how difficult and confusing even simple probability problems can be. Once you have grasped this issue, you may suspect how unlikely it is that even world-leading statisticians can fully understand the meaning behind EBM's large-scale clinical trials.

Medical decisions rely on incomplete data and thus involve *probability*, which is a measure of the chance a particular event will occur. When faced with probability, many people are worried that the subject is too difficult. However, we can let you into a secret: even mathematicians find the concept challenging. The simplest probability problems can be hard to understand, so don't worry if you find parts of this chapter difficult, or even astounding.

One of our aims is to help readers become familiar with science and decision-making. Medical decision-making involves working with limited knowledge, a unique patient, and an uncertain environment. In making a diagnosis, a doctor selects the most probable disease and uses this assessment to guide treatment. Physicians do what they can to reduce the risk of getting the diagnosis wrong. For example, although a particular lump is likely to be a benign cyst, it may turn out to be a tumour. Since the consequences of misdiagnosis could be catastrophic, the physician may ask for tests to exclude this possibility.

Hold on to your hat—you might find these following sections mind-bendingly strange.

Probability – Case 1

Let us start with a simple example. A doctor is sitting in her office, when a mother of two enters the room, accompanied by her elder child, a boy. What is the chance of her second child also being a boy?

The answer is, of course, a 1 in 2 chance. The other child could be either a boy or a girl.

We know nothing about the second child and, assuming an equal number of boys and girls in the population, there is a 50-50 chance that the second child is a boy. (The probability that the second child is a girl is also 1 in 2.)

Probability – Case 2

Next, another mother of two comes into the doctor's office. The mother is accompanied by one of her children, a boy. Now, what is the chance that her other child is also a boy?

This time, the answer is 1 in 3! There is only a 33% chance that the absent child is also a boy.

If you find this result surprising, you are not alone. This example is a classic exercise in probability and logic. Because probability is a measure of ignorance, even the slightest change in the question can change the outcome. The difference between Case 1 and Case 2 is subtle: the first mother was accompanied by her *elder* child, but the second mother was with an *unspecified* child. In these two examples, it makes a difference whether you know the accompanying boy is the elder child, or not. The extra information in Case 1 allows us to exclude two possible combinations, because we know that the elder child is not a girl. In Case 2, we are more ignorant, because we don't know the order of the children, so we cannot exclude as many options.

Combinations for Second Child (100 two child families)						
	Boy-Boy	Boy-Girl	Girl-Boy	Girl-Girl		
Case 1	25	25	25	25	A: Elder child is a boy	50
	25	25	25	25	B: Second child also a boy	25
					Chance of B, given A:	1 in 2 (50%)
Case 2	25	25	25	25	C: Any one child a boy	75
	25	25	25	25	D: Two boys	25
					Chance of D, given C:	1 in 3 (33%)

Probability of two boys in two-child families if:
Case 1: The elder child is a boy, is 50%, 1 in 2, or 50-50
Case 2: At least one child is a boy, is 33%, 1 in 3, or 25-75

Detailed Explanation

This problem was introduced because it is both simple and deceptive. The problems are almost identical but the results are different. Since this issue goes to the heart of the EBM problem, we now provide clarification.

In Case 1, the mother has two children. The possible combinations for two children (elder-younger) are: boy-boy (BB), boy-girl (BG), girl-boy (GB), and girl-girl (GG). For a mother with two children, all these are equally likely. However, we know that the elder child is a boy. Only two options include a boy first, BB and BG. Of these two options, only one has two boys. Thus, there is one chance in two, or 50-50, that the second child is a boy.

In Case 2, however, there is a subtle difference. In this case, we do not know whether she has brought her elder or younger child to see the doctor. We know that the mother has at least one boy, because he is with her. We therefore know that she does not have two girls (GG). There are three remaining possibilities for her two children: BB, BG, and GB. In only one of these three options, the absent child is a boy. So, the chance of her other child being a boy is 1 in 3 (33%).

In case this still seems bizarre, we will give yet another explanation. With the first mother, since we know the *elder* child is a boy, we know the order of the children. We are therefore considering the first-born and second-born children independently. This is equivalent to asking two questions: the sex of the first child (1 in 2, or 50-50) and the sex of the second child (1 in 2). We are told the answer to the first question, but this provides no information about the second question. Thus, there is still a 1 in 2 chance that the second child is a boy or a girl.

In Case 2, there is only one question - to determine the sex of the other child, given that at least one of them is a boy. In this question, we do not know the order of the children. Another way of looking at this is to say that the chance of the mother having one boy and one girl (BG or GB) is twice that of having two boys (BB), so the absent child is twice as likely to be a girl. Only one of the three possible combinations includes two boys, so the chance of that is 1 in 3 (33%).

If, at this point, you remain more confused than convinced, try not to worry—one of the main objectives of this section is to show that probability can be hard to understand, a point you doubtless appreciate by now! Even the apparently simplest of questions can be tricky.

Probability – Monty Hall problem

We can now look at a slightly more complex puzzle. This entertaining problem is a conundrum that once again illustrates how statistics and probability reflect the amount of ignorance a question entails. This one has fooled even leading mathematicians.

The Monty Hall problem is a modern classic, based on the US television game show *Let's Make a Deal*, hosted by Monty Hall. The problem is easy to state, though remarkably difficult to understand. If interested, you can go through the mathematics carefully to understand this intriguing problem. However, we include it here to show how even apparently simple questions in probability can stump world-class intellectuals.

Suppose you are on a game show and have the choice of opening one of three doors (doors One, Two, and Three). Your prize is behind the door you select. You have been told that an automobile is behind one door. However, behind each of the other two doors is a goat. You would prefer to win the car!

There is no reason to value any particular door, so you choose door One. Next, Monty Hall, who can see behind the doors, opens door Two, revealing a goat. He then asks, "Would you like to swap your door for door Three?"

The question is – should you switch doors?

Most people assume that there is an equal chance of the car being behind either door One or Three, because there is no way to know which of the two doors hides the car. They conclude that the knowledge we have about both doors is the same, so switching would make no difference: it is a 50/50 choice, similar to heads or tails when tossing a fair coin. For this reason, many people decline the offer to switch doors, preferring to stick with their original choice.

However, a more thorough analysis of the problem indicates that you should switch. Indeed, if you switch from your initial choice (door One) to the door that Monty left closed (door Three), you double your chance of winning the car.

If you stay with your first choice, you have the same 1 in 3 chance (one of three doors) that you had originally. Surprisingly, though, the door that Monty left closed has a 2 in 3 chance of hiding the car. The reasoning is relatively simple: there was initially a 2 in 3 chance that one of the doors that you did not choose (doors Two and Three) hid the car. Since Monty has now opened door Two to reveal a goat, the 2 in 3 chance on those two doors now applies to door Three only. Therefore, you should switch.

When this problem was published, in the September 1990 edition of Parade magazine, many readers complained that this answer was wrong. It is claimed that over 1,000 PhDs argued that the published solution was mistaken. They thought the probability was still 50/50.

Andrew Vazsonyi, a PhD mathematician,[88] told the problem to Paul Erdős, one of the 20th century's most celebrated mathematicians.[89] Erdős published more research papers than any other mathematician in history. Most mathematicians can tell you their "Erdős number". An Erdős number of one means you

Tarnished Gold

published a paper with Erdős, two means that you have published with someone who co-authored a paper with Erdős, and so on. Albert Einstein had an Erdős number of two. Erdős himself had an Erdős number of zero. He published in many areas of mathematics, notably probability.

Vazsonyi, the subject of this tale, had an Erdős number of 1. When he asked Erdős about this problem, Erdős initially replied that the answer was 50/50. Vazsonyi was amazed that the great Erdős had got it wrong. He went through the methods from his undergraduate quantitative techniques of management course, and demonstrated that switching doors was the right thing to do. It doubled the chance of winning from 1/3 to 2/3. Erdős was not impressed with Vazsonyi's explanation and said, "You are not telling me *why* to switch!" and then "What is the matter with you?"

When Vazsonyi admitted he did not know why, Erdős remained unsatisfied. Erdős was a mathematical genius. Yes, he had been confused (like many others) by a simple problem in probability. He was willing to accept that the decision to switch was correct, but he wanted to understand why. We would like readers of this book to apply a similar thought process to "evidence-based" medicine. EBM is usually wrapped in complicated statistical methods, which seem to confer authority. We are not interested in equations or complicated statistics. Yes, we can understand that palaver—but it does not explain why! We want to look at EBM in a simple and fundamental way. We want to know how medical decisions should be made and, as Erdős might demand: why?

The answer to why switching doors is more likely to yield the prize car is actually quite simple. As in our first example of the mothers with two children (Cases 1 and 2 above), the secret is that probabilities are measures of ignorance. When first presented with the three doors, you were completely ignorant as to which door hid the car. The probability associated with each of the three doors was therefore 1 in 3. There was one chance in three that the car was behind any door you chose.

After choosing a door, but not yet opening it, you still had one chance in three of having selected the car. The chance that the car was behind one of the other two doors was two chances in three (2 in 3). Nevertheless, although you were ignorant and had no information about the location of the car, Monty Hall knew what was behind the doors: he had complete information about them.

Once Monty opened one of the other doors and showed a goat, the problem changed. The only way he could *always* show a goat (and, of course, he never gives away the location of the car) is if he knew what was behind both doors. Once he shows a goat, you have gained information and so the probability becomes two chances in three that the car is behind the remaining door (door Three). Now ask yourself, would the outcome be the same if Monty had no knowledge and had opened the second door at random?

Monkey puzzle

For over 50 years, a version of the Monty Hall problem infected the psychological literature with a logical error.[90] In 1956, psychologists at Yale University performed an experiment that was similar to the Monty Hall problem.[91] In one form of the experiment, a monkey is given a choice between three different coloured M&M chocolates: red, blue, or green.

First, the monkey is asked to choose between two of the M&Ms, say red or blue. If the monkey chose red, it was given a choice between the remaining colours, blue and green. More often than not, the monkey would reject the blue M&M again, and select the green one. The psychologists assumed this to be "choice rationalization": if a human rejects something, they tell themselves they didn't like it in the first place. In so doing, they avoid the uncomfortable feeling of having made a mistake. Monkeys are rather similar to humans and the explanation that they wanted to avoid feeling bad about making a mistake seemed reasonable.

In 2008, economist Keith Chen showed that the explanation for this celebrated experiment was flawed.[92] The monkeys' rejection of the blue M&M is rational. The problem was that the psychologists had assumed that all three colours had the same value to the monkey. In reality, this is unlikely to be true: monkeys (like humans) would probably prefer some colours over others. If so, the monkey's selection of colours was sensible.

The explanation is similar to that for the Monty Hall problem. By opening one door to reveal a goat, Monty provided the contestants with information, thus changing the probabilities associated with the different doors. Similarly, the monkey's first choice of M&M colour gives us some information: it tells us which of those two colours the monkey prefers. The monkeys' initial choice of a red

M&M could reflect a slight preference for red over the rejected blue, for example. In the second choice (green or blue), the monkey favours green over blue because, as shown in the table below, there are two chances in three that it always preferred green M&Ms to blue ones.

Preference order (123)	1st colours offered	Monkey's 1st choice	2nd colours offered	Monkey's 2nd choice
RGB	RB	R	BG	G
RBG	RB	R	BG	B
GRB	RB	R	BG	G
GBR	RB	B	BG	G
BRG	RB	B	BG	B
BGR	RB	B	BG	B

Possible colour preferences and consequent choices

As is the nature of these apparently simple probability problems, the discussion and analysis continue with increasing complexity.[93,94] The reader might be relieved to think that the monkey was acting only on its preferences, and not solving the Monty Hall problem!

The Monty Hall problem is important, however, because it shows how challenging simple probability problems can be. This problem confused many scientists and mathematicians, even the brilliant Paul Erdős. Its solution depends critically on how much information each of the participants in the experiment possess. A full understanding of the Monty Hall problem and its related issues goes beyond statistics, into the theory of games and cybernetics.

As we have seen, we require a sophisticated theoretical analysis to understand even a simple game of what lies behind three doors. "Evidence-based" medicine, however, involves far more than this: studies include thousands of subjects, huge numbers of variables, and enormous numbers of interactions. It also involves many participants, each of which has some knowledge, or information, of the disease, treatment, experimental design, preferences, and financial constraints.

If leading mathematicians can struggle to analyse an experiment involving just three doors, and psychologists can misinterpret the results of a monkey's choice of three M&Ms, we can see that the potential for confusion and misunderstanding in the far more complex field of EBM is enormous.

Deceptive clinical trials

One of the main problems with conventional clinical trials is that the significance of the result is affected by slight variations in the experimental design. The number of subjects used, the sequence of patients, and the stopping rule can all influence the results.

As stressed above, the probabilities provided by statistical tests are a measure of uncertainty or ignorance. Through a series of examples, we have seen that the answers to questions (about children, cars and goats, or M&M's) can vary, depending on the information provided. Likewise, the significance of medical trials can change with the intentions and knowledge of the experimenter.

Most people do not realise that the most innocent decisions in the design of an experiment can change the result. To illustrate this, Professor Don Berry has described a hypothetical clinical trial, in which there are ten patients: seven who were treated successfully and three whose treatment failed.[95] He explains two scenarios: in the first (A), the researchers decide in advance to include ten patients in the study. In the second (B), they decide to keep the experiment going until they have had three failures; in the event, these failures just happen to occur after ten patients.

Let us suppose that in both scenarios, the sequence of outcomes was SSFSSFSSSF, where S is a success (cure) and F is a failure (patient died). This means that, regardless of the decision mechanism for ending the study, both scenarios involve ten patients: seven successes and three failures, in the same order. Nothing in the numbers or the sequence and procedure of the experiment has changed. Nevertheless, because of the choices made before the start of the experiment, the standard probabilities are different, despite the outcomes being apparently identical.

The experimenters' initial decision to use all 10 subjects (Scenario A) or to end the trial after three failures (Scenario B) gives different probabilities for exactly the same results. Bizarrely, the calculated probability for Scenario B is much smaller than that for Scenario A. To stress the point: the results are identical, using the same measurements, from the same patients, made by the same researchers, in the same experiment; the only difference is the initial idea behind the trial. The probabilities for Scenario A are:

Number of patients (out of 10) cured by the treatment assuming a 35% success rate (p=0.35)											
Successes	0	1	2	3	4	5	6	7	8	9	10
Probability	0.013	0.072	0.176	0.252	0.238	0.154	0.069	0.021	0.004	0.001	0.000

Suppose the established success rate for our treatment is 35%: we might therefore assume that the most likely outcome for a trial of ten patients would be that three or four patients would be cured. It would be less likely, though possible, that either two or five patients would be cured, and so on.

In EBM statistics, a result is said to be significant when its probability is less than one in twenty. The chance of something happening one time in twenty may be expressed as a percentage (1/20 x 100%), giving a 5% probability. In scientific papers, the fraction 1/20 is often expressed as a p-value decimal: p=0.05.

In scenario A, with 10 patients in the study, the possible outcomes range from 10 successes and no failures, through to 10 failures and no successes. We can calculate the likelihood of each number of successes, from none (p=0.013; or 13 in 1,000 - very unlikely) through to ten (p=0.00003; or 3 in 100,000 - exceptionally unlikely). The chance of having exactly seven cures, as in Don Berry's scenario, is twenty one in a thousand (p=0.021).

In this case, the chance of seven or more cures is p=0.026 (from the table 0.026=0.021+0.004+0.001+0.000). This value (26 in 1,000) means that if we repeated the trial 38 times, we would expect to get one result where seven or more patients were cured, just by chance.

Since the results of scenarios A and B were identical sequences of seven cures and three failures, we might assume that the probabilities would also be the same. However, this assumption would be wrong. In EBM, the probabilities do NOT apply just to

79

the results of the trial: they apply to the whole experiment! Bewildering as it may seem, the estimated probability is a result of the precise design of the experiment, the particular results, and even *what was in the experimenter's mind.* Note that we do not mean to imply mind over matter or some other psychological effect here, merely uncertainty arising from the method of calculation and design of the experiment.

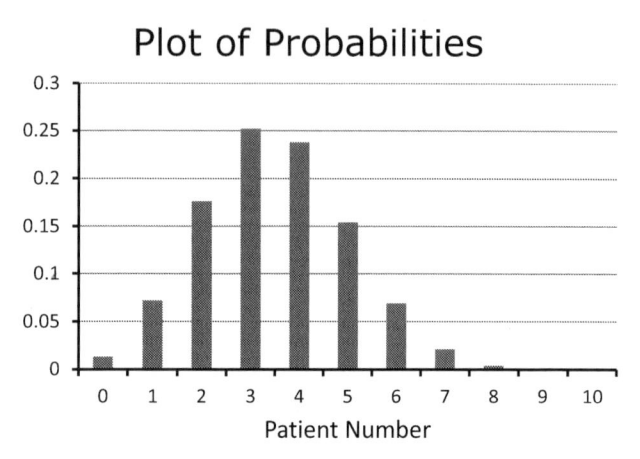

Plot of Probabilities

Visual plot of the probabilities in our table of 10 subjects in Scenario A with a 35% probability of cure

To see what this means, let us consider the possible outcomes for scenario B. Since there have to be three failures, we can start with an outcome of three failures and no successes. This would mean that Patient 3 was the last failure, and the trial was then stopped. Another possible outcome would be that one patient was cured and Patient 4 was the last failure. Or, two patients were cured and Patient 5 was the last failure, and so on. Theoretically, the experiment could go on forever, if patients kept on being cured.

In scenario A, the probability associated with the actual outcome was 21 in 1,000 (p=0.021). However, the corresponding probability for scenario B is only about one fifth of this or 4 in 1,000 (p=0.004). The reason it is so much smaller is that scenario B offers far more options than scenario A. In scenario B, the number of patients was not known before the experiment started, because the plan involved keeping going until three patients had died. In A, there must be ten patients, whereas in B, there might be only three, or there could be an infinite number. Each extra option reduces the likelihood of getting exactly seven successes and three failures. Thus, the estimated probability of this particular result is lower under the conditions of scenario B.

If we imagine a Martian sceptic, overlooking every aspect of the experiment with absolute rigour, he would not see anything different. The experiments are identical, though the probabilities are not. The only difference was information hidden away inside the doctor's head! Our Martian could not reliably calculate the probability of the result using EBM's methods without reading the experimenter's mind.

Implications

Don Berry's thought experiment suggests that an EBM experimenter's intentions can greatly change how we interpret the results obtained in an experiment. This was a very simple clinical trial. Its different probabilities indicate that the typical EBM clinical trial lacks consistency and reliability. Using the current statistics, any change in the experimental design (as may often happen), such as a patient dropping out, deciding to end the study early, adding a new patient, or so on, means the reported probabilities will be incorrect. As we have seen, EBM's statistics apply only to a specific and precise design.

Unfortunately, the problems go deeper than this. The probability may not be valid, even if the recipe and statistics for the trial are apparently specified in advance, and outwardly carried out precisely to order. As with the inspection made by our hypothetical Martian, while there may be no observable difference between trials, we cannot be sure what the researcher intended.

In practice, clinical trials can be messy. There will be a variable number of patients, some will refuse to sign up, some will guess that they are receiving the treatment, and others may lie or not cooperate. Subjects may die or leave the experiment abruptly. The experiment may be terminated early at the request of an ethics committee. A researcher may move to another university. In the real world, such changes are commonplace.

Before the reader becomes convinced that all statistics are suspect, we should explain that it is possible to design reliable experiments with unambiguous probabilities. The internal thoughts of the researcher do not really change reality. One approach is to use Bayesian methods. We will describe a simple but solid trial later.

Knowing the odds

It may be surprising to realise that schoolchildren use probabilities all the time, with little difficulty. It is only when the process is formalized in school that they seem to find it hard to understand. Even young children have little problem accepting, for example, that tossing a coin is a 50-50 bet, with a 1 in 2 chance of either heads or tails. The trick is to stick to counting possibilities—use fractions and odds rather than relative figures like percentages and decimal p-values. Straightforward fractions and odds will simplify the process.

The "Grand National" is the world's most famous steeplechase race, held every spring at the Aintree Racecourse, Liverpool, England. On Grand National day, it is common for British children and adults to have a favourite horse, and to quote and compare odds for the race. A horse with odds of "one hundred to one" (100/1) generally has less chance of winning than a favourite at "seven to one" (7/1), but if it does win, the reward will be greater. In 2009, a French horse called *Mon Mome* won the race, with a starting price of 100/1. A one dollar bet on *Mon Mome* would have netted you $100, plus your original dollar stake. The year before that, the race was won by the joint favourite, *Comply Or Die*, starting at only 7/1; so, a one dollar bet on *Comply Or Die* would have won you just $7, plus your $1 stake.

Betting is popular in many fields, including football, cricket, the World Series, or who will top the pop music charts at Christmas. It involves an appreciation of both probability of winning and risk of losing. However, in betting, the outcomes are clearly stated. A dollar stake on a twenty-to-one bet will give you a return of $21 ($20+$1) if you win. The 20-dollar gain is balanced against the potential loss of one dollar.

Many people only bet infrequently, perhaps placing a small yearly wager on the Grand National, without real consideration of the chance of winning. In such cases, the choice of horse may be based on apparently irrelevant factors, such as the horse's name, rather than any great understanding of its form. Those placing bets may choose a horse with a funny name, or one with a particular meaning to them. Their idea is to have a stake in the race, providing a psychological attachment to a particular runner, to add interest and increase enjoyment. If they win, that is a bonus.

Strange as it may seem, in the absence of expert knowledge, choosing a name you recognize can be an effective strategy. This approach is called the *recognition heuristic*. Professor Gerd Gigerenzer and colleagues have investigated name recognition in choosing companies on the German and international stock markets.[96] The results showed that well-recognized companies outperformed those that were less familiar. Moreover, when choosing international stocks, the beneficial effect of the recognition heuristic was strongest for those groups who were most ignorant of the market. Random participants using the heuristic outperformed two managed funds. To quote Gigerenzer's group:

> ...the collective ignorance of 180 pedestrians in downtown Munich was more predictive than the knowledge and expertise of American and German fund managers.

Medical probabilities

Unfortunately, in medicine, probabilities are not given as fractional odds, such as 1 in 20 (or 20/1, as in horseracing), but in the rather confusing p-value notation. In medical and scientific experiments, a less than one in twenty result is noteworthy (the standard p-value of less than 0.05, i.e. $p<0.05$). So, in EBM, a significant result means that it is not particularly likely to be a fluke. However, by definition, that same result might occur by chance roughly once in every twenty cases.

We need to include a disclaimer here, because of the confusion about probabilities: the p-value is actually the chance of finding the observed result if the samples were taken randomly from a common population. If we did not state this, EBM statisticians might accuse us of being misleading or lacking understanding. We might have been talking about the wrong kind of fluke! Here we prefer a direct interpretation, as it can increase understanding. However, it is good to remember that, in an important way, the p-value says nothing about the underlying reality. We have already shown that the calculated EBM p-value is not a property of the results but of the whole experimental setup including, potentially, the experimenters' prejudice or viewpoints. Despite this, the p-value is at the heart of EBM, as it is the primary outcome of significance testing.

Originally, Sir Ronald Fisher (1890–1962) proposed p-values as an informal estimate of the evidence. He suggested the p-value should be used along with other data for and against the idea. Fisher's relaxed approach to interpretation is in line with Bayesian statistics. In particular, the evidence for the idea before the experiment was performed may dominate current results. This realisation is standard practice in tests of, say, extrasensory perception, where positive results at 5% levels of probability would be treated with extreme caution. *Lindley's Paradox* occurs when, despite an experiment returning a significant p-value, the weight of pre-existing data suggests the result is incorrect.[97] If it disagrees with solid experimental results, such as established biochemistry, a gold standard EBM clinical trial may be significant and obey all the rules, and yet be preposterous.

Sometimes, a result is described as being "highly significant". This means it has less than one chance in a hundred of being a fluke. This is equivalent to *Mon Mome* winning the 2009 Grand National at 100/1—an unlikely event, but, as we have seen, unlikely events sometimes happen. The odds of a highly significant result happening *by chance alone* are at least 100 to one against (i.e. $p<0.01$).

Let us return briefly to the topic of betting, where probabilities are more easily understood. Imagine Alice wants to bet on a heavyweight called Joe Boxer, to win a world title fight. The bookie offers odds of 100 to 1; these odds suggest Joe has only a small chance of winning. However, if a commentator were to claim that these odds meant that Joe has been "proven" to be going to lose the fight, Alice would be rightly surprised, as Joe (just like *Mon Mome*) still has a chance of winning, otherwise there would be no point in Alice placing her bet.

Odds of 20 to 1, 100 to 1, or even more, do not mean that Joe Boxer has been *proven* to lose the fight, before it begins! It means that the bookie taking the bet believes he is going to make a profit by offering those odds. In EBM, however, a result with these odds may be described as "proven" or (more often) a group of studies that do not meet this criterion will be described as "unproven".

For example, an editorial in the Journal of the American Medical Association (a bastion of EBM) opens with the following:

Tarnished Gold

> There is no alternative medicine. There is only scientifically proven, evidence-based medicine supported by solid data or unproven medicine, for which scientific evidence is lacking. [98]

Proponents of EBM may object at this point and say that "proof" depends of the outcome of at least one large-scale clinical trial. It isn't the odds that matter, they may add, but the quality of the study, how well controlled was the experiment, and, especially, how many subjects were involved. However, these arguments are rather confused. Either the trial was a fluke, or it was not. To claim any kind of *proof*, based on probabilities, would mark these EBM proponents out as an easy target in a betting shop, investment bank, or casino.

Confusing the doctors

EBM presents the results of tests in a way that is deliberately misleading. Such presentation makes minor effects appear much more important than they really are. The presentation of probabilities in EBM misleads both doctors and patients.[99] Never trust a report that provides its results only in the form of a percentage risk or a relative value.

The concept of risk involves both the likelihood of an event and its consequences. In the United States, the risk of dying from a lightning strike is reported to be 6 deaths per 10,000,000 people per year.[100] Technically speaking, the idea of risk applies to benefits, as well as harmful events, though this is not usual in everyday speech. Now, suppose the risk of winning a lottery is 1 in 10,000,000: in this case, a person would need to purchase 6 tickets a year, to have as much chance of winning the lottery as of being struck by lightning. People readily pay to play the lottery, but may not be as eager to part with even small amounts of money as insurance against lightning strikes. Perhaps they think the probability of being hit is so small, it is not worth insuring. In the case of the lottery, the risk of losing your stake is high, but the stake is small, so its loss is not catastrophic. A person might get great pleasure imagining and discussing what they would do with the lottery win, but prefer to avoid thinking about being fried by a lightning strike.

In EBM, risk is expressed in relative terms. Suppose a hypothetical large-scale study of a new drug reports a 50% decrease in heart attack. The report is accurate, but highly misleading. Only half the number of people receiving the drug had a heart attack, compared to the controls. But this form of presentation does not tell us anything about the actual incidence of heart attacks in the population.

Since it is a large-scale EBM trial, let us say that 1,000 people received the drug and the same number were used as controls. Of these 2,000 people, suppose that four of the controls had a heart attack, compared with two members of the treated group. In this case, the reported 50% decrease actually means a reduction from 4 in 1,000 to 2 in 1,000.

The reported 50% reduction in risk sounds like a big, important effect, and may be used by marketing specialists to imply that everyone at risk should be using this new drug. However, the actual risk (down from just 4 in 1,000 to 2 in 1,000) is tiny, regardless of whether or not you take the drug. While a person might be willing to pay several hundred dollars a year for a drug to halve their risk of death from heart disease, they might not be so eager if they realized how small the real reduction in risk was. Certainly, the chance of heart attack is greater than that of being struck by lightning in the earlier example, but the same argument applies. If the risk is sufficiently small, it is not worth the cost of insuring or medicating against it.

Percentage risk reduction is great marketing for persuading ill-informed people to take a new drug. Physicians may also be deceived, unless they take the trouble to read the original research paper with great care. Unfortunately, doctors tend to be busy and short of time. Such misrepresentative numbers benefit pharmaceutical companies and are picked up and hyped by the media. However, reports that do not include the actual incidences of the disease are misleading: they are worthless and should be ignored.

Don't be misled–always use frequencies

We will reinforce the point about percentages here using Bayes' theorem or, as it might be popularly described, applied common sense. With Bayes, the risks are referred back to the original population.

To avoid being misled, we suggest the reader should *always* convert percentage values into frequencies, when considering clinical trials. Let us consider a real case of misrepresentation, concerning statin drugs. A recent study of the beneficial effects of the statin drug rosuvastatin (trade name Crestor), claimed that it resulted in almost half the risk of heart attack (46%) and stroke (52%).[101] At face value, a person should take this drug, as it appears to lower their risks by large amounts. However, looking more closely, it is apparent that the results are deceptive.

The actual risk of heart attack in the treated population was 0.17% (17 heart attacks in a population of 10,000). This compares with a risk of 0.37% (37 heart attacks in a population of 10,000) for the untreated controls. So, the actual decrease in risk was 20 fewer heart attacks in 10,000 people (0.2%). The figures were estimated over a period of 100 person years. The number needed to treat was 500; that means 500 people would need to take the drug to prevent a single heart attack! Furthermore, all 500 would be at risk of any side effects the drug may have.

Large EBM studies are particularly prone to this misrepresentation of unimportant results. This statin drug might seem a lot less useful if the data was presented using absolute values, such as "by taking this drug, patients will gain a 1 in 500 (0.2%) reduction in their risk of having a heart attack." A person might be happy to pay $1,000 a year, for a drug that cuts their risk of heart attack by half. They might be far less willing if they realised the real reduction in risk was only two in a thousand. This means that the cost per heart attack saved is $500,000. Given the absolute figures, the person could make a rational choice and spend their limited funds on more effective ways of reducing their risk of disease. The person's health and wellbeing might benefit more from a gym subscription, improved nutrition, or even a holiday.

Measuring benefit

A key measure to indicate the degree of benefit from a drug is the *number needed to treat* (NNT).[102] This is the number of patients that must be treated in order to obtain some specified benefit, such as an improvement of vision in a person with cataracts. The NNT is a direct indication of the utility of a drug. For example, if an anti-cataract drug has an NNT of 5, you would typically have to treat five people to improve the vision of a single patient. Ideally, you would prefer a drug with an NNT of 1, so it would work for every patient. By contrast, if the NNT is high, then many people have to be treated in order to help just one. In this case, the financial costs and risk of side effects to the majority might outweigh the benefits to the one.

The much hyped and popular statin drugs, used as preventive medicine, have a number needed to treat of between about 50 and 200.[103,104] To make these numbers more palatable, they are often fudged. The NNT is spread over, say, 5 or 10 years, rather than a standard one-year period. So, the benefit is multiplied by the time period, making the drug seem more effective. The patient pays for this "benefit" in a continuing cost of medication and associated side effects. Unfortunately, doctors often fail to inform patients that their chance of being helped by the prescribed drug is remote.

Medicine needs to return to direct measures of outcomes, probabilities, and benefits, and stop misleading the public about the likely effects of treatments.

Main Points

- Probability is confusing.
- Even a simple experiment or game can confound leading mathematicians.
- EBM trials are far from simple; misinterpretation is almost inevitable.
- EBM's statistics apply to the whole experiment, not just the results.
- EBM's methods cannot deal with its overcomplicated clinical trials.
- Results in EBM can be deceptive.
- Decision science and Bayesian statistics can help make things clear.

> If your result needs a statistician then you should design a better experiment.
>
> Ernest Rutherford

Understanding Results

An approximate answer to the right problem is worth a good deal more than an exact answer to an approximate problem.

John Tukey

Clinical trials are generally large complicated affairs, but can be viewed as simple tests. Here we will describe a basic form of medical test used for screening. Screening is used to detect health problems, such as cancer. Test findings may use EBM data from clinical trials and epidemiology. The general view appears to be that medical screening should be part of EBM.[105,106,107] In this book, we are concerned mainly with the application (and misapplication) of such data to individual prediction.

We will use medical screening as an example, to outline some critical aspects of clinical trials. Medical authorities increasingly request people to have health screening checks, though they are often of little value and can sometimes be positively harmful. The statement that medical screening based on current methods is generally useless should not be considered heretical. The Bandolier Group, an Oxford University associated team dedicated to "evidence-based" healthcare, has a blacklist of medical screening tests for which they consider evidence is lacking.[108] These include:

- Chest X-ray in older patients, smokers and travellers
- Haemoglobin for anaemia
- ESR for inflammatory infective or malignant disease
- Liver function tests in blood
- Renal function tests
- Calcium, uric acid or glucose in blood
- Cholesterol and HDL/LDL ratio
- Mammography in women over 40 years
- Ultrasound examination of the ovaries

- Examination of the aorta in men over 55 years
- Bone density in women
- Resting ECG and exercise ECG on a treadmill
- PSA in men over 50 years
- Helicobacter pylori

We congratulate Bandolier on this blacklist. Unfortunately, Bandolier then ruined their critical success and responded to establishment reproach by providing a whitelist of screening tests that they claim may be useful: [109]

- Breast cancer screening for women over 50 years (but qualified with two references)[110,111]
- Cervical cancer screening for women over 20 years, though not more often than every five years for maximum cost-effectiveness
- Screening for high blood pressure according to the British Hypertension Society guidelines
- Identifying cigarette smokers and advising them of the benefits of stopping smoking

We find we can agree once again with Bandolier—but only on smoking. Cigarette smokers can be identified definitively: they are the ones sucking on little white sticks, with a fire at the end. Any individual who decides to give up smoking is likely to benefit both financially and in health terms. However, smoking is a matter for personal choice and the health issues are common knowledge. If we were feeling generous, we might concede that blood pressure monitoring could sometimes be useful. We will now explain why medical screening is so controversial.

CT scans cause cancer?

Magnetic resonance and x-ray CT scanners are routinely used to investigate symptoms. However, whole body CT scanning is sometimes carried out to search for early signs of disease in healthy people, before symptoms appear. Presumably, the rationale is that the early detection of, say, cancer may allow treatment to be started before the disease has had chance to progress. People assume they will benefit, otherwise the screening would not be increasingly popular.

It is easy to see why radiologists and medical technology companies might value the screening. To quote Karen Horton, Professor of Radiology at Johns Hopkins University School of Medicine, "To be truly successful at whole-body CT screening—defined by finding very early-stage lesions, not simply by making money—it is necessary to invest in the latest CT technology."[112] Dr Horton seems to imply that some of her medical colleagues might consider a high tech CT scanner as a cash-cow, regardless of therapeutic benefit. Nevertheless, she recommends the latest technology, because it will find the smallest, early-stage lesions.

One disadvantage of whole body scanning, particularly for patients who cover their own costs, is that it is expensive. Ironically, it is also rather risky, as it delivers a large dose of x-rays to the patient, which can lead to the development of cancer. The risk varies with the dose and age of the patient. A single CT scan to the abdomen will increase the risk by a little less than 0.1%, i.e. up to one extra cancer per 1,000 people. This may sound reassuring; however, multiple images are collected in whole body screening and the process may be repeated every few years. An optimistic estimate is that such screening may result in an additional two cancers for every hundred people who undergo lifetime screening.

The use of CT scans is increasing; by 2006, the estimated number in the US was 62 million scans a year.[113] Between 1980 and 2005, the number of scans increased twenty-fold. These scans were estimated to be responsible for 1.5-2% of all cancers. That means that of every fifty or so cancer patients, one will have developed the disease because of a scan. While imaging can be of great benefit for the sick, overuse is clearly dangerous. Perhaps one third of CT scans in children—who are most susceptible to harm—could be replaced or not performed at all.[114] High levels of x-ray exposure can hardly be recommended for screening apparently healthy individuals.

A further and perhaps surprising disadvantage is that CT scans, as recommended for screening by Dr Horton, could be *too accurate*. Dr Robert Stanley, a former Editor-in-Chief of the American Journal of Roentgenology, has described the problem of detecting tumours using radiological techniques by comparing it with mapping islands.[115]

Stanley asks his readers how many islands there are off the coast of Maine. Of course, it depends on how closely we look and how big an island we include in the search. A small-scale map of the coast, in a world atlas, may not show any islands. But if we look closely at a local map of the coast near Bangor (north of Boston), we will see several islands that were not visible on the atlas. Some of these islands even have names, and locals may be able to tell you what even smaller islands are called. Looking more closely, we might notice large rocky outcrops that are visible only at low tide; Stanley asked whether these rocks qualify as islands. The point of the story is that the closer we look, the harder it becomes to decide what is an island and what is not.

A famous mathematician, Benoît Mandelbrot, once asked a similar question: how long is a coastline? He noticed that the length of a coastline increases, depending on the level of detail chosen. As a result, Mandelbrot discovered fractals, a revolution in mathematics and computer science.[116] These lead to wonderfully complex computer graphics, which, like a coastline, appear more and more detailed as you zoom in and examine them ever more closely.

Stanley's islands are analogous to Mandelbrot's fractals: they suggest that the closer you look for disease, using successively higher levels of resolution, the more you will find. You may initially think this is good. Unfortunately, this process may reveal symptomless diseases that might never have caused trouble, even if the person lived to be over 100 years old. Once the "problem" has been found, the patient will probably be investigated further and treated, with all the risks that implies.

Stanley goes on to ask how many people have cancer of the kidney. His reply is that the answer depends on how closely you look and how you define cancer. For example, in autopsy studies of people who had died with no apparent kidney disease, the number of tumours depended on how closely the tissues were examined. Look closely enough and you will find tumours, even in healthy people.

Testing the tests

Medical screening tests are intended to find out whether or not a person has a particular disease. However, the results are not always as accurate or unambiguous as we might hope. Let us assume the test provides the result *diseased* or *healthy*, and that these results could be either correct or incorrect. An incorrect result means the test could indicate someone has the disease, when they are healthy (or *vice versa*).

Health Screening Test – Possible Results				
		Patient is really ...	
		Diseased	Healthy
Test says:	Diseased	True positive	False positive
	Healthy	False negative	True negative

Simple binary trials of this kind are completely general. Any information resulting from a scientific experiment can be described in binary "yes/no" or "true/false" terms. Thus, we can use this type of table as a basis to evaluate any set of medical experimental results. The implications of such test results are as follows:

- True positive: the person has the disease, which is correctly identified by the test. They can receive appropriate treatment.
- False positive: the person is healthy, but the test suggests they are not. They may be given extra tests, uncalled for treatment, or even surgery. In the worst case, the patient may die as a result of procedures they did not need.
- False negative: the person has the disease, but the test fails to identify it. They will not be treated and may be lulled into complacency. In the worst case, they may die of the disease or spread it to other people.
- True negative: the person is healthy and the test confirms it. Patients wish to achieve this outcome. They will feel reassured and will not receive any treatment.

Jargon

A simple binary (true or false) medical test has four possible outcomes; this is easy enough to understand. Unfortunately, there is a substantial amount of jargon associated with this simple table, which we will explain briefly and then disregard. The first piece of jargon applies to a result where the test is positive but incorrect (false positive); this is called a *Type 1* error or an *error of the first kind*. A *Type 2* error, or *error of the second kind*, is when the test is negative but incorrect (a false negative).

We will use the terms false positive and false negative to indicate inaccurate test results, where the patient is wrongly diagnosed as ill (false positive) or wrongly declared to be healthy (false negative), as the terms are a little more descriptive.

False Positive	Type 1 error	Error of the first kind
False Negative	Type 2 error	Error of the second kind

A number of additional and somewhat confusing terms have been used to describe this simple two-by-two table. The *sensitivity* is the proportion of correct positive results; a sensitivity of one means a positive test result is always accurate. Similarly, a test's *specificity* is the proportion of correct negative results; a specificity of one means a negative test result is always accurate. We will avoid these terms and include them here only for the sake of completeness.

Sensitivity	Proportion of correct positive results If Sensitivity=1, then a positive test is always accurate
Specificity	Proportion of correct negative results If Specificity=1, then a negative test is always accurate

Medical screening

Nowadays, it is common for people to receive letters asking them to attend a medical examination to be screened for a disease, such as prostate or breast cancer. Most people are surprised by the suggestion that having the test might do them more harm than good. However, the evidence implies that, unless you have a good reason to think you have the disease, screening tests are quite likely to be detrimental. On this basis, a rational person would reject most medical screening tests.

Let us take the example of screening for cancer, a disease which strikes fear into the hearts of doctors and patients alike. Cancer screening is intended to provide an early indication of disease. However, a truly immature cancer is tiny, starting with just a single cell about ten millionths of a meter across. It may double in size every 100 days or so, in which case it would take something in the region of ten years to reach one centimetre in diameter. By the time screening can detect the illness, the cancer has been growing for years and contains billions of cells. Thus, there is a reasonable probability that it has started to spread.[117]

Although both mammography and PSA (prostate specific antigen) screening for breast and prostate cancer respectively are popular, there is little direct evidence to support their benefits. Prostate testing can result in harm as well as benefit, as it may cause men to be rendered incontinent and impotent, following unnecessary surgery.[118] However, we will use mammography as our example.

Rational screening decisions

A careful look at mammography will show how to approach screening tests more rationally; this is essential knowledge. At the start of the 21st century, a review of breast cancer screening concluded: "Screening for breast cancer with mammography is unjustified. If the Swedish trials are judged to be unbiased, the data show that for every 1,000 women screened biennially throughout 12 years, one breast-cancer death is avoided whereas the total number of deaths is increased by six."[119] Hard as this result is to believe, it claimed that for every life saved, six extra lives are lost.

We need to begin by clearing up some of the prevailing myths. Mammography screening tests do not reduce the incidence of cancer. These tests are not for people with symptoms, but for the wider population. Even if a mammogram reveals a small tumour, that tumour may not go on to develop into a disease. An example is called *ductal carcinoma in situ* (DCIS), which may not progress to malignant disease.[120] If left untreated, some women with DCIS do not develop breast cancer. There is not much data on this, as most women are treated, but what there is suggests that over a time span of approximately 25-30 years, less than half of untreated low-grade lesions become invasive.[121] Following a mammogram, however, such DCIS patients may be classed as cancer patients. They might undergo invasive treatments such as surgery, followed by radiotherapy and chemotherapy. Consequently, an illness they possibly did not have is misleadingly labelled as "cured", helping to support the claim that the treatment is effective.

Since some of the tumours found by mammography may be harmless, early detection is not necessarily of benefit to the patient. Moreover, contrary to popular belief, early detection does not automatically mean that the risk of death is reduced. Reality is often surprising. For example, the leading cause of death in 63,566 older women diagnosed with breast cancer was not cancer, but heart disease.[122]

Screening example

This example shows what happens when people undergo screening for breast cancer. For illustrative purposes, we have drawn from data presented by Dr David Eddy in 1982.[123] There may be more up to date results, but these will serve our purpose. The exact numbers vary with the study but our concern is with understanding the principles. Initially, our analysis follows that of Professor Gerd Gigerenzer, eminent European decision theorist.[124] It will be used as a guide to medical tests and experiments, particularly screening.

From the table below (people with cancer column), we can see that if 1,000 patients with cancer have the test, 792 cases will be detected accurately. This means the test is about 80% accurate, which is a reasonable level of accuracy for a medical test. Similarly, if 1,000 healthy women take the test, 904 will be correctly cleared.

Thus, the test is about 90% accurate in identifying healthy people. Unfortunately, this means that 208 cases of cancer will be missed in every thousand. Furthermore, 96 out of 1,000 healthy women who take the test will be told, wrongly, that they might have cancer.

	People with Cancer	Healthy People
Number Tested	1,000	1,000
Positive	792	96 (false positive)
Negative	208 (false negative)	904

The relevance of these figures depends on the incidence of the disease; let us say it is one in a thousand. If we test 1,000 women, perhaps one will have the disease. However, since there are far more healthy people in the population than ones with breast cancer, then there will be many false positives. According to these data, there will be 96 false positives compared to just one woman who actually has the disease. For this reason, people should not worry unduly, even if test results suggest they have cancer. Of course, not being disturbed when told your mammogram is positive, i.e. suggests cancer, may be easier said than done, so it is important to understand that a positive result is not the automatic death sentence that patients often assume it to be.

Although the incidence of breast cancer in the general population is low, other groups have a higher incidence of the disease and are at greater risk. These include women who are having a mammogram because they have already found a lump. Before the test, it is known that about 1% of such lumps turn out to be malignant. The actual chance of a patient with a positive test having a malignancy is only about 0.077.[124] In other words, out of every 1,000 people who have a lump and have tested positive, only 77 will have a malignant cancer. So, the positive test result has increased the likelihood that the patient has cancer from 1% to 8%. Thus, the risk of cancer is still quite low, even for a woman who has found a lump and then received a positive test result.

Does mammography save lives?

From four randomized trials, involving 280,000 women in Sweden, the relative risk reduction for breast cancer mammography was reported as 25%.[125] Sounds good, doesn't it? However, look what happens when this result is converted to direct odds. Gigerenzer reports that the apparently impressive 25% was actually tiny: a reduction of just one death in a thousand—that is from four in a thousand to three.[124] Put this way, the result sounds a lot less striking. It is easy to appreciate why breast screening has long been controversial.[126]

Despite the controversy, the World Health Organization suggests that breast cancer screening can save lives.[127,128] In the UK, the National Health Service still promotes mammography.[129] A paper from the Institute of Cancer Research claims that mammography has reduced breast cancer mortality in the UK by 1,400.[130] This is extremely hard to estimate, as the incidence varies from year to year and there are numerous possible influences. The paper compared the actual death rate with an arbitrary predicted value. It was really claimed that screening *and other factors* had resulted in substantial reductions in mortality from breast cancer.

There are excellent reasons to reject such ideas. We note, in passing, that the Institute of Cancer Research showed a graph of mortality but truncated the axis, starting at 40 per 100,000 rather than 0. This is one of the approaches to magnify an apparent effect, as described by Daryl Huff in his excellent little book *"How to Lie With Statistics"*.[131] With this in mind, we have simply redrawn the graphs for the highest and lowest mortality groups properly here. We have also computed the trend lines through the data. If the screening were effective, there would have been a correspondingly large reduction in mortality following its introduction. Despite the official claims, we find no reduction in deaths!

Breast Cancer Mortality per 100,000

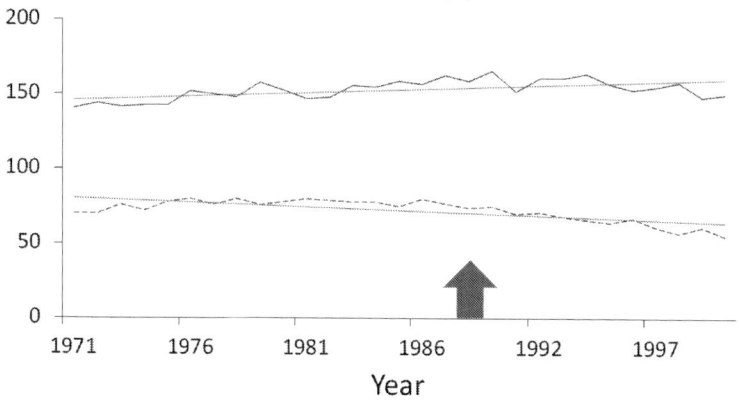

The solid line is for women aged 75-79 years while the dotted line is for women aged 50-54 years. The trend lines are shown in grey. The arrow indicates the introduction of screening in 1988, which had no apparent effect.
(Institute of Cancer Research data)

When the data are presented without bias, the lack of benefit from screening is apparent. Here we simply drew an appropriate chart. As a first step in counteracting this kind of bias, we suggest people dealing with a medical decision start with a decision tree. This powerful technique allows you to understand medical questions. It also provides a simple way of applying Bayesian statistics.

Building a decision tree

Building a decision tree is equivalent to asking a series of questions. The decision tree is a diagram that illustrates the series of available options. We will use similar figures for mammography to those given by Stuart Sutherland in his book *Irrationality*,[132] to show how one can be created. Here is our decision tree for mammography screening. The diagram shows a decision tree for a positive screening test.

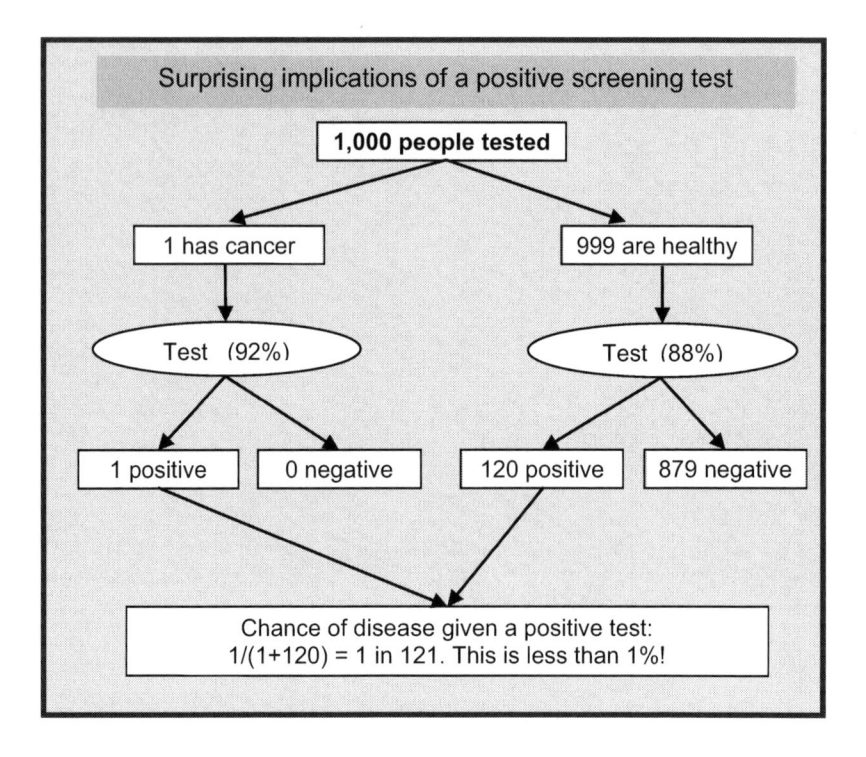

```
┌─────────────────────────────────────────────────────────┐
│        Surprising implications of a positive screening test │
│                                                         │
│                  ┌─────────────────┐                    │
│                  │ 1,000 people tested │                │
│                  └─────────────────┘                    │
│                    ↙            ↘                       │
│         ┌──────────────┐   ┌──────────────┐             │
│         │ 1 has cancer │   │ 999 are healthy │          │
│         └──────────────┘   └──────────────┘             │
│                ↓                    ↓                   │
│         ⟮ Test (92%) ⟯      ⟮ Test (88%) ⟯              │
│            ↙      ↘            ↙        ↘               │
│   ┌──────────┐ ┌──────────┐ ┌──────────┐ ┌──────────┐   │
│   │1 positive│ │0 negative│ │120 positive│ │879 negative│ │
│   └──────────┘ └──────────┘ └──────────┘ └──────────┘   │
│            ↘                   ↙                        │
│          ┌───────────────────────────────────────┐      │
│          │ Chance of disease given a positive test: │   │
│          │ 1/(1+120) = 1 in 121. This is less than 1%! │ │
│          └───────────────────────────────────────┘      │
└─────────────────────────────────────────────────────────┘
```

These are the steps to build such a tree:

- To begin with, we choose a large population size, say 1,000 people, and write down this number. Choose a number big enough that you do not need to use fractions.
- Next, we split the large population into two groups: healthy (999) and sick (1), according to the incidence of the disease (1 in 1,000).
- Then we apply the test to each of the two groups. We treat the healthy and sick groups separately, according to the test accuracy for each group. In this case, the test is reported to be 92% accurate for sick people and 88% accurate for healthy people. So, rounding off the numbers, our sick person tests positive and 879 out of 999 (88%) of the healthy people test negative.
- We write down the results of the testing:

Sick (1 person)		Healthy (999 people)	
Positive	False Negative	False Positive	Negative
1	0	120	879

- Then we combine the results, to find the chance of having the disease if the test is positive:

    Number of people testing positive = 1 + 120 = 121
    Proportion of true positives = 1/121

- This means that less than 1% of women with a positive mammography test actually have breast cancer. The other 99% have suffered the stress and cost associated with a positive test, when they were never ill at all.

Building a decision tree can be a little tricky at first. Often, problems arise because people do not convert the probabilities to actual numbers of people. Always start with a large population as it simplifies the arithmetic. In this example, we needed a population that was large enough to contain at least one person with cancer. Since the incidence was 1 in 1,000, that means we needed at least 1,000 people. If we wanted to be able to consider false negatives, we would need to start with even more: a population of about 10,000 would be needed to yield one false negative.

It is also important to think about the order of the questions. We started with the incidence of breast cancer, in order to know how large a population was needed. The incidence tells us how many people would be in the cancer or healthy groups, splitting our population into two uneven groups. The next question concerns the accuracy of the test for either healthy or sick people: we applied the relevant accuracy to each group, to find out how many people would be diagnosed accurately or wrongly.

An additional trick is to favour those questions that split the groups into roughly equal numbers, such as splitting 10 subjects into two groups of 5. With a little practice, the process becomes straightforward. Clearly, this was not possible here, as healthy people vastly outnumber people with breast cancer. Here "healthy" means "not having breast cancer". Of course, the screening tells us nothing about other diseases or conditions.

This decision tree tells us that a woman who tests positive still has a very low probability of having breast cancer. The likely outcome, however, is that she will be invited to repeat the test. She would probably be interested to know the implications of this. You may care to repeat the decision tree, starting with 121 people (120 healthy and 1 with cancer). If you do this, you will find that 15 people test positive for a second time, but only one of these has the disease. In other words, the chance of having breast cancer, even after two positive tests, is less than 7%. The vast majority of second test positive results (93%) are still inaccurate.

Decision trees are applicable across the whole of medical decision making. So, for example, the question of whether or not to have a surgical operation or to take a statin drug can be expressed as a decision tree. Decision trees are deceptively powerful, simple to understand, and need no special training to interpret. Even children are able to understand decision tree solutions, after a short explanation of how they work.

Decision trees can be useful for difficult problems. The process of building a tree throws light on the situation and its associated risks; it also allows immediate comparison of the different alternatives. Probabilities can be estimated when they are not known accurately. Even working with guesstimates can give insight into an important decision.[133] Complex statistical methods are not needed to construct a tree, just a little arithmetic. Despite this simplicity, decision trees allow people to do their own Bayesian analysis of important choices.

The real meaning of clinical trials can be settled by using decision trees. However, you are unlikely to find a decision tree interpretation in published EBM trial results—it would highlight deficiencies. Similarly, if patients and doctors demanded an unbiased decision tree for every screening test, they would understand the implications and, in many cases, might rationally decline the offer of screening.

We suggest that readers consider applying decision trees to all their important medical decisions. Such action would remove irrationality and leave doctors and patients with the freedom and autonomy to choose the option they consider best. Unfortunately, in our experience, the necessary information to interpret a screening test is unlikely to be available in the clinic, despite it being essential to making a rational decision.

When is screening sensible?

Before giving any test, doctors need to know three facts. Rational doctors should know the incidence of false positives, so they can avoid the risk of telling healthy people they are ill. They also need to know the incidence of false negatives, to help them avoid failing to detect an illness. Furthermore, unless they also know the incidence of the disease in the relevant population, the test result will be meaningless. It should be clear that if the risk of disease is low, screening is generally counterproductive.

Similarly, patients wishing to protect themselves would ask the doctor proposing a test for the same background information; namely: test accuracy (false positives and false negatives), the chance that they have the illness (disease incidence), and the reason for thinking the test is appropriate in their particular case. This would allow them to make a rational decision about whether or not to take the test.

If patients were to start asking for such information, medicine would be forced to become genuinely evidence-based. In an ideal world, the doctor would be able to provide patients with appropriate data. The doctor would also know the real meaning of a positive or negative test result, and be able to explain it to the patient. The follow-ups and treatments would have similarly quantified risks. Unfortunately, we do not yet inhabit an ideal world: many doctors, let alone patients, find the results of these kinds of tests hard to understand.

In one study, researchers demonstrated that staff and students at Harvard Medical School found test results difficult and failed to interpret them correctly.[132] Subjects were asked about the results of a diagnostic test. The medics were told that the illness occurred in one person per thousand, and the accuracy of the test was 95%. This meant that 5% of healthy people (50 in 1,000) would test positive. Therefore, only 2% of those with a positive test would have the disease.

If a person had a positive test result, the medics were asked, what is the likelihood of that person having the illness? About half of the subjects claimed there was a 95% chance that the patient had the illness. This meant they had ignored the fact that the incidence was low, meaning there would be far more healthy people testing positive (50 in 1,000) than people with the disease (1 in 1,000). If you doubt this, we recommend you draw a decision tree and check the figures for yourself.

Heuristics to help decide whether or not a test is sensible

Diagnostic tests are useful if:

- The patient is in a particularly high risk group
- The risk is large
- There is good reason to believe the patient has the disease
- The patient has symptoms
- The test is exceedingly accurate.

A very accurate test would overcome the problems of diseases with a low incidence. If the test is accurate, a low risk patient who tests positive will probably have the disease. However, medical tests are performed on biological systems and highly accurate diagnostic tests are rare.

Risk includes both the likelihood of having the disease and the magnitude of its consequences. It is important not to overlook the counterbalancing risk of being wrongly treated as a result of a faulty diagnosis.

A diagnostic test is not sensible if:

- There is no particular reason to believe the patient is at risk
- The patient is not in a high-risk group
- The patient does not have symptoms
- The test is not accurate.

There is a final *caveat* to this decision making process. People need to consider the likelihood of too little information being made available. The medical authorities proposing the test should be able to provide minimal test statistics, including the rates of false positives, false negatives, and incidence of the disease. In addition, they should have statistics about particular high-risk groups, to whom the test might be applied.

However, in the small number of cases where we have tried to obtain such information, the data has not been available in a useful form; we have been forced to estimate it ourselves from the medical literature. In the absence of such information, patients may use guesstimates. Typically, assume a good clinical test is 70-90% accurate for both the sick and the healthy and then estimate the range of incidence in the population. An internet search can act as a guide. Then present the calculation or decision tree to your doctor and ask for clarification or corrections.

Main Points

- Medical tests illustrate the problems with clinical decision making.
- Medical screening is rarely helpful.
- Screening tests are mostly useless and sometimes harmful.
- A decision tree can help resolve test results and guide clinical decisions.
- Guesstimates can be useful when medical data is sparse.
- Always use a decision tree for important medical decisions.

> Risk estimates are even more important in evaluating screening and preventive care, since individuals are counselled to seek these services. For this counsel to be ethical, not only must the action not be harmful, but it must have a reasonable chance of benefiting the person.
>
> Lester B. Lave

What Is Evidence?

Bayesian statistics is difficult in the sense that thinking is difficult.

Donald Berry

Clinical trials are simple practical tests and clinical research methods are essentially straightforward. Here we outline a form of clinical trial that overcomes most of the problems with EBM. Clinical research methods are essentially straightforward. By looking at medical evidence in more detail, we can describe expert diagnosis, and design a modest Bayesian clinical trial. Such clinical trials can be robust, simple, and inexpensive. In principle, a family doctor can do one in a standard clinic. Importantly, it is scalable to the required size and easily combined with other data. In short, a humble Bayesian trial is at least as powerful as EBM's overhyped large-scale randomized clinical studies.

A modest clinical trial

Small experiments can be more effective than large-scale trials. A clinical trial, straightforward enough to be performed by a family doctor, is robustly scientific and can be replicated with equal ease.

In EBM, a clinical trial typically compares two groups of patients: the treated and the controls. The test is to see whether the two groups differ significantly. It is often stated that a "not significant" result between treated and control groups means there is "no evidence" that the treatment works.[134] This is not true. Any difference constitutes evidence, whether significant or not. The difference may not have reached an arbitrary criterion of significance, but it is nevertheless information, with an associated probability.

Since it is not valid to apply results from groups to individual patients, we need a new approach that will allow us to treat each patient individually, and predict which treatments will be effective. It turns out that the design of such a trial is particularly straightforward. We note the results in a sequence of patients and use them to predict how well the treatment will work.

Let us consider a modest example. Dr Carlos is a general practitioner, who wants to know which of two drugs will lower his diabetic patients' blood glucose levels more effectively. Drug A is old and inexpensive, has been off-patent for several years, and there are a number of generic suppliers. Drug B is new and costly, and its pharmaceutical company claims it is a breakthrough in the treatment of diabetes.

Dr Carlos gets ethical approval to test the two drugs on a sequence of patients. This is fine, because both drugs are acceptable therapies and are believed to be relatively safe. Then he sets the criteria for his experiment. If the drug lowers glucose by three points, Dr Carlos defines the result as a success (S); otherwise, he classes the test as a failure (F).

Dr Carlos sets up a spreadsheet on his computer and waits for the first diabetic patient. As suitable diabetic patients arrive, he measures their glucose levels for a month. Then the spreadsheet randomly assigns each patient to receive drug A or drug B. After a specified period, say a second month, Dr Carlos measures the patient's blood glucose levels again. The level is entered into the spreadsheet, which notes the success or failure and calculates the probability the drug will lower the blood glucose by the specified amount. The results might look like this:

SSFFFSFSSSFFFFFFSFFF for the first 20 patients on drug A
and
FSSSSSSFSSSSSFSFFSSS for the first 20 patients on drug B

With drug A, there are 7 successes in 20 patients. We might roughly estimate the probability of the drug being effective at 35% (or 7/20). Similarly, we can immediately see that drug B seems more effective, with 15 successes in 20 patients, which makes it 75% (15/20) effective. So, we can see that drug B appears preferable to drug A, all other things such as side effects and cost being equal (which may not be the case).

We can now go a little further and let the spreadsheet calculate the probabilities. This allows us to check how likely it is that patients will benefit from each of the drugs, by calculating every possible probability, using Bayes' theorem. The result (called a probability density plot) looks like this:

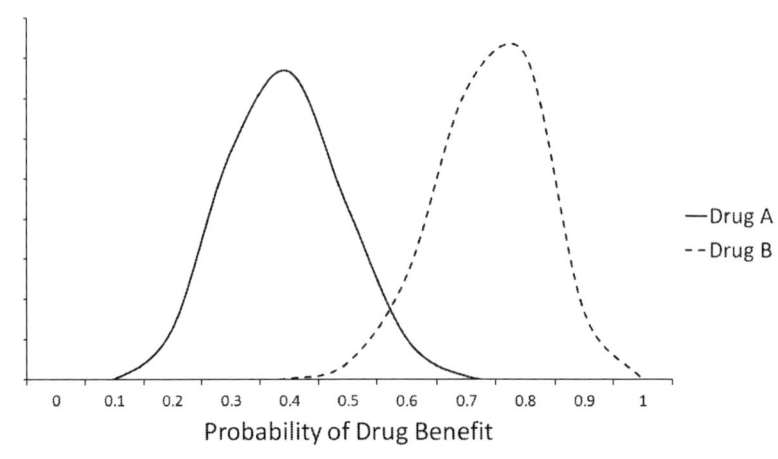

[Figure: Probability density plot showing two curves — Drug A (solid) peaking around 0.35, and Drug B (dashed) peaking around 0.75 — with horizontal axis "Probability of Drug Benefit" from 0 to 1.]

The horizontal axis is the probability of benefit. All probabilities are listed from 0 to 1. Zero means the drug is completely ineffective, while one indicates it works in every patient. Some probabilities are more likely than others, and this is represented by the height of the curves. So for example there is no chance that drug A always works (probability of drug benefit 1) as some patients failed to respond. As expected, the peak of the curve for drug A indicates the probability of the drug working in about 35% of the patients, while drug B peaks at approximately 75%. These values indicate the chance the next patient will benefit from the treatments.

From these calculations, Dr Carlos can gain a greater understanding of the benefit of the two drugs for his patients. Dr Carlos will not need to consider the usual gobbledegook surrounding the p-value, such as it being "the probability of a result being observed that is more extreme than the one we found, assuming the treatment was ineffective." The result just tells Dr Carlos which of the drugs is more likely to work with the next patient. The relative effectiveness of the two treatments is now obvious.

Using the Bayesian approach, Dr Carlos can immediately see the likely benefit to an individual patient. He knows that the study is reliable as, unlike EBM trials, Bayesian statistics are not highly sensitive to the experimental conditions. Dr Carlos can communicate the information visually to other doctors, who can repeat the study and add supporting data or, perhaps, report when they get a different result. Any number of patients can be included. Doctors could collaborate in teams, combining results. This type of clinical study is cheap, provides rapid results, and is at least as valid as the "best" EBM offering.

The significance of results from EBM experiments can vary with the design of the experiment, as described previously in the chapter *Beating the Odds*. By using a Bayesian approach, Dr Carlos knows the meaning of the experimental results depends on his initial assumptions, but these are not as critical as they are with EBM. This is because the probability of benefit is recomputed after each patient. Any problem caused by the experimenter's initial ideas rapidly diminishes as the trial progresses.

In our example, Dr Carlos assumed that there was no initial information about the two drugs he was testing. If he wanted an idea of performance at the start of his trial, he could have used published data to get an improved starting point. It would not make a lot of difference to his eventual findings, however. The effect of the initial assumptions quickly fades as information from patients accumulates. It is also possible to compute how the results would change for any variation in initial assumptions.

The central problem in medicine is one of prediction. During diagnosis, a doctor predicts the patient's disease and which treatment will offer the greatest benefit. The reason medical statistics are not already based on Bayesian analysis, pattern recognition, and other robust forms of prediction, is that these techniques require more computing power than traditional methods. Many of the statistical techniques used in EBM were designed when computation was carried out using a mechanical desk calculator. Today, even a cell phone may have more computing power than an early supercomputer. It is thus time for medicine to be based on something a little less primitive!

Dr Carlos' trial enables him to calculate the probability that either of his drugs will help an individual patient. A drug that benefits only a small proportion of patients will fail this test. If the doctor is persistent and studies a large sequence of patients, an ineffective drug will still give a similar low probability of helping the next patient. The estimate of the chance of benefit will become more precise as the number of patients increases; however, small numbers of patients will cover the practical issues of a practicing physician.

The cost-benefit implications of finding the probability of benefiting a patient are obvious. A drug that provides a minor benefit to only one patient in 100, as promoted by current methods, will be seen as a waste of resources. Physicians like Dr Carlos will be guided to use solutions that are more effective.

Busy doctors need straightforward methods. One criticism of EBM is that it is complicated and difficult to understand. Dr Carlos entered his results into a spreadsheet and performed no calculations. He could see the difference between the drugs on a visual display. Real science gives direct results, which clarify the information. Our simple Bayesian trial illustrates this well.

Evidence or information?

Before we can appreciate the advantages of this simple trial, we need to get back to the nature of evidence. Most computer-literate people know that information is measured in *bits* and is described as *data*. Dr Carlos's hypothetical trial produced two series of 20 bits, specified as a list of successes (S) or failures (F). As we go on, some readers may be wondering what a list of ones and zeros has to do with medicine. But look at Dr Carlos's simple trial. If we substitute 1 for S and 0 for F, then the sequence of patient outcomes SSFFFSFSSSFFFFFFSFFF becomes 11000101110000001000—a sequence of 20 bits. Perhaps surprisingly, all decision making can be expressed as the problem of predicting whether the next symbol will be a one or a zero.

Medical knowledge involves concepts and ideas, which are not easily defined, and it is debatable whether they can be represented fully as information. A sequence of bits, such as 0000 or 0101, contains information. However, information is not the same as knowledge or wisdom. Current computers contain and process information, though they have little, if any, capacity that people would recognize as wisdom. Our modern electronic society is overloaded with information and data processing, but is deficient in genuine knowledge.

Decimal number	Binary number
0	000
1	001
2	010
3	011
4	100
5	101
6	110
7	111

As with Dr Carlos's results, the outcome of any clinical trial can be represented as a series of binary digits. Viewed in this way, the trial is searching out and separating order from apparent disorder. Information can be defined as the number of bits needed to represent a set of data. Suppose we count the integers from 0 to 7. Using binary notation, it takes 3 bits of information to represent all of these values.

Order and disorder

> Uncertainty is the only certainty there is, and knowing how to live with insecurity is the only security.
>
> John Allen Paulos

People generally have a reasonable understanding of the terms *random*, *disorder* and *noise*, but may not realise how these concepts relate to information. To begin with, the more disordered a set of data is, the greater is the information needed to describe it. Consider the sequence 1,1,1,1,... In Dr Carlos's clinical trial, this would describe a perfect treatment that is always successful, i.e. S,S,S,S.... To specify this sequence, we need simply to indicate that it is a "list of 1's, continuing forever". Since a short phrase can specify the complete sequence, we say that its information content is low.

By contrast, if we tossed a fair coin, it would give a random sequence of heads and tails, say, h,h,t,h,h,t,t,h,t,... We can represent this in binary notation as 1,1,0,1,1,0,0,1,0,... using 1 for heads and 0 for tails. Surprisingly, perhaps, the information content of this list is high. Since each throw is random, we cannot predict the result of the next throw, so to describe the list we have to write down every digit in the sequence. When we say that the information content is high, it means it takes more bits to describe a random sequence than an ordered one.

To see how Dr Carlos's hypothetical trial relates to practical medicine, suppose a doctor has given penicillin to the last 10 patients suffering from a particular illness, and they recovered. Should the doctor prescribe the drug to the current patient with the same illness, yes (1) or no (0)? If the doctor thinks that the patient is likely to recover more quickly with the drug, he might prescribe it.

Similarly, the answer to a question of the form "Should we operate?" is an inference that depends on the experience and outcome of previous surgeries. Either the surgeon operates (yes, i.e. 1) or does not (no, i.e. 0). In an uncertain world, the surgeon predicts which treatment is most likely to be effective and acts accordingly. An operation occurs (1) or does not (0).

Medical and surgical decisions can always be represented in terms of a binary string, as in Dr Carlos's trial. If you are wondering what this is all about, please be patient; these binary sequences of zeros and ones will provide the basis for a new understanding of science and all medical trials.

Variety and uncertainty

> There is nothing to it. All one has to do is hit the right keys at the right time and the instrument plays itself.
>
> Johann Sebastian Bach

You may think that Dr Carlos's simple trial is too small to be important in today's world of mega-studies and meta-analyses. However, we ask you to put this preconception on hold for the time being, while we delve more deeply into the nature of information, variety, and uncertainty.

Randomness, uncertainty, and disorder are measured in terms of what is called their *entropy*. In computing and information science, the term entropy describes the amount of information in a system. In physics, entropy specifies increased levels of disorder or randomness. Each discipline may define entropy in a slightly different way but it consistently relates to disorder and is one of the most fundamental concepts in science.

Perhaps the most powerful rule in classical physics, the second law of thermodynamics, states that isolated systems increase in disorder with time. Their entropy increases, which means they become more random and their information content rises.

As Michael Flanders and Donald Swann described in a comic song, the second law of thermodynamics lays down the following rule,

> That you can't pass heat from a cooler to a hotter,
> Try it if you like but you far better notter,
> 'Cos the cold in the cooler will get hotter as a ruler,
> 'Cos the hotter body's heat will pass to the cooler.

A characteristic of living organisms is that they circumvent entropy. Although life is hard to define, most people are able to recognize it when they see it. They would surely agree, for example, that a frog or a flower is living, whereas a stone is not. At first, living creatures appear to break the second law of thermodynamics: they can become more ordered with time. Living cells absorb energy from their surroundings and use it to create complex structures, biochemistry, and behaviour. The overall effect is a loss of energy. This process can be interpreted in terms of information: living organisms increase their internal organisation, at the expense of increased disorder in their surroundings. As a result, the environment's increased entropy is balanced by the organism's increased organisation.

This information conversion produces the variety of living creatures we find on earth. The increase in order associated with living creatures is usually expressed in terms of an organism's use of energy. Despite this, an organism's transfer of information is, in some ways, more fundamental than its energy use. The unit of life, a living cell, is a negative entropy machine. We recognise living things because of the way they embody and use information.

If you remember the twenty questions (20Q) game described earlier, we can measure the information content of a sequence or list, by finding the smallest number of binary questions needed to specify it completely. Each yes-no question specifies a bit and we thus measure information content and variety in bits of information. As a rule, the best questions, those that provide the

113

maximum information, are the ones that split the data into two equal sets.

To take a simple example, we will ask you to think of any whole number between one and one hundred. To determine this number, we will need to ask a maximum of seven binary questions. We first ask if the number is greater than 50, which allows us to find out which half of the data contains the number. Then we ask a second question, to split the data in two again: if the number was less than 50, we would ask if it was greater than 25. With each response, our information about the size of the number is increased. In fact, if we split the data into equal sized groups, each question adds one bit to our information. Since we need to ask at most seven questions to isolate any number up to 100, the information content of the numbers from one to one hundred is seven bits. One way to find the number of questions needed is to divide the range of numbers (100) repeatedly by two, until the result is one or less. This is a reasonable rule of thumb approach to determining the amount of information, or number of questions, required to solve the problem.

In fact, seven bits would allow us to find a whole number between one and 128, so our information estimate is a little larger than necessary. The actual information content needed to find a whole number up to 100 is 6.64 bits. The use of fractional bits of information provides greater accuracy in our estimates, but is less easy to explain in words.

Ross Ashby's concept of variety is another way of describing information. We use variety and information content interchangeably. The concept of information is extremely powerful in science.[135] The bit is the basis of mathematical logic and computing. Information is fundamental to the sciences and holds the ultimate position in rational explanation.

Having enough variety

> Half of science is asking the right questions.
>
> Roger Bacon

If a physician is diagnosing a patient and there are 100 possible diseases, the doctor would need to ask a minimum of seven yes/no questions to reach an accurate diagnosis. If we now assume the doctor has forgotten one of the questions and can only ask the first six, the result will include two diseases, as the question needed to discriminate between them will not be asked. The patient will be given a differential diagnosis of, say, influenza or the common cold. If the doctor was more forgetful and was unable to ask the last two questions, the differential diagnosis would contain four possible illnesses, for example, 'flu, common cold, meningitis, or pneumonia.

If a doctor does not have sufficient variety in his questioning, he will be unable to determine the diagnosis accurately. This brings us back to Ashby's law or "only variety can destroy variety." In this case, the physician needs a variety level of seven bits, in order to determine which of 100 diseases the patient has. If the physician does not have the right questions, i.e. has an effective variety of less than seven bits, the accuracy of the diagnosis will decline. The physician must have sufficient relevant information to reduce the uncertainty in the symptoms and provide an accurate diagnosis. Note here that the appropriate seven questions are always enough to separate the diseases, whether they are common, similar, or complicated. The only issue is which questions are needed.

Doctors spend a long time in medical school accumulating knowledge and, hopefully, methods of reasoning. This long period of study is to increase the variety in the physician's mind. With a large amount of variety, the doctor can tackle the massive levels of uncertainty in normal physiology and disease processes. It seems a truism to state that a more learned and intelligent doctor can potentially provide greater help to patients. However, there is something far more fundamental at work.

Every rational action in medicine must conform to Ashby's simple law. Any action or process that does not have sufficient variety is flawed.

Scientific methods

As far as is practicable, rational medicine is based on science. Science works in a simple way. A person has an idea and tests it. If the test confirms the idea, it is provisionally accepted, at least until another experiment is performed. When an experiment contradicts or refutes the idea, it is modified or discarded. This process is called induction and is equivalent to the use of Bayes' theorem. Bayes updates current beliefs (ideas or hypotheses) with new evidence (the results of tests or experiments).

Hypotheses and theory are the main way in which we understand medicine. Theory simplifies, explains, and helps researchers to progress. The germ theory and the theory of circulation, for example, were core elements of scientific medicine. Germ theory led to the development of antibiotics and numerous other ways of combatting infection. William Harvey's theory of blood circulation paved the way for modern techniques, such as cardiopulmonary bypass machines, used in heart surgery.

Medicine, like other sciences, needs core theories. We use the circulation of the blood and the germ theory of disease as critical examples from history, to show how a theoretical breakthrough has advanced medicine. Germ theory became established with the work of Robert Koch in the 19th century. However, the germ theory had been described centuries earlier. In 1546, Fracastorious proposed that epidemics were caused by "spores" or tiny particles, which could transfer infection by contact or through the air.[136] It is often the case that theoretical advances in medicine have a long history before they are properly investigated and become accepted. Fracastorious' spores were influential and eventually morphed into Koch's germs. More recently, the theories of genetics and DNA have revolutionized our understanding of the biology that underlies medicine.

The development and understanding of theory is of major importance to medicine and underlies its practical applications. A good theory is one that fits the known facts and makes useful predictions; such theories are the ultimate aim of science. By contrast, evidence-based medicine is largely free of basic theory. It contains plenty of (flawed) statistical models, but little that relates to individual patients, health, and illness. As we have stressed, EBM is an *ad hoc* collection of results of large-scale social science type experiments. The resultant information is of the form "drug A is clinically proven to work in anorexic women aged 43-57 years old with disease B, but not in adolescent males with disease C." Diseases are attributed to more-or-less vaguely associated risk factors, but there is a shortage of theoretical models, to explain *how* things actually work.

The theory-based trial-and-error method of science is powerful. It is the most potent way we have of understanding the physical world. Science is the process of inductive reasoning based on observation and experiment, and described by Bayesian statistics. In the next chapter, we outline the simplicity of science, for comparison to EBM and its statistical complexity.

Main Points

- EBM's complicated clinical trials are just simple practical tests.
- Understanding tests leads naturally to Bayesian statistics.
- EBM's clinical trials are no more reliable than a simple Bayesian trial.
- The main problem in medicine is one of prediction.
- A simple Bayesian trial overcomes most of the problems with EBM.

Don't be afraid to take a big step.
You can't cross a chasm in two small jumps.

David Lloyd George

The Search for Simplicity

> The more probable the message, the less information it gives. Clichés, for example, are less illuminating than great poems.
>
> Norbert Wiener

EBM claims to use the "best" evidence. Here we show that simple evidence is preferable to complicated evidence. To achieve this, we need to look more closely at simplicity and chance. Perhaps surprisingly, they are intimately connected.

EBM claims that complicated meta-analyses and large-scale clinical trials provide the gold standards for medical research. By contrast, basic science suggests that simple experiments provide a high level of confidence and are an efficient way of searching for cures. Simplicity is a surprisingly subtle idea, which is central to an understanding of medical science. In this chapter, we explain the power of simplicity and the corresponding weakness of overly complex solutions. Our description will take us on a short detour away from medical science. The new tools we pick up along the way will allow us to gauge the scientific basis of EBM.

Throughout scientific history, simpler theories have been preferred. Darwin's theory of evolution, for example, is a statement of how living creatures change with succeeding generations; the notion of "evolution by natural selection" wraps up a tremendous amount of information in one short statement. Evolution provides an incomplete but unifying model for biology. Darwin's theory is powerful and it would be difficult to understand modern biology without his ideas. However, a person does not need to read the whole of his book, *On the Origin of Species*,[137] in order to grasp the theory. The power of Darwin's theory is that it is concise and straightforward. A similarly elegant theory is the double helix model of DNA (deoxyribonucleic acid), which arose from the work of Rosalind Franklin, Raymond Gosling, Frances Crick, and James

Watson.[138,139] The symmetry of the proposed structure of DNA is starkly beautiful, yet simple.

Our aim is to show that EBM's *ad hoc* recipes for clinical trials can be replaced by a return to the elegance and simplicity of earlier medical pioneers. We will also begin to show how methods such as Dr Carlos' humble Bayesian trial that we described in the last chapter provide a more powerful approach than current "evidence-based" medicine.

Parsimony

The principle of parsimony has a long history and goes back over two thousand years. It follows from the work of Aristotle, who said that, all things being equal, we may assume the superiority of techniques that need the fewest assumptions or hypotheses. This might be regarded as an early warning against multiple risk factors and multifactorial explanations.

In the 13th century, Thomas Aquinas, Dominican priest and eminent medieval philosopher, wrote "If a thing can be done adequately by means of one, it is superfluous to do it by means of several; for we observe that nature does not employ two instruments where one suffices."[140] Soon after, a 14th century English monk called William of Occam came up with a description of the rule that now bears his name: *Occam's razor*.[141] Little detail is known about William of Occam's life, though he is credited with explaining the benefits of simplicity. He was keenly interested in natural philosophy (the precursor of modern science) and in the work of Aristotle.

Occam's razor implies that, given a choice of explanations, we should choose the simplest that is consistent with the facts. In applying this to the development of scientific ideas, the aim is to make as few assumptions, and use as few causes, risk factors, or variables, as possible.

Simplification

The process of simplifying problems is arguably one of the greatest achievements of science, though in practice it is surprisingly challenging. We can show how difficult is it to be simple using the history of mathematics. The main aim of modern mathematics is to find short elegant proofs. For a mathematician, proving a statement involves deriving it logically, from basic given facts, called axioms. Fermat's last theorem, one of the most famous ideas in mathematics, illustrates this process well.

Pierre de Fermat was a 17th century French lawyer and mathematician. Fermat commonly stated theorems and claimed he had a proof for them; sometimes, though not always, he described the proof. Despite this, many mathematicians thought it unlikely that he could really have proved some of his claims, because they were exceedingly difficult: their solution needed mathematical tools that were not available in his time. However, Fermat was a genius and it is possible that he did have the proofs he claimed. Whenever Fermat had made such claims, later mathematicians eventually showed that he was correct, by generating a proof.

Fermat's last theorem is perhaps the most famous in mathematics. For those of a mathematical bent, it states that you cannot add two powers of integers together to obtain another integer of the same power, if the power is greater than two. (This is not important to our argument.) Most young maths students at some point examine the problem and many try to find the elusive proof. In 1995, after more than 300 years of failed efforts, an English mathematician, Andrew Wiles, achieved a proof of Fermat's theorem while working at Princeton University.[142] Wiles' proof is a triumph of modern mathematics and his technically difficult paper runs to 108 pages of the Annals of Mathematics.

Nevertheless, Wiles' achievement leaves some mathematicians a little uneasy. Fermat, in the margin of his 1670 edition of Arithmetica, claimed "I have discovered a truly marvellous proof of this, which this margin is too narrow to contain." After three centuries, mathematicians have now shown that all Fermat's claims were correct and have even found a proof for his last theorem. However, there remains a lingering doubt that his *marvellous* proof, which was perhaps just too long to fit in the margin of a page, has eluded re-discovery. Many mathematicians think Fermat might have made a mistake and his short proof may not have been valid. Wiles' proof was long. We now must wait to see if anyone can produce a short proof, or else show that a shorter proof is impossible.

The point of this story is to illustrate just how much value is attached to short, elegant descriptions. Occam's razor, with its demand for simplicity, has been a determining rule for mathematicians and scientists for hundreds of years. Even when simple theories are less accurate than more complex ones, they may have greater practical value. For example, the special theory of relativity, derived by Henri Poincaré and Albert Einstein, provides slightly more accuracy than the simpler Newtonian physics. However, this level of accuracy is often irrelevant. Even at speeds approaching the sound barrier, use of relativity theory for engineering calculations would be pointless. Newton's physics was good enough to get NASA into space and is more than adequate for most practical purposes. Incidentally, there is a joke that NASA spent millions researching a pen that would work in zero gravity. The Russians had a simpler solution: they gave their astronauts pencils.

Measuring simplicity

The pre-eminent 20th century philosopher of science, Karl Popper, described science as testing ideas by means of experimentation, and rejecting those that fail. Popper understood the power of simplicity, though he thought the principle of Occam's razor lacked substance. This was because in Popper's time, there was no objective way of determining which of two explanations was simpler, so use of Occam's razor was bound to be subjective. However, things have changed since then.

Deciding the relative simplicity of two theories is not as straightforward as it might appear. For example, some students find biochemistry easy, while others are confused by the long names and acronyms. In any subject, what is simple to one student might be difficult to another. Popper thought that without the ability to measure how simple something was, Occam's razor was merely subjective. Despite these objections, Popper considered simple ideas more useful and testable than more complex ones.[143]

One way of comparing two mathematical proofs might be to count the number of symbols used in each. Practical computer engineering uses a similar approach; the number of lines in a program is used to measure software output, or as a crude estimate of quality. A programmer might say he had written 1,000 lines of code, but perhaps that code is too long—he has used 1,000 lines, when 25 would have done just as well. Like mathematicians, programmers appreciate concise, elegant code. Given the choice between two programs that do the same thing, the shorter one is usually preferred. Short computer programs tend to run faster and are usually much easier to debug.

This comparison to computer code gives us a way of generalizing our ideas about simplicity, since any statement that can be made, in any language, can be represented as bits in a digital computer. Thus, we could count the number of bits needed to store a statement, and use this as a measure of its information content.

Of course, the length of a statement can vary, depending on the form of representation used. Despite this, the two versions contain equivalent amounts of information: it is just expressed more concisely in one language than another. To explain this further, we can represent the same statement in many different ways. For example, "one and one makes two" contains 21 characters (including spaces), whereas "1+1=2" contains only five, although they both mean the same thing.

Fortunately, we can measure the information content of a string directly. An early American computer scientist, Claude Shannon, explained how the information content (or variety) of any string can be computed.[135] We define the information content as the smallest number of bits needed to convey the message in a string.

A bit complicated?

There is an intimate relationship between chance and simplicity. The amount of information in a statement depends on how simple it is. Complicated strings contain more information. Paradoxically, as we have seen, random strings contain the most information. Since many people find this counterintuitive and confusing, we will provide a little detail.

Within a computer, a statement is just a string of zeros and ones. It is possible that any such string could be generated by chance alone. For example, we might toss a coin and record 1 for heads and 0 for tails or, in a clinical trial, record a successful treatment as 1 and a failed treatment as 0.

Suppose we found a string of 100 bits on a computer disk, we might want to know whether the string consists of random data or was placed there by an intelligent being. Astronomers face similar problems, when examining signals from outer space. The Search for Extra-terrestrial Intelligence, carried out by the SETI Institute in

California, involves looking at light or radio signals from stars and planets. One problem is how to recognize a message from an alien who uses a different language. The standard answer is that signals from aliens would probably show some form of order. A scientist who found a signal switching repeatedly between 100 zeros and 100 ones might intuitively assume that it was produced by a non-random action. A person might expect a purely random string to contain a mixed-up sequence of zeros and ones. So, searching for aliens entails looking for patterns in the signals from space.

Strangely, a simple sequence of 100 zeros is just as probable as any other sequence. Indeed, any sequence of zeros and ones is as likely to occur as any other. However, in practice, random sequences look disordered and lack simplicity. This perceived disorder is because there are many more mixed-up sequences than simple patterns. We expect a string selected at random to appear messy or disordered. So, if we find a simple pattern, we naturally conclude it is not random, and a SETI researcher might think that it could, just possibly, originate from an alien intelligence.

We need to understand why simple patterns are so important. Suppose Alice tosses a fair coin 99 times and each time it comes up heads. Alice then asks Professor Bob to bet one dollar on the next toss of her coin coming up tails. Alice will give Bob two dollars if he wins. Since Professor Bob knows probability theory, he knows that a fair coin has an equal chance of coming up heads or tails: each toss is independent, so the previous results are irrelevant. If the coin is fair, it always has the same 50/50 chance of coming up heads or tails. According to the theory of probability, Professor Bob should accept Alice's bet.

In the real world, Professor Bob would be wise to choose heads, or else be prepared to lose his money.[33] If the coin really were fair, a sequence of 99 heads would occur only about one time in 500,000,000,000,000,000,000,000,000,000 tosses. (The probability is about 2×10^{-30}.) That means once in five hundred thousand trillion trillion coin tosses. Now, the universe is reportedly only about 13.7 billion years old. So, even if Alice had repeated the experiment by throwing coins every second since the beginning of the universe, she would never have expected to see 99 heads in a row, using a fair coin! The following quotation describes it well:

> If a coin falls heads repeatedly one hundred times; then the statistically ignorant would claim that the 'law of averages' must almost compel it to fall tails next time, any statistician would point out the independence of each trial, and the uncertainty of the next outcome.
> But any fool can see that the coin must be double headed.
>
> Ludwik Drazwk

Despite the subtlety, the point we are making here is quite modest. Just 100 bits, or coin tosses, can give rise to silly probabilities: results that would not be expected in the whole of human history. By direct analogy, a small clinical trial with 100 patients in each group can be equally powerful. The critical requirement for such a trial is that an individual patient has a good expectation of receiving benefit from a treatment. That is, for a small trial to be valid, the number needed to treat should be small. Importantly, if this is not the case, the results are correspondingly of little relevance to the patient!

KISS

"Keep It Simple Stupid!" is a heuristic used in many business and self-help books. The aim is not to over complicate issues. This is shortened to KISS, which some more politely describe as shorthand for "Keeping It Short and Simple". This version may be particularly profound.

We need to find a way of deciding if something is simple or not. Consider writing a string of one million ones, which we have abbreviated here, for obvious reasons:

11111111111111111... ...11111111111111111

This is a long string, but it is also simple, because all you need to tell someone how to write it down is the instruction: "Write a million 1's." However, if we want to write down a random number, the process is not so easy. Suppose we toss a coin one million times and write 1 for heads and 0 for tails. The result might look something like this:

0010110101011101100001... ...10101110

There is no short way to tell someone how to write this random string. The shortest way is to give them the whole string to copy, digit by digit. Since the next zero or one occurs at random, there is no rule for predicting what comes next. If such a rule existed, the sequence would not be random.

Our SETI researcher is looking for a string is that is unlikely. He assumes the aliens have the sense to send a simple pattern, so someone picking it up will recognize it as an intelligent signal, a message. Short patterns are more likely to arise by chance. By contrast, long complex patterns often come from large complex processes. Being more specific, in repeatedly tossing a coin, short patterns, such as two heads in succession (HH), will occur more often than a long complex pattern, say THHTHTHHTHHTT, where T indicates tails. If you doubt this, notice that the longer string contains the shorter string (HH) three times.

Simplicity is easy to recognize when we see it. However, telling a philosopher that something looks simpler than something else is hardly likely to be convincing.

Complications

There is another approach to simplicity. The opposite of simplicity is complexity. So, if we find out how complex something is, we also know how simple it is. In 1960, Ray Solomonoff, an American computer scientist of Russian descent, described a way of measuring complexity.[144] Five years later, an established Russian mathematician, Andrey Kolmogorov also showed how this could be done.[145] Solomonoff was the first and should have received the credit. Despite this, we describe this phenomenon as *Kolmogorov complexity*. This process of giving credit to the more prominent researcher is common in science and medicine, and is known as the Matthew effect:

> For to all those who have, more will be given, and they will have an abundance; but from those who have nothing, even what they have will be taken away.
>
> Matthew 25:29

Anyway, because of Solomonoff and Kolmogorov, we now have a way of measuring complexity. The Kolmogorov complexity of a sequence of characters (known as a *string*) is the length of the shortest program that can print it.[146] In other words the shortest description of the string. So, as we explained, a repeated sequence of 1's is not complicated, because the program to print it can be short and simple: something like: "keep printing 1".

Without the program (e.g. "keep printing 1"), the string would not be printed. For this reason, the program to print the string is called its cause, because it causes the string to be output. In this way, the shortest program to print a string is its *logical cause*. The logical cause is the simplest (or shortest) possible way to reproduce that string.

A computer program is itself just a list of zeros and ones. This means we can consider a computer program as just another string of data. We do this whenever we load or save a program in a computer. If we have no information about it, a very short binary string, with just one bit, has a 50/50 chance of being either a zero or a one. This is analogous to how a coin lands, as either heads or tails. Two bits can take four values [0,0][0,1][1,0][1,1] and each pair of values has a one in four chance of occurring. In tossing a coin twice, you may get 2 heads, 2 tails, or one of each (head/tail or tail/head). The longer the sequence, the less likely you are to get a specific pattern. Getting a particular long sequence, like Alice's sequence of 99 heads, is astronomically unlikely.

We now have a way of checking how simple something is. Simple short sequences are common and will occur often when tossing a coin. We can restate Occam's razor rather awkwardly as—given any two ideas, the one with the lower Kolmogorov complexity is to be preferred. Karl Popper would be reassured, because we can now compare scientific ideas and show which is best.

Unlikely ideas

When EBM says it uses the best evidence, people seem to accept the claim as reasonable and clear. Here we go a little further and define best as the *most probable*. For example, a doctor wants to give the best drug: the one most likely to benefit the patient. A scientist wants to develop the best theory: the one with the greatest chance of describing reality.

So, to validate EBM, we want to find the best, i.e. most likely to be correct, evidence. Therefore, the evidence we need to find is the simplest and most probable. Now things become just a little weird.

An idea has a probability all on its own: which relates to the prospect that it might arise by chance.

An oft-made assertion suggests that if you give a monkey a typewriter for an infinite amount of time, it will eventually produce Shakespeare's Hamlet. There are several versions of this idea—for example, you might employ an infinite number of monkeys and typewriters for a short period of time, perhaps a year. There is a *theory of the infinite monkey*,[147] and most people can see that it presents some underlying truth. However, people reading Hamlet in the real world will suspect that the author was more intellectually gifted than a monkey.

The text of Hamlet, like any other idea, is a string of characters that we can enter into a computer. Once in the computer, we can use Kolmogorov's complexity to find its associated probability. It reflects the likelihood of a particular string occurring by chance. Not surprisingly, the chance of the text of Hamlet occurring by chance, or of a monkey hitting the keys of a typewriter in the required order, is extremely low. Surely, that is the moral of the story of monkey and his typewriter.

Archie's greatest success

My first, worst, and most successful clinical trial.

Archie Cochrane.

The most successful trial of EBM's founder was a simple small experiment. Back in the 1930s, EBM pioneer Dr Archie Cochrane studied psychoanalysis. Psychoanalysis is a philosophical belief system, rather than a science. Studying it seems to have resulted in Cochrane's disillusionment with all theories that were not based on experiment. His experience of psychoanalysis helped him take a more scientific approach to medical knowledge. Ironically, however, Cochrane's most fruitful trial seemed to break all the EBM rules.

In the Second World War, Cochrane was captured by the Germans and found himself acting as a medical officer in a prisoner of war camp at Salonica, Crete. He was in charge of around 8,000 inmates, some of whom had swelling on and above the knee, probably caused by malnutrition. This kind of swelling is known as pitting oedema: after pressing the swollen skin with a finger, the indentation remains for a while after the pressure has been removed. Cochrane also had this and other symptoms. The diet in the camp was poor, providing only four or five hundred calories a day. Breakfast was imitation coffee, lunch a bowl of vegetable soup, and supper two slices of plain, presumably white, bread.

People living on such a diet might expect acute vitamin deficiencies. Deficiency of vitamin B1, B2, or C could have caused the swelling. Cochrane vaguely remembered that wet beriberi, caused by deficiency of vitamin B1, could cause swelling. Remembering the experiments of his medical hero, James Lind, on vitamin C and scurvy, Cochrane decided to investigate.[148] He bought some yeast (rich in B vitamins) on the black market, and found 20 volunteers. Cochrane numbered the prisoners and separated them into two groups, using a simple rule: odd numbers in one ward, even numbers in a second ward. One group was given two spoonsful of yeast each day and the other was given vitamin C tablets (Cochrane did not specify the dose). He measured fluid intake and frequency of urination. There was no clear response for 3 days but, on the 4th day, the results were "conclusive"; the yeast (vitamin B) supplement was successful in relieving the symptoms.

In addition to this experiment, Cochrane also performed what he later described as "unsatisfactory tests". He asked the patients how they felt: nine out of ten receiving yeast felt better, but none of the ten control subjects did. Cochrane made the subjects walk for half an hour and convinced himself that the yeast supplement had visually reduced the swelling. The results were sufficiently obvious to be deemed conclusive and Cochrane managed to get the Germans to provide yeast for the prisoners. The incidence of leg swelling among the yeast supplemented prisoners was lowered from 12-30 per thousand each week to between 0 and 6 per thousand. The treatment was a success.

Unfortunately, Cochrane later thought his simple trial was unsound. Firstly, he realized the swelling was not classic wet beriberi. For some reason, this made him dismiss the idea that the problem was a vitamin deficiency. He thought the yeast supplied protein to the blood, lowering the swelling by simple osmotic pressure. However, it is doubtful that the yeast would provide enough additional protein for this effect. Then, he suggested that the randomization was inadequate. Nevertheless, numbering off the patients to alternate groups could be a suitable procedure under these circumstances. Coin tossing might have produced improved selection but, at that time, randomization in trials was rare. Finally,

Cochrane thought the trial was poorly controlled. For example, he put the groups in separate wards. Some difference between the wards might have caused the improvement. Perhaps one had more sunlight, generating warmth and vitamin D in the skin, for example, or any of a number of possibilities.

Cochrane described his prisoner trial long after it happened, in 1984, when large controlled trials were becoming popular. As he learned more statistics and experimental techniques, the apparent deficiencies of his first trial became apparent to him. Consequently, he found it amusing that his little trial had been so effective. In his words, "it was amazing what a little bit of science and a little bit of luck achieved." We feel this attitude is rather sad, because Cochrane had displayed a shrewd and courageous approach to the design of his trial, especially given the circumstances within which it was conducted.

The details of his experimental method provided a rational way of making the decision. Cochrane was addressing an illness in a prison camp. Under such conditions, a large-scale randomized multi-centre (i.e. prison camp) trial was not only impossible but inappropriate: the war would have ended before it was complete. The later, statistically sophisticated Cochrane seems to have forgotten the purpose of the experiment. In this case, the aim was quickly to test a hypothesis that would suggest a treatment for the illness and then to help the patients. His trial was an appropriate size. He implemented an arbitrary method of selecting his subjects. On the negative side, the experimental controls were potentially biased and his methods for determining the outcome were slightly suspect. However, the young Cochrane wanted a big effect. He was looking for a result substantial enough for it to be "conclusive" so he could help his men. Most importantly, the trial was a success and the prisoners benefited.

Cochrane describes his early experiment ironically, as his first, worst, and most successful clinical trial. Regrettably, his study of simple statistics appears to have removed his rationality. The experiment may have been his first trial. It may have been the worst, according to the rules of EBM. However, it was his *most successful* trial. Sadly, he later wrote that he still did not know why the treatment worked.

It is unfortunate that his later trials, which were supposedly technically correct, would almost inevitably be less successful and useful. Had Cochrane remembered that statistics is only a secondary experimental tool and studied decision theory, we might now have gained a more scientific medicine. There is no cookbook for the design of an effective experiment. Physicists, chemists, and biologists design specific experimental methods that are appropriate to the problem they are addressing. A simple definitive observation can be conclusive. Cochrane's later methods and beliefs were irrational. His little trial, though not without flaws, was basically sound and was, by his own admission, his most successful.

A lack of control

Cochrane's successful trial brings us back to Ashby's law of requisite variety, and the Goldilocks principle. Effective answers to medical questions should be neither too complicated nor too simple; they should be just complex enough.

EBM, as we have seen, provides complicated solutions to simple problems: large-scale trials, adorned with multivariate statistical analyses, are typical. Such methods *over-fit* problems. Over-fitting is a problem when Occam's Razor is ignored.[149] Accuracy is lost when you have an approach that is too complex for the problem at hand: such methods give deceptive results by "explaining" the noise or error in the system. In EBM, over-fitting means the trial appears more accurate that it really is and the results are not useful for clinical prediction.[150,151]

EBM presents what its specialists consider are highly accurate and sensitive solutions, derived through use of what they claim are the most advanced techniques. However, EBM's multiple risk-factors may fit the background noise and obscure the solution. With sufficient risk-factors, you can get an explanation for anything: your over-fitting will be complex, ostensibly accurate, and wrong.[152]

When we do not know the cause of a disease, it is reassuring to assume it is associated with numerous factors. The factors can be studied and measured, giving the illusion of progress and understanding. We have already described two medical examples where numerous risk factors and confusion were superseded by establishing a simple cause: tuberculosis and peptic ulcer. A third example is pellagra. Pellagra was a severe epidemic illness in the US, characterized by the four D's—dermatitis, diarrhoea, dementia, and death. Essentially, deficiency of niacin (vitamin B3) made people psychotic, but the disease was attributed to numerous other factors, such as spoiled corn or infection. Dr Joseph Goldberger was head of the Public Health Service's pellagra investigations. Goldberger observed that pellagra occurred among the inmates of mental hospitals but not the nurses and other staff. This suggested that pellagra was a dietary disease, rather than an infection. After detailed experimental work, Goldberger showed that pellagra was a result of an inadequate diet. Regrettably, he died in 1929, before it was confirmed that most cases of pellagra were due to symptoms of a deficiency of niacin.

Conversely, some proposed solutions to medical problems may be too simple. Surgical removal of a lump in the breast is a well-defined answer to the problem of breast cancer. In many cases the surgery will fail, as cancer cells have migrated to other parts of the body and will seed secondary tumours. Just like the over-fitting in EBM, too modest a model will also fail.[153] The difference is that, in practice, it is relatively easy to refute compared with a large-scale trial. Albert Einstein expressed a similar approach to scientific investigation "Everything should be made as simple as possible, but not simpler."

Despite scientists' aim for simplicity, some problems are intrinsically complicated. In the 1940s and 1950s, when digital computers were in their infancy, some scientists began to see the world in terms of systems. One of these was Norbert Wiener, a child prodigy who graduated high school aged eleven, gained a degree in mathematics at fourteen, and was awarded his PhD at only eighteen. Wiener developed cybernetics[154] which would later give birth to various other disciplines, such as artificial intelligence, control systems, and robotics. However, with this separation, a little of the refreshingly anarchic nature of cybernetics was lost.

Since its inception, cybernetics has tended to ride roughshod over specializations: cyberneticists simply looked at anything and everything as a logical system. To them, there were no boundaries between disciplines, though they believed that specialist areas must be rational, if they were to be taken seriously. The kind of areas they addressed were widespread and varied, and included the functioning of the brain, business management, cell physiology, medicine, ecology, economics, military strategy, and the avoidance of conflict between nations.

By contrast, scientific specialization has generally tended to increase over recent centuries. Indeed, modern scientists look back wistfully to the days when it was possible to be familiar with the whole of science. Similarly, in the medical field, we have heard older members of the profession bemoaning the loss of the truly general surgeon or physician. Whether for good or bad, there seems to be little doubt that today's experts are becoming focussed on ever narrower stretches of their discipline. With scientific specialization comes the inappropriate idea that a domain belongs to its specialists and that other scientists should keep out.

Cybernetics' early reputation suffered, because it was born during times of weapons research and is associated with cold war military systems. It also has multiple uses in artificial intelligence and robotics, though it can be applied more widely in biological systems. For example, cybernetics was used to show that the known plant hormones were insufficient to explain the control of development in plants.[155] The difference between adaptive and non-adaptive evolution has also been modelled using Ashby's law.[156] This law found a particular niche in business analysis and management. Stafford Beer, a management scientist, was one of the first to apply Ashby's law to organizational management.[157]

By way of an example, let us suppose a doctor wishes to travel from New York to Boston, and asks his assistant to arrange the trip. In order to arrange the journey by train, the assistant would need to collect information from the doctor, such as the day he wanted to travel, the time he needed to be in Boston, and so on. Additional information needed includes the location of the local rail station, if it would be practical to travel to Boston by train on that day, and the train timetable. All this data contributes to the requisite variety that is needed to carry out the task. However, if the doctor asked "Is this the cheapest way of travelling to Boston from New York?" the information (or variety) gathered so far would be insufficient. For an accurate reply, the assistant would need additional information about the costs of rail, automobile, air, and boat travel, not to mention the possible use of a bicycle.

The implications of Ashby's law can be profound. In 1995, a failure to appreciate Ashby's law led to a terrible collision, known as the Fox River Grove level crossing accident.[158] A Union Pacific train crashed into the rear of a school bus, at a railway intersection on US Highway 14. The bus was transporting students to a local High School. The train destroyed the bus, ripping its body from its chassis. Five students died immediately. A further 23 students were injured and two of these subsequently died from their injuries.

How did this happen? The bus's route meant it had to go across a level crossing and, immediately afterwards, go through a road junction, with traffic lights. The crossing itself was equipped with two sets of traffic lights, one for the motor vehicles and a similar system to warn the train drivers.[159] However, the Illinois Department of Transportation designed and placed the road signals, whereas Union Pacific controlled the railway signalling. Both sets of signals appeared adequate to the engineers working with their part of the system, but there was a mismatch in the timing of the lights. If a bus approached the level crossing just as the lights were changing, there was not enough time for the bus to get across the level crossing and through the road junction traffic lights. In this case, the bus crossed the railway but was immediately stopped by a red light at the road junction.

On the day of the accident, a substitute driver (normally a safety director) was in control of the bus, and was unaware of its exact length. Unbeknown to her, about three inches (7-8 centimetres) of the rear end of her bus butted out into the train's path, as she waited for the road traffic light to change.[160] Despite this overhang, the rail signal changed to green allowing the train through.

Originally, the road signals had been set with a larger margin of safety, but they had been modified shortly before the accident. Thus, the controls did not cover every possible set of road and rail traffic conditions. The horrified children saw the train and yelled frantically at the driver to move, but the inexperienced driver froze, unable to decide what to do amid the panic, trapped between the red light and the rapidly approaching train.

In this example, the control system includes the bus driver herself. Several important pieces of information were absent from the controls. The lights for the road junction and level crossing were not properly synchronized and allowed vehicles to get stuck between the two sets. The gap between the railway and road junction was too short for long vehicles, so the controls did not allow for the bus. The driver was unaware that the back of the bus was over the tracks. The students tried to help, but the driver was overloaded and inexperienced, and could not take in what they were saying. The train driver slammed on his brakes but did not realize what was happening with enough time to stop before his train hit the bus.

It is clear that this was an accident just waiting for the right conditions, since, even if she knew the length of the bus, the driver could not have avoided the collision without running through a red light. In terms of Ashby's law, the control system for trains and traffic at this complex junction lacked the requisite variety. A disaster was almost inevitable.

Ashby's law, which is central to control and systems theory, arose from a consideration of biochemical and physiological control mechanisms in animals. Perhaps shockingly, a search of PubMed, the online medical database listing numerous scientific journals, gave a single result for a search on the phrase "Ashby's law" and found only five papers for "requisite variety".[161] This paucity of research is an indication of the narrow scope of the medical sciences, and particularly their statistical methods.

Ashby's law stipulates that the minimum amount of information needed to give an accurate answer is *exactly* the amount needed to specify the problem. Any less information means your solution will be inaccurate, whereas any additional information would be redundant, potentially adding confusion and errors, in the form of noise.

However, an effective solution requires more than simply having the minimum information: it must model the problem. Earlier, in our simple Bayesian clinical trial, Dr Carlos studied a sequence of treated patients. The experiment was similar to the process experienced by a typical physician, who sees a series of patients in normal practice. Thus, the design of the trial was a close copy of normal clinical practice. This modelling was not accidental: to be informative, the trial needed to model the problem accurately.

Ross Ashby and Roger Conant's *good regulator theorem* states this explicitly.[44] Here, *good* means a simple and effective solution. *Regulator* means control, as in a treatment that cures an individual patient by dealing with the illness. A good clinical trial is necessarily a simple model, which represents the individual patient, the illness, and the treatment. The original good regulator dealt with perfect answers but can be generalised to cover any effective solution.

Solutions are often obvious, if the problem is described in the right way.

> Solving a problem simply means representing it so as to make the solution transparent.
>
> Herbert Simon

Our simple Bayesian clinical trial is a clear and direct description of the problem: Dr Carlos wants to use the drug that is most helpful to his patients. To do this, he needs to treat and analyse each patient individually in the clinical setting. In this context, Ashby and Conant's theorem implies that a useful scientific trial needs to model, that is copy, the clinical situation. The individual patient is the key.

This brings us back to EBM's clinical trials, which model the behaviour of *large groups*. The doctor needs to predict the individual patient's outcome, not what a group of patients will do on average. When you model the individual patient, the group behaviour emerges automatically. However, the reverse is not true: group statistics do not provide the information needed to help a particular individual.[162,163]

Suppose that, on average, a drug saves one life from a group of 100 patients. This sounds useful, but what if it had really saved 20 lives and killed 19 people? The EBM doctor prescribing this drug based on the group statistics thinks he is being helpful because on average he is saving a life. However, the doctor has just killed 19 people. Had 19 of the patients not been treated, they would still be alive. Working on EBM's aggregate results, the doctor saved a single life, but properly studied and applied at the individual level, 20 people could have lived.

We have described the superiority of Dr Carlos's simple Bayesian clinical trial. The design of the trial models the doctor-patient relationship: a simple predictive experiment, based on individual patients. Before we continue to outline the problems with EBM we will now explain how Bayes and the scientific method combine to produce the real power of science.

Main Points

- Simplicity is the aim of science.
- An effective trial is an experimental model of the clinical situation.
- Simple small trials can be performed and repeated with ease.
- Simple Bayesian trials have requisite variety and model the individual patient.
- A predictive clinical trial must model the individual doctor and patient.

> That's been one of my mantras—focus and simplicity. Simple can be harder than complex: You have to work hard to get your thinking clean to make it simple.
> But it's worth it in the end because once you get there, you can move mountains.
>
> Steve Jobs

Science is Induction

> Inductive inference is the only process known to us by which essentially new knowledge comes into the world.
>
> Sir Ronald Fisher

In this chapter, we describe what a perfect prediction system for medical science might look like. Earlier our simple clinical trial demonstrated the core requirements for clinical medicine. Diagnosis and treatment depend on making accurate predictions about an individual. Doctors need to be able to predict whether a treatment will work with a particular patient. As described here, scientific prediction is a form of inductive reasoning.[164,165] Although the analysis in this chapter arose in computer science, it goes to the heart of current difficulties in the field of medicine. Where medicine has a claim to being scientific, it fits the requirements described here.

Closed minds

A clinical trial is not done in isolation: it occurs within an environment of current ideas, known as a belief system. The belief system is the whole of our current knowledge. Furthermore, in order to prevent bias in our clinical trials, it is essential to apply an important rule.[166] It is this:

> Do not discount any ideas, unless you know they are impossible.

We must stress that, in this context, "impossible" does not mean the same as "highly improbable". In science, even the most highly improbable idea might turn out to be correct, if it is consistent with the data. Discarding a weak hypothesis could mean you throw away the answer you are seeking. We are reminded of the words of fictional detective, Sherlock Holmes, who said that "when you have eliminated the impossible, whatever remains, however improbable, must be the truth."[167] Eliminating the impossible, by means of experimental refutation, is essential to scientific progress. If we also reject what we currently consider a little unlikely, we may miss an important new idea.

The concept that you need to consider all possible data is by no means new; it originated with Epicurus, an early Greek philosopher of science, who lived between 341 and 270 BC. Epicurus provided one of the first descriptions of the scientific method. He thought that nothing should be believed, unless it came from direct observation and logical deduction. Epicurus generated many philosophical principles, in particular, his *principle of multiple explanations*. This says that if several theories are consistent with the observed data, we should keep them all.

In common parlance, Epicurus tells us not to jump to conclusions. Suppose, while out walking your dog, you found a dead body on the common. On reporting the death to a police officer, you would not know how the man had died. He could have been shot, stabbed, poisoned, electrocuted, perished from a heart attack, or succumbed to hypothermia. To determine the most likely reason for the death, the most probable explanation needs drawing out from all the potential causes. Even a detailed autopsy might produce an open verdict, in which the cause of death would be unstated or unknown.

Why, you may ask, is it so important not to reject the most improbable ideas—surely, it would make our work more efficient and save us from chasing up lots of blind alleys? This may be true, but given that we do not know the results of our research until after we have done it, elimination of an apparently minor hypothesis can have a huge impact. We cannot risk throwing the proverbial baby out with the bathwater. Earlier in the book, we described the well-known example of the black swan, which people originally thought was fictitious, as all the swans they had ever seen had been white. Over the centuries, many so-called heretics have been greeted with suspicion, despite their correctly challenging a prevailing dogma.

In 1799, for example, a sceptical response greeted the first specimen of a duck-billed Platypus shown in England.[168] The scientists of the day thought it was clearly a hoax, as they were convinced that there were no egg-laying, beaked mammals, with webbed feet! Critics cried fraud, and searched for the taxidermist's stitches, which they believed must be there. These researchers were not particularly closed-minded—rejection of something new is a natural reaction, which most of us have experienced at some time or other. As scientists, however, we must strive to keep our responses open and find ways to overcome our initial knee-jerk rejection of unexpected findings.

Although available data and the current belief system contain some information about the real world, knowledge is always incomplete. A young researcher starting a PhD, after first being overwhelmed by the mass of literature, may be shocked to realize the limitations of human knowledge. We simply do not have all the information we would like, even when it concerns well-established findings. Science is a world of approximation. Humility is needed, as our information about the world is limited, and we must proceed by trial and error.

The methodology of EBM, with its emphasis on the "best" evidence, prunes out apparently unlikely data and ideas. Its reviews and meta-analyses often exclude the vast majority of case studies, observations, and uncontrolled trials, claiming, for example, that such studies are in some way methodologically inadequate and therefore provide weak evidence. Such reviewers may claim that the evidence removed could be biased. Unfortunately, by omitting even somewhat unlikely hypotheses (and they reject far more than this), this supposedly rigorous approach impedes the attempt to find solutions to medical problems.

The Bayesian clinical trial in the earlier chapter showed how easy it is to perform medical research. Our imaginary trial was small, simple, inexpensive, and easy to replicate. It modelled the clinical problem with minimal assumptions and no selection of data. Similarly, observational and case studies can be unselective, cover outliers, and allow replication, at insignificant cost or difficulty. Ever since Newton described his falling apple (an observation that would surely be rejected by EBM as mere anecdote), people have known about gravity. Even a child could repeat Newton's experiment and get the same result—though it took a genius to interpret it.

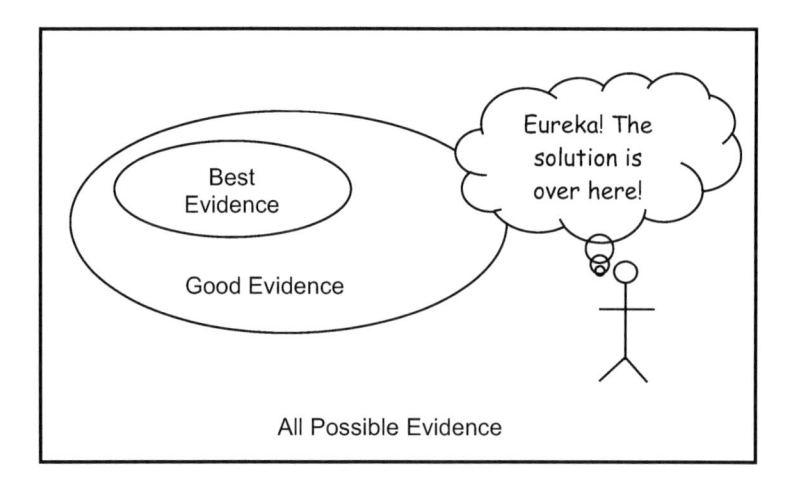

In searching for the solution to a scientific problem, we may need more than the "best" evidence.

Lethal bias

The use of "best evidence" necessarily involves bias and results in a decreased ability to find the solution. To those who are used to working with EBM, this suggestion may appear counterintuitive. It appears obvious to supporters of EBM that, if you wish to solve a problem, you should use the best data you have. This is a fatal mistake.

To take an analogy, let us imagine that Bob has lost his keys. Bob has not left the house since he last used the keys, so they must be within the building. He thinks the most likely place is the kitchen, either in his jacket pocket or on the table. Bob wants to look in the kitchen, as this uses the best evidence. Alice tells him he should start in the kitchen but should also extend the search, as the keys could have been left anywhere in the house. If you were offered a bet, say $100, on who would find the keys, would you bet on Bob finding the keys by looking only in the kitchen (i.e. using only the best evidence) or on Alice, starting in the kitchen but then searching the whole house (i.e. using all the evidence)? Clearly, Alice has the advantage: if Bob's keys are anywhere other than the kitchen, he will not find them.

An open mind

In order to find Bob's lost keys, Alice might need to search every room in the house. They could have fallen out of his pocket in the hall. It would be nice if the keys were in the more likely place, but life is not like that—things are often found where you least expect them to be. Searching the whole house is the only assurance that they will be found. Children sometimes learn this lesson quite early, when looking for lost toys, hidden treats, or presents.

This example illustrates why, as Epicurus explained, we should keep all available data and all ideas. It does not make scientific sense to exclude information from experiments, trial results, or clinical observations. Even if an experiment is performed badly, the data it produces may still be relevant. A classic example of an experimental failure that resulted in an outstandingly important observation was Alexander Fleming's discovery of penicillin. In 1928, he noticed a mould growing on an accidentally contaminated Petri dish, which led him to discover the antibiotic.

> One sometimes finds what one is not looking for.
>
> Alexander Fleming

Obviously, including "all the evidence" requires a degree of common sense. There is no need to include absurd suggestions, such as the moon being made of green cheese. We can exclude an idea if it is impossible. There are no cows or other mammals on the moon to provide milk for the cheese. NASA and its astronauts brought back samples and claimed that it was not made of cheese. The moon does not have a suitable atmosphere. It is not green. It does not have the observed mechanical and gravitational properties of known types of cheese. Moon rock has a different chemical composition to cheese, and so on. Each observation reduces the probability that the moon is a big green cheese, to the extent that we can rationally consider it impossible.

Some theories may be improbable, silly, or just plain nuts; this is not really a difficulty. They just have a low probability of being correct. We are reminded of Hickham's dictum for doctors, "patients can have as many diseases as they damn well please."[169,170] Similarly, diseases can have many possible solutions or therapies. It is not acceptable to exclude a hypothesis or a clinical trial because it appears to be somewhat *unlikely* to be true. A clear, unambiguous, and definitive refutation is required. Otherwise, such exclusion is prejudice and restricts progress.

Sceptics

A scientific education involves learning intelligent scepticism. In other words, scientists are trained to evaluate evidence critically. However, although criticism of the work of others is essential, it is a limited and ultimately unfulfilling part of the scientific process.

The most exciting part of scientific achievement is creative; it involves building theories to explain the available data. The great scientists are famous for their inventive genius. Alan Turing created his universal computer, Michael Faraday explained electromagnetism, Charles Darwin and Alfred Russel Wallace originated the theory of evolution, Benoît Mandlebrot introduced fractals, and Linus Pauling described chemical bonding. Critical thought is needed, however it is a secondary consideration for great science. Darwin's opinion was clear:

> I am not very sceptical... a good deal of scepticism in a scientific man is advisable to avoid much loss of time, but I have met not a few men, who... have often thus been deterred from experiments or observations which would have proven serviceable.

Despite Darwin's warning, some modern scientists have made an excellent career of simply being critical. Indeed, scientific scepticism might be considered a safe default position. The sceptic's aim seems to be to judge the current mood and not to criticize the prevailing scientific paradigm. Performing low-grade experiments, or clinical trials, is also important: an unspectacular clinical trial that confirms current ideas is innocuous, as it is unlikely to attract the wrath of fellow sceptics.

Importantly, as a sceptic in the field of medical research, it is essential to make sure you obey all the customary rules of statistics. You should perform standard, large-scale, randomized, placebo-controlled clinical trials. If this is not practicable, because of cost or other issues, a run-of-the-mill scientist can always carry out a meta-analysis. Despite its impressive sounding name, a meta-analysis typically involves a simple and repetitive search of the literature and the application of a software package. You may note our reserve, as we (almost) refrain from the using the term cookbook science!

In the foothills of the scientific establishment, dwell what we might call activist sceptics. These are typically not capable of adding to the scientific acquisition of knowledge, so they make a career of supporting the *status quo*. Activist sceptics are bullies, who remain on particularly safe ground. They pick on soft targets, such as homeopathy, creationism, or aromatherapy, and proceed to ridicule them. Such scepticism is a low-grade intellectual activity, which can unfortunately be harmful to science and the dissemination of knowledge.

The French mathematician, Henri Poincaré, put it well,

> ... doubt everything or believe everything: these are two equally convenient strategies. With either we dispense with the need for reflection.

Repeating experiments

In science, we learn by induction, which is a process of trial and error. We use our initial observations to construct a hypothesis, which we test using an experiment. If we keep repeating experiments and continually get the same answer, we might assume that our result is a fact and things will always turn out that way. However, as we introduced with the story of the black swan, such inductive reasoning has a problem.

Bertrand Russell, the eminent British philosopher and mathematician, explained the issue with a short story about a turkey farm.[171] Suppose that each day, the turkeys wake up, are fed, and their cages are cleaned; they learn to trust the nice humans who look after them. The repeated helpful behaviour of the people reinforces their expectations and the turkeys feel confident in their belief. Indeed, life is good: this is an open organic farm, the fence is old, and the turkeys could escape if they wanted. However, they are content, and growing large and fat—they have no need to escape the care of their friendly protectors. Unfortunately, the turkeys' belief system is limited; no matter how often they experience another day's kindness, it does not add to their knowledge. This becomes apparent one winter morning, when the unwitting birds are rounded up and butchered, ready for Thanksgiving or Christmas dinner.

Using induction, Russell's turkeys repeatedly tested their hypothesis that humans are harmless and kind. Each day, their prediction was correct. Scientists work in a similar way: a scientist has an idea and tests it, by carrying out an experiment. However, a scientist who believes that the results of his experiment *prove* his theory is thinking like a turkey. In principle, no amount of experimental support can provide conclusive evidence that an idea is correct. By contrast, a single counter example (such as one occurrence of Thanksgiving) can destroy the idea and any associated belief. Bertrand Russell's turkeys bet their lives on the idea that humans are always caring. Unfortunately, modern "evidence-based" medicine bets your life on analogous "clinically-proven" ideas.

Science and mathematics have changed fundamentally over recent decades and understanding of induction has increased. We are now aware that some things are unpredictable, even in theory. Newton's work enabled scientists to calculate a path to the moon and back but, despite the advantages of supercomputers, we now know our ability to predict something as mundane as the weather will always remain limited.

Induction is unable to deliver the certainty that some people might wish for, hence we have to use a slight variation. We saw above that a single refutation can destroy an idea; this concept is powerful. Science benefits most when using experiments and observations to attempt to *disprove* or *refute* hypotheses. If someone reports doubtful results, another scientist can copy the experiment or, perhaps, design another one, to show the previous results are wrong. The authority of science stems from the replicability of experiments.

Clearly, it is easier to repeat small, low-cost experiments than the massive clinical trials favoured by the pharmaceutical industry. Suppose that prominent doctors from a dozen leading medical centres published a massive study of 10,000 patients, costing 30 million dollars. Unless you are unusually wealthy and scientifically trained, replication would depend on government support or a research grant from a drug company. The chance of you gaining such funding is approximately zero, particularly if you are not a recognised member of the scientific establishment and a supporter of the *status quo*.

The award of a substantial grant to conduct a large-scale clinical trial will boost the career of a medical researcher. There is little kudos in performing a small trial, on just a few patients—anyone can do that. Large clinical trials attract respect. Despite this social favouritism, however, small focused studies are more likely to result in important discoveries.

Paradoxically, the larger and more expensive a trial, the more cautious we should be in accepting its results. Since replication of large trials is so difficult, we need to know that competent scientists performed the experiment carefully. We need to be far *more* critical of big studies and not be taken in by the large numbers or statistical mumbo-jumbo. This is the opposite of the usual EBM claim, that small trials are unsound and large-scale trails provide the "best" evidence. Once again the scientific rule is: trust but verify.

Back to Bayes

The scientific method is a rational approach to finding out how the world works. Science is Bayesian; it uses experiments and inductive reasoning to update our beliefs.

A doctor's diagnosis and treatment are also Bayesian undertakings. If a patient (Alice) has a disease, such as influenza, there is a chance that she will have a particular symptom, such as a high temperature. However, a more valuable question is: if a patient has a symptom, such as a high temperature, what is the chance they have the 'flu? In other words, it is useful to look at the problem in reverse. This use of symptoms to diagnose an underlying disease is essentially similar to the scientific process of evaluating theories, based on experimental evidence.

Many doctors are unaware that they solve Bayesian problems in their day-to-day activities. In diagnosis, the physician selects the illness that is the most likely cause of the symptoms. Bayes developed his theorem for just these sorts of problems. As a result, we can find out how new evidence (e.g. a skin rash) affects our current belief (that the patient has the 'flu). Despite Bayes' theorem being a logical and simple way of analysing diagnostic inferences,[172] medical science has largely ignored it.

One problem with Bayes' theorem is that it is considered subjective. Bayes treats probability as an indication of how confident we can be in our current beliefs. Certainly, the term belief gives the impression of subjectivity. Nevertheless, Bayes is exceptionally practical and useful.

For example, a doctor considering the relevance of a high temperature to a diagnosis may start with a list of possible diseases and risks. Medical students start by learning such "differential diagnoses" verbatim. Inexperienced doctors use their medical training and experience to refer to a list when examining patients, whereas experienced doctors may not think consciously of such lists—they have internalized them through years of practice. Like the Bayesian concept of strength of belief, this initial list of diseases, or starting data, could also be considered subjective, as it might vary from one doctor or hospital to another.

A universal solution?

Fortunately, there is a solution to this problem: a genuine gold standard, which applies to medical science, diagnosis, and treatment of disease. In some ways, this process is the ultimate method for addressing scientific problems and related decisions. It is known as Solomonoff Induction and is the benchmark for scientific decision-making.

We encountered Ray Solomonoff earlier in the book, when discussing simplicity. According to Solomonoff,

> algorithmic probability can serve as a kind of 'Gold Standard' for induction systems.

Solomonoff gave us a mathematical description of the scientific method. He combined Occam's razor, Epicurus' principle, and simplicity, to develop an ultimate form of induction. Basically, Solomonoff Induction tells us:

- Keep and use all the data, though the simpler the better
- Perform repeated experimental tests
- Use each test result to update your ideas, using Bayes' theorem.

Solomonoff Induction computes the probability of each theory or hypothesis, which might help provide a solution to a problem. A doctor treating a sore throat might have a list of such ideas, some probable and some (for the purposes of this explanation) much less so. Some possible "theories" for treating a sore throat include:

- Penicillin cures sore throats.
- Gargling with 1% hydrogen peroxide cures sore throats.

- A clinical trial with 1,000 adult male patients shows tetracycline cures 67% of sore throats.
- Granny says wearing a woolly scarf cures sore throats.
- And so on…

Even quite improbable ideas, like the scarf your Granny told you to wear, are included, to satisfy Epicurus' principle of multiple explanations. However, an idea is excluded if shown to be completely impossible.

Clearly, some theories are more likely to provide a solution to the problem than are others. It is natural in such cases to list the theories in order, by assigning each a probability. We can assign less likely theories an extremely low probability of being correct. So, based on a clinical trial, "penicillin cures sore throats" might have a probability of 0.80. (A probability of 0.5 means a random result, while a probability of 1 would mean it would always work.) Here the 0.80 (or 80%) probability means the penicillin will benefit 4 out of 5 throat infections. Patients would expect doctors to prescribe treatments in order of likelihood of success, as they would prefer the one with the greatest chance of curing their illness and the least side effects.

You may have noticed that our list of theories included the results of a clinical trial on 1,000 patients. The list can include anything that might help provide a solution, whether actual experimental data, statistics, or whatever. We simply include them in a list of hypotheses: they are ideas that might solve the sore throat problem.

We described earlier how we can calculate whether a statement is simple or complex. Short simple statements are more likely and complex strings are less likely. This gives us a starting point for fully understanding the scientific method.

To show how this might work in practise, we will consider a simple Bayesian trial on a sequence of patients. In a new clinical trial, Dr Carlos again studies sore throats but has multiple possible solutions, rather than just the two drugs A and B. Dr Carlos thinks penicillin has the highest probability (0.8) of being effective. He tests the idea by treating a patient's sore throat with penicillin. If the patient responds positively, the doctor calculates a new probability for penicillin, which increases from 0.8 to, say, 0.81 (or 81%). This will increase the likelihood of the doctor selecting penicillin for the next patient with equivalent symptoms. Perhaps, however, the patient rejects the antibiotic and elects to try Granny's recommended scarf. The doctor may have thought that this had only a one in a ten thousand (0.01%) chance of being effective. When Granny's treatment fails again, the associated probability might be lowered to one in 100 thousand (0.001%). The doctor is learning by trial and error—or induction.

The doctor's problem is to predict and use the "best" treatment for the patient. It turns out that the most effective way doctors can search for effective treatments for sore throats is to use induction. This also means they are testing the treatments scientifically. Now, an effective method to find the best treatment has some restrictions:

- To be admissible, the approach must approximate to that of Bayes.[173] An admissible method means that no other technique is always "better" than it is. The Bayesian approach is admissible.
- The method used should be an approximation to Solomonoff Induction. In some ways, Solomonoff Induction is the perfect universal learning method for such problems. It can start with an absolute minimum of data and predict any computable result.[174]

Ray Solomonoff explained that the scientific method is powerful because it approximates to his induction process. Solomonoff Induction tells us what an *ideal* prediction method would be like. An effective technology would be similar to Solomonoff Induction and have some specific properties:

- It uses all the data, rather than just the "best" evidence
- Simple solutions, experiments, or trials are preferred
- It allows easy replication and repeated testing
- It uses Bayesian methods or a close approximation
- Nothing is ever proven.

Solomonoff provides a guide to the quality of research methods. Similarly, a brilliant doctor will intuitively diagnose and treat patients using something similar.

EBM is the one major instance of a "scientific" methodology that breaks all these rules. The EBM approach is diametrically opposite in both theory and practice to the real scientific gold standard.

Both useful and incomputable

I pointed at the moon and some fool looked at my finger.

Zen saying

Solomonoff Induction is truly inspiring and powerful, and merits a little explanation. One objection to Solomonoff Induction is that it is not computable and appears, at first glance, to be unworkable. However, a similar and related advance seemed equally unserviceable.

Alan Turing was an English mathematician who showed that some problems were not computable. He solved a major mathematical problem by an unusual method: instead of providing a standard proof, he invented a computer.[175] His computer was imaginary, a paper model; it was really an idea for a theoretical computing machine. His machine design was impractical, it worked by mechanically reading and modifying symbols on a strip of tape. Turing didn't actually build his machine, but he did give the world a new way to think about computing. His ideas formed the basis for modern theories of computation.

The digital computers we use today are Turing machines and, in a theoretical sense, they are all equivalent. There are differences in the implementation and they don't manipulate symbols on a strip of tape, but computers ultimately perform the logic decreed by Turing. A Turing machine can compute anything that is computable. Given enough time and memory, all modern digital computers are equally powerful; anything that is soluble with the most powerful supercomputer can be solved with a small laptop, or even your digital watch. This is interesting but also impractical—you should not attempt to use your digital watch to check the output of a supercomputer, as you might not live long enough to finish.

Arguably, modern computer science began with Turing's imaginary machine. Turing's later accomplishments included being the prime mover in cracking the German Enigma codes during the Second World War and being a founder of artificial intelligence. He conceived a form of code breaking, based on Bayesian methods,

149

which was used from 1941 until 1943.[176] However, he is perhaps best known as an inventor of modern computing.

Alan Turing's theoretical computer, the Turing machine, paved the way for the development of computers as we know them. In a similar way, Ray Solomonoff has described a perfect induction system. Solomonoff Induction is a touchstone for checking the value of other methods. A touchstone is a hard stone used to scrape across gold jewellery. The gold leaves a coloured residue mark on the stone and the assayer applies acids that react with metals other than gold, which enables the grade to be determined. In a similar way, we can use Solomonoff's methods to check if a claimed "gold standard" is tarnished.

Solomonoff Induction can be used to address any scientific problem. It does not provide a cookbook, but a description of what makes an effective method. An excellent scientific technique will have the characteristics of Solomonoff Induction. Put it this way, if your desktop computer were not a Turing machine (i.e. Turing complete) you may soon consider it useless and take the item back to the shop. Similarly, we can reject EBM, because it fails to look or work like a good (Solomonoff) induction machine.

Rational medicine

Science, as described by Karl Popper, is an approximation to Solomonoff Induction. However, many people object to Popper's ideas, because individual scientists do not behave in this ideal way. They have pet theories, are irrational and eccentric. Some scientists will be overly sceptical, while others are a little too imaginative. Individual scientists are human and typically do not behave according to Popper's ideal ideas. Thomas Kuhn and other philosophers have suggested that science is a social phenomenon of paradigms (theories) and revolutions.[177] Contrary to the philosophical ideal of refutation, many scientists are actually trying to show their ideas are correct.

Objections such as these mistake the study of scientists and people with the science itself. The philosophy of the social construction of reality competes with the idea that there is an external reality to be discovered. Social construction is for sociology. Science is discovering real things about an independent external world. It does not matter how many sociologists or philosophers explain that gravity is not real, we have the impression that gravity simply does not care. A heuristic might be: do not jump off a bridge, just because a philosopher says you can fly.

Scientists are human, they can have pet beliefs, become confused, and suffer groupthink, just like anyone else. Nevertheless, the progress of science is a result of the process of hypothesis, experiment, and refutation. Human activities are messy and chaotic, and there will always be variation in the methods of individual scientists. However, a scientist who is trying, apparently unscientifically, to "prove" his idea is simply maximizing its associated probability. What one oddly behaving group of scientists does at any one time in history does not negate the overall progress of increasing knowledge. Science not only works because of the scientific method: it *is* the scientific method and the results generated by it.

Main Points

- Prefer simple ideas.
- The real scientific gold standard is Solomonoff Induction.
- EBM is a poor induction methodology.
- EBM is not science.
- Simple Bayesian trials are fundamentally dominant.
- A good doctor is more help to patients than the whole of EBM.

What most experimenters take for granted before they begin their experiments is infinitely more interesting than any results to which their experiments lead.

Norbert Wiener

Doctoring Evidence

What is wanted is not the will to believe, but the will to find out, which is the exact opposite.

Bertrand Russell

Many highly intelligent and well-educated people believe in EBM, which is widely considered a solid and appropriate form of medical science. Here, we continue to show that this faith is based on an illusion, and that EBM is unscientific.[178] We need to develop the explanation gradually, as the flaws in EBM are subtle but profound.

"Evidence-based" medicine arose gradually, following the introduction of randomized controlled trials in the 1940s and 1950s. In 1972, Archie Cochrane published a book called *Effectiveness and Efficiency: Random Reflections on Health Services*.[179] In this, he promoted the use of controlled clinical trials and epidemiology. Partly as a result of his little book, Cochrane's international reputation grew and, by the year 2000, there were 15 Cochrane Centres in 13 countries.[180]

Cochrane wanted an international collaboration for the systematic review of evidence from clinical trials. His book seems to have acted as a focus for EBM. In particular, he inspired international reviews of medical data by the Cochrane Collaboration (posthumously named in his honour), an organization dedicated to "evidence-based" medicine. According to the Collaboration, Cochrane believed that controlled trials provide information that is more reliable than other sources of evidence.[181] This assertion is untrue. Cochrane considered those treatments that demonstrated direct and obvious effects to provide the most reliable evidence,[179] as do we. The top of Cochrane's list of evidence was "Those therapies, with no backing from RCTs [randomized controlled trials], which are justified by their immediate and obvious effect, for example insulin for acute childhood diabetes." In other words, Cochrane agreed with us that reproducible *direct measurement of clear effects* constitutes more powerful evidence than a clinical trial.

EBM was introduced formally in a second book, in 1985,[182] and a journal called *Evidence-Based Medicine* was launched in 1995. The Lancet greeted the new journal with some disparagement, pointing out that

> Cochrane, a fierce individualist ever at war with people who thought they knew best, would hardly welcome the elitism of much evidence-based medicine, and he would certainly scold the founders.[183]

Indeed, had Cochrane not died in 1988, we would not be surprised to hear that he had written a book explaining how EBM had got it wrong.

EBM is not well defined. Where definitions do exist, they frequently disagree with observed practice. A typical definition is:

> Evidence based medicine requires the integration of the best research evidence with our clinical expertise and our patient's unique values and circumstances.[184]

This definition of EBM includes reference to clinical expertise. It appears to mean that the doctor evaluates the results of EBM studies and applies them in clinical practice. However, EBM provides data that is more suitable for use by governments and large organizations than by practicing doctors. For governments and other major organizations, limiting the scope of doctors' responses tends to mean that treatments are standardized. This suits politicians, protecting them from claims that different patients get dissimilar treatment. However, it may also mean that the doctor's role becomes restricted to the provision of set treatments, largely determined by EBM.

Gaining administrative control over healthcare may be a primary driving force for the uptake of EBM. In 2006, Dr Bernadine Healy, former Director of the National Institutes of Health, criticised EBM, suggesting that "The autonomy and authority of the doctor, and the subsequent variability in care, are the problems that EBM wants to cure."[185] Others have suggested that EBM has a fascistic structure.[186] Even people defending EBM have implicitly made the case for controlling doctors: a response to Healy states "That is the purpose of EBM: to base our treatment decisions on the best available science rather than on prevailing opinions or 'expertise.'"[187] Note that this hardly agrees with the claim that EBM integrates the best research evidence with clinical expertise. When

EBM is put into practice, authoritarian guidelines tend to take precedence over a doctor's knowledge.

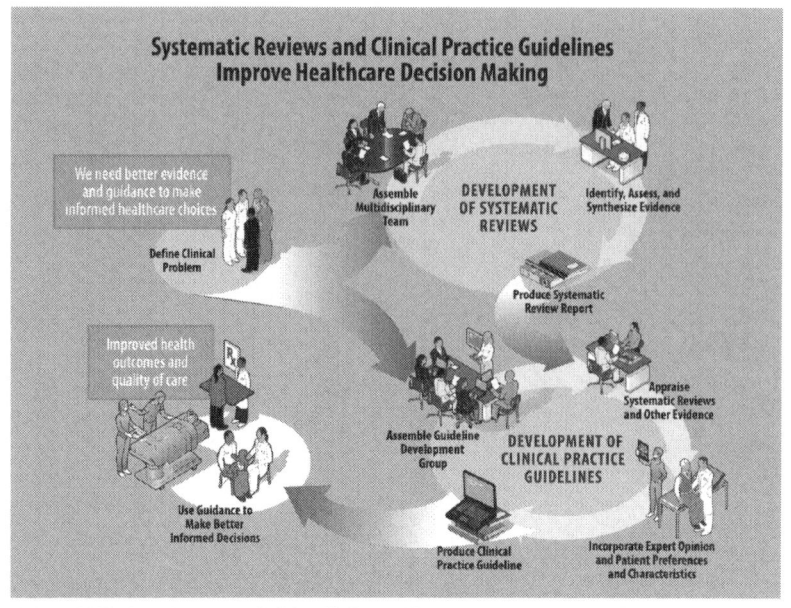

The US Institute of Medicine illustrates how EBM provides clinical guidelines[188]

The suggestion that EBM is applied according to a patient's "unique values and circumstances" inevitably requires a doctor's expertise. We know of no mechanism that would enable population statistics to address a patient's individuality. In a rational world, EBM guidelines would merely provide a doctor with general background information.

Central control

The fundamental philosophy of EBM is central control. A group of experts instruct others as to what medical evidence is and how it should be considered. However, such central planning always fails. This is an immediate result of Ashby's law: a group of experts clearly have less variety than an entire profession and their patients.

Back in 1945, a Nobel Prize winning economist, Friedrich Hayek, explained the issue in an essay entitled *The Use of Knowledge in Society*.[189] Hayek argued that a centrally planned market could not match the efficiency of an open market, because each expert knows only a small fraction of what is known collectively. Free market economies work when they invoke a form of the *wisdom of crowds* and, in principle, can use all of the available information. Central planning fails because the bureaucrats only have aggregate statistical data; the result is a highly inefficient and ineffective economy or organization. Not surprisingly, bureaucrats and their medical equivalents love EBM, because of its central planning aspects. Given an opportunity, apparatchiks will take control and exercise their power. Those who support authoritarian control would do well to remember the fate of the former totalitarian regimes, based on central planning.

EBM is highly supported by the medical industries, particularly pharmaceutical companies. An economist's game theoretic view of corporate medicine is that it is a way of extracting profit from the sick. We are not making an ethical statement here. Corporations are legally responsible for maximising their shareholders' profit. In contrast, preventive medicine lowers profits, as it reduces the number of sick people. To a drug or medical technology company, preventing or curing a disease does not make financial sense. Long-term treatment is more lucrative than a cure for chronic illnesses, such as cardiovascular disease or diabetes. Importantly, the return on research and development has been falling for years. In real terms, funding for research and development has dropped consistently since 1950.[190]

Defence of the status quo is another example of game theory's rational self-interest in action. Those who are making profits defend corporate medicine. Financiers want to keep making money. Bureaucrats want to keep their jobs and be promoted. The continued existence of many medical organisations requires a steady or increasing flow of funds.

The agency problem

The *agency problem* describes a form of conflict of interest according to which agents work for their own advantage, rather than their clients' benefit. An agent is a person or organisation whose job is to act on behalf of another. An estate agent or real estate broker, for example, will sell your house for you. Other examples include literary agents, lawyers, doctors, accountants, and surveyors. A doctor is an expert agent, responsible for looking after the health interests of patients. Similarly, a clinic or hospital is an agent tasked to help support the health of a community.

People use professional agents to overcome the limitations of their knowledge in specialist areas. It is no longer possible for a single person to be an expert in all fields—the speed of change in an area can render even specialists obsolete. Since people cannot cover all subjects in detail, their ability to behave rationally is restricted by their relative ignorance, learning capacity, and lack of time. In the field of decision-making, we say that each person is in a state of *bounded rationality*.[191]

Given that people cannot always make decisions based on full knowledge, they have to do the best they can without it. This form of decision-making is called *satisficing*. We satisfice when we seek a simple solution to provide a satisfactory, though not necessarily perfect, outcome. For example, if Alice goes shopping for a new pair of shoes, she could try on every pair in the mall, before going back and selecting her favourite. Alternatively, she could buy the first acceptable pair that fits. In the first case, she may end up with slightly preferable shoes, but if she takes the second option, she will buy an OK pair of shoes and have enough time to look for a new dress to go with them.

Agents are often pulled in several directions and have to decide whether to work in the best interests of clients, employers, or themselves. The agency problem implies that agents all too often work primarily for their own benefit. For example, suppose a lawyer could handle a divorce quickly by mediating, but would get paid more if he encouraged the parties to argue. Ethically, the lawyer should do what is best for his client but, in the real world, people tend to do what is in their own interests. This is not a new phenomenon—Charles Dickens described it well in his nineteenth century novel, *Bleak House*, in which lawyers stretched out an inheritance case until all the money has been consumed.

The benefits to an organization of acting in its own interests ultimately outweigh those of behaving responsibly. An agency that acts for itself can have an advantage in a competitive environment and may soon replace one that does not. For example, a drug company acting largely for the benefit of patients is likely to lose value compared to one that maximizes its profits and increases its market share.

The agency problem in medicine is often disguised, because many people want, or even need, to think of a doctor as acting entirely in the patients' best interest. The key factors driving medical agents may be less than helpful for individual patients. The prime consideration for medical journals, for example, often becomes funding, without which they could cease to exist. Advertising by drug companies is a major or even primary source of income for journals. Pharmaceutical companies are agents for their staff and shareholders, and use EBM as advertising to promote their drugs.[192] In short, corporate medicine operates using agents and suffers from multiple conflicts of interest.

Conflict of interest is inevitable when people or organizations are allowed, encouraged, and trusted to look after the interests of others.[193] The agency problem is non-discriminatory—it applies to almost any business or organisation you may deal with: your financial advisor, the garage that services your car, the charity to which you have just given a donation,[194] and the hospital that treats you as a patient.

Organizations sometimes attempt to address the agency problem by internal regulation. They may have methods for vetting potential employees. Bonuses may be given to staff for productivity and good behaviour. The organization can fire aberrant employees. Governments may establish watchdogs, such as the US Food and Drug Administration (FDA), to oversee the behaviour of medical and food related organizations. Of course, these are simply additional agents and, before long, they start acting in their own interests.

One way to evaluate agents, organisations, and medical systems—such as EBM—was provided by Stafford Beer. Beer coined the term *POSIWID* or "the purpose of a system is what it does."[195] According to Beer, POSIWID "stands for a bald fact, which makes a better starting point in seeking understanding than the familiar attributions of good intentions, prejudices about expectations, moral judgements, or sheer ignorance of circumstances."

Suppose a system appears to be malfunctioning. Perhaps medical aid to a third world country is lowering health care standards, while enriching both the local politicians and medical corporations in the donor country. Many might conclude that the political system is not working and these are side effects. Applying POSIWID, we can conclude that we have uncovered the real purpose of the aid, unless the politicians can provide a valid and convincing alternative explanation.

EBM provides governments and other large organisations with central control of medicine. Large pharmaceutical companies make massive profits on the back of EBM trials. Selected medical researchers obtain major research funding, prestige, and career enhancement. Epidemiologists and statisticians have risen from technical support to become arbiters of medical science. Low-grade people administering cookbook medicine gain respectability and legal protection. Patients however get little, if any, benefit as resources are wasted. The purpose of EBM is what it does.

Cookbook medicine

> There are no routine statistical questions, only questionable statistical routines.
>
> Sir David Cox

One of the things we noticed when researching this chapter was that proponents of EBM go to great lengths to state that it is not "cookbook medicine".[10,196] The sensitivity of supporters to the charge of cookbook medicine reflects the popularity of the term with critics,[197,198] who accuse EBM of straitjacketing doctors.[185]

Supposedly, EBM requires a bottom-up approach that integrates the best external evidence with individual clinical expertise and patient-choice. Thus, supporters claim, it *cannot* result in slavish, cookbook approaches to individual patient care.[10] This is clearly an overstatement: any doctor *could* take a cookbook approach to EBM. As Shakespeare might have said, EBM "doth protest too much".[199]

In its formalised version, EBM has introduced guidelines for experimentation and practice; people could take them as recipes for research.[200] However, we agree with the supporters of EBM to this extent: "evidence-based" medicine cannot provide an adequate medical cookbook, as it does not provide sufficient information.

Cookbooks act as a guide, offering instructions for competent cooks, who may improvise variations. Expert cooks will use a recipe as a heuristic, providing a useful outline. They might modify it by adding raisins and a splash of Calvados to enhance an apple pie, for example. Equally, a lesser cook may be able to produce an acceptable, if uninspiring, apple pie, by following the instructions slavishly. Cookbooks have their value, to both beginners and fully trained chefs.

Despite their training, doctors can be intimidated by complex mathematics, or unable to respond to arguments such as their direct observation not being valid evidence under the rubric of EBM. It is important that a doctor is able to appreciate the meaning of a clinical trial's results. With EBM, doctors are supposed to assess the information critically. However, the critical appraisal process in EBM takes a formalised approach.

Critical appraisal

In EBM, doctors judge studies according to how well they meet the rules. Critical appraisal is used as a mechanism to support EBM. If you disagree with EBM, you are faced with Joseph Heller logic. In Heller's Catch 22, a World War 2 bomber pilot who was insane would continue to fly missions, unless he claimed he was unfit because of insanity. However, claiming insanity was a sane thing to do. Any person claiming to be unable to fly missions because he was insane was therefore sane and had to fly! In a similar circular argument, people are expected to criticize EBM's clinical studies using EBM's rules.

EBM has its own selective internal logic. Part of this—the process of arbitrarily excluding unwanted information—is a characteristic of cult science. There are examples throughout the history of medicine. Historian David Wootton, author of Bad Medicine, describes how doctors maintained the status quo long ago, in the face of the germ theory:

> Once doctors decided they need pay no attention to microorganisms, they immediately ensured that they would never have to encounter evidence suggesting they had made the wrong choice.[201]

EBM specifies its own critical appraisal techniques. These are an attempt to help doctors to evaluate scientific studies, such as clinical trials. This kind of appraisal is another set of rules.[202] The rules define questions that a doctor might ask, such as "were the patients in a clinical trial randomized?" The rules amount to little more than a reiteration of the EBM requirements. In this context, critical appraisal involves acceptance of the rules of EBM: the method generates a selective (we are tempted to say cookbook) criticism of a study. The circular logic of critical appraisal defines a poor study as one that does not agree with the rules of EBM.

Initially, the word evidence in EBM was applied to the use of statistical information, such as population studies. With time, the word has also come to encompass financial and other considerations, which are not necessarily in the best interests of patients. Hiding considerations of quality and financial interest behind terms like medical evidence may be dangerous and unethical.[203] These aspects may offer important evidence to the medical agency but would not be useful for a particular patient. Notably, financial considerations were a core consideration of Archie Cochrane, in his initial suggestion for a medicine constrained by statistics.

Definitive evidence

Archie Cochrane provided a tentative ordering of medical evidence. Definitive results provide the most reliable evidence. The term *definitive* involves direct, large, obvious effects. For example, the guillotine was used in France to execute by decapitation. Removing a prisoner's head was claimed to result in death—a definitive effect, if ever there was one. There were no randomized controlled trials of the procedure. Moreover, there were no controls of any kind: the only evidence presented was from case reports.

Among such reports, there was some doubt as to how quickly decapitation brought about death. Some observers reported severed heads blinking and showing responses for several seconds. A Dr. Beaurieux interrogated the detached head of Henri Languille, guillotined in 1905, reporting that it responded to his voice. An 1887 report, by Drs Regnard and Loyein in the British Medical Journal, suggested that no consciousness remained two seconds after decapitation of one individual, though reflexes remained for up to six seconds.[204] Unsurprisingly, apart from ghost stories, there are no reports of people surviving guillotine decapitation in the long term.

According to a strict "evidence-based" interpretation, these reports of guillotine deaths are mere anecdotal case study reports; since no clinical trials have been performed, no reliable evidence has been provided. The guillotine is therefore an "unproven" method.

There were no controls to show that the deaths were caused by a factor other than decapitation. In EBM, the executioner's black hood might be considered a risk factor, as would the crowd of onlookers, potentially explaining the death. (The deaths occur when the executioner's hood is worn in public, but not otherwise.) Reports from forensic medicine of suicide by decapitation would also be taken as weak evidence.[205] However, we do not suggest replication and hope that the reader accepts these anecdotal case reports as genuinely definitive. We do not believe people will survive decapitation.

Along similar lines, Drs Gordon Smith and Jill Pell published a spoof review suggesting clinical trials of the use of the parachute to prevent death when falling from an airplane.[206] Their tongue-in-cheek conclusion explained,

> As with many interventions intended to prevent ill health, the effectiveness of parachutes has not been subjected to rigorous evaluation by using randomized controlled trials. Advocates of evidence-based medicine have criticized the adoption of interventions evaluated by using only observational data. We think that everyone might benefit if the most radical protagonists of evidence-based medicine organized and participated in a double blind, randomized, placebo-controlled, crossover trial of the parachute.

Cochrane suggested that a doctor's opinion is the worst kind of observational evidence. Expert opinion is clearly suspect; indeed, physicist Richard Feynman amusingly defined science as "belief in the ignorance of experts."[207] Though spoken partly in jest, Feynman implies that scientists should suspect all authority and reach their own conclusions. Note that rejection of expert opinion does not preclude the use of specialist decision-making skills. A doctor's opinion on the efficacy of some new drug may lack rigor. Nevertheless, choosing a particular drug for an individual patient currently requires human decision-making.

How good is the best evidence?

The EBM concept of evidence strength was not based on science. We were unable to find any scientific rationale for it, until we realized that "evidence" in EBM referred not to science but to a form of legal approval.

EBM Hierarchy of Evidence		
Level		Origin
1	"Best Evidence"	Evidence obtained from a systematic review of all relevant randomised controlled trials (e.g. meta-analysis)
2		Evidence obtained from at least one properly-designed randomised controlled trial
3		Evidence obtained from well-designed pseudo-randomised controlled trials
4		Evidence obtained from comparative, observational, and similar studies
5		Evidence obtained from comparative studies with historical controls
6		Evidence obtained from case series
7	"Weakest Evidence"	Expert opinion, physiology, bench research, or "first principles"

The hierarchy of evidence table lists types of clinical evidence, in terms of assumed importance. We present a table modified slightly from those provided for EBM by the Australian Government National Health and Medical Research Council,[208] the Bandolier group,[209] and the Oxford Centre for Evidence Based Medicine.[210] There are several published evidence hierarchies, which differ slightly in terms of the technical details. However, the simplified table presented here provides a consistent outline.

In this table, the evidence is ranked according to perceived quality. In EBM, higher quality relates to increased numbers of patients and to the use of certain statistical methods. The greater the number of controls and constraints in the method used to obtain the data, the higher the quality rating. This is because controls are used to try to avoid bias and error. Also, quantitative data and measurements are preferred.

In EBM, what is considered the best evidence (Level 1) is that which arises from a systematic review of a number of randomized controlled trials. A meta-analysis is a systematic review. These reviews can cover large populations and thus are often assumed to provide the best evidence.

Clinical trials themselves are sometimes judged to provide slightly lower quality evidence (Level 2) than meta-analyses. However, to qualify as such relatively excellent evidence, they are required to be "properly designed", "randomized", and "controlled". Each of these terms relates to approaches to prevent bias in trials. In Level 3, we find clinical trials that are not completely randomized, or have some other technical deficiency.

Level 4 evidence refers to evidence provided by comparative or observational studies. In these, the allocation into groups is not under the control of the investigator. For example, when comparing cancer patients with healthy controls, the experimenters may not have been able to set up two identical groups (treatment and control) and follow both until enough people get cancer. Instead, they try to match patients who have already presented with cancer to others who have not. This weaker kind of control is sufficient to lower the acceptability of the evidence.

If the controls are from a different period in time (Level 5), the perceived quality of the evidence is reduced further. For example, if a study involved the effects of radiation from telephone use in 2010, then it would be inappropriate to use subjects from 1958, as cell phones were not available in those days.

Case studies are ranked low in the evidence hierarchy (Level 6). These are reports of interesting or potentially important observations, made by physicians. Although the number of patients is low, case studies allow possibly rare drug side-effects to be reported early, for example. Reports of death by decapitation would also fall within this group.

Finally, at Level 7, we find explanations based on experimental research, physiology, physics, mathematics, pharmacology, and expert opinion. These are ranked as the lowest quality of evidence. For example, an explanation based on biochemistry and biophysics, which explains why you should not expect to live after a guillotine has removed your head, is supposedly the weakest form of evidence!

The EBM-mantra

The fundamental building block of EBM is the following:

a well-designed, large-scale, double-blind, randomized, placebo-controlled, clinical trial.

This list of words is what we will refer to as the EBM mantra. In the context of EBM, authors who describe a study in this way hope to broadcast the quality of their evidence. The mantra can also provide a quick defence of the EBM position. To reject a study, it can be used in a shortened form, for example:

"There's no placebo!"

"It's not a randomized trial!"

Thus, the EBM mantra provides practitioners of EBM with a shorthand way to dismiss undesirable results. In our experience, such shortened references to the mantra provide the main strategy for those defending EBM. It apparently carries great power: a simple reference to the mantra may be enough to brush away criticism.

Mantra-consistent clinical trials

A clinical trial is a practical test of a medical treatment or procedure. To take an analogy, before an aircraft enters passenger service, a test pilot will fly it and engineers will carry out an extensive series of tests, to be sure it is safe. Similarly, when new drugs are developed, doctors test them in a series of clinical trials before releasing them into general medicine and health care.

Clinical trials are a core element within EBM. Essentially, such a trial is a test of an intervention. If a drug is going to be useful in treating a disease, it needs to have an effect on patients. There may be excellent theoretical reasons for believing it will be effective; the drug might cure the disease in Guinea pigs, rats, mice, and rabbits, for example. However, we cannot know that it will work on humans without testing it on real patients.

In addition, clinical trials can help discover whether a drug has side-effects. Some side-effects are species specific: a particular drug could be harmless in mice and rabbits, but might turn humans blue. Tested on mice, the drug would appear safe. However, a clinical trial would allow researchers to explore whether it was safe for humans or, in this case, it turned them blue. Thus, a clinical trial can suggest that a drug is free of common, obvious, and major side effects.

Since EBM puts such stress on the mantra attributes, we might assume that the EBM research procedure would itself have been subjected to well-designed, large-scale, double-blind, randomized, placebo-controlled trials, to demonstrate its superiority over other kinds of research. However, there is only limited direct evidence to support EBM's claims of the advantages of mantra-consistent studies over other forms of clinical trial.

For example, it is often assumed that observational studies will overestimate the effects of treatment. This is because an observational study is not randomized and the investigators simply witness what happens to the patients. However, when well-designed observational studies are compared to mantra trials,[211,212] differences cannot be objectively validated without a definitive measure of reality.[5] If one study shows great benefit and another harm, how are we to know which is correct? An independent and accurate assessment is needed for comparison and validation. Despite this, studies consistent with the EBM mantra can be refuted by observational studies. For example, observational demonstration of a rare but serious side effect could refute a claim that a drug is safe.[213]

We will briefly consider the different parts of the EBM mantra. Firstly, the phrase "well-designed", which in this context indicates that the clinical trial obeys the major rules of EBM. However, the term well-designed is not clearly defined: it refers to a subjective impression that the study is structured soundly.

The "large-scale" attribute usually means that there are many subjects or patients. A rule of thumb might be that to merit this prefix the study should include 1,000 patients or more. Practitioners of EBM may consider the value of scale self-evident, since, by the law of large numbers, an enormous number of subjects will provide a more precise result than is usually obtained in a small study.[214] EBM mistakenly generalizes this to large studies are "best".

The next stipulation in the mantra is that the study should be "double-blind". A blind study is one in which the patients do not know if they are taking a drug or an inert tablet (*placebo*), which has no expected physiological effect. "Blinding" the patients helps to prevent psychological and other bias entering the study. Double-blind means that neither the patient nor the doctor knows whether the subject is receiving the drug or the placebo. The doctor and the patient do not learn who has received the drug until the experiment is complete, so they are not influenced by the knowledge. By using the double-blind approach, EBM has a mechanism to prevent some forms of bias.

It is possible to take this blinding procedure even further. In a triple-blind protocol, the statistician or person analysing the data also does not know which patients received the treatment. However, triple blinding is not often used. We note that triple-blind trials would be less susceptible to bias by data manipulation than are double-blind trials. It is possible for commercial influences to vary the analysis to prejudice the analysis of clinical trials in favour of a new drug, for example. If used, triple-blind trials and independent analysis would make this source of bias more difficult.

Randomization usually means that patients are allocated to receive either the treatment or the placebo according to chance alone. They could be placed into the respective groups by tossing a coin, but more sophisticated methods of random allocation may be used.[215,216] The aim of randomization is to try to make sure that there is no systematic bias, such as putting all the healthy patients into the same group.

Placebos and bias

Placebos are a way of controlling for unwanted psychological influences on patients in a study. For example, we could imagine that if a doctor tells a patient that a drug will help, and the patient believes this, it is possible that this belief would affect the outcome. For that reason, a dummy pill is used to make such influences less likely. Often, a placebo is an innocuous tablet that has no effect; it is sometimes called a sugar pill. There are ethical issues associated with this procedure. If a doctor leads a patient to believe that a sugar pill is really a drug, the uncovered lie might destroy the patient's trust in the doctor, for example.

If patients receiving the drug return to good health during the study, it could simply be that the study lasted six months and they would have recovered naturally within two months. In such a case, the patients receiving the placebo would also improve, so the experimental group's return to good health will not be wrongly attributed to the drug. It is not often realised that placebo control is only important when the trial is not measuring definitive outcomes.[217] There is no need for placebo controls in a study of the guillotine: the subject's decapitation and death constitute a definitive outcome, and would be unlikely to result from psychological expectations.

Despite the intentions of researchers, the use of a placebo can introduce bias into clinical trials. A trial will generally state that a drug was compared with a placebo but may not describe what the placebo contained. Without knowing the specific content of the placebo, it is impossible to verify any claims. Consider the following studies of migraine treatments, which illustrate the problem.

In the first study, a low dose of vitamin B2 (25 mg riboflavin) was used as a placebo and compared with the treatment, which consisted of a combination of 400 mg vitamin B2 with 300 mg each of feverfew and magnesium.[218] All three substances are believed to prevent migraine. In this experiment, both the "placebo" and the treatment appeared to lower the incidence of migraine. The authors sensibly suggested that their low dose riboflavin was an effective treatment, rather than an inert placebo. This result is not surprising, as the body can only absorb about 27 mg of riboflavin in one dose.[219] So, the placebo might reasonably have been expected to have equivalent effectiveness to the treatment.

Similarly, a placebo that causes the illness that is being studied would bias the results; even if the treatment did nothing, it would appear better than the placebo. In studies of the food additive monosodium glutamate (MSG) as a migraine trigger, the placebo control was also a trigger.[220] Aspartame, a known migraine trigger, was used as a masking sweetener for both the MSG and the placebo. These studies did not test MSG against an inert placebo, rather, they covertly compared the difference between two migraine triggers.

The inappropriate use of placebos litters the medical literature. By choosing a therapeutically active substance as the so-called placebo, a researcher can minimize the apparent benefit of a treatment. Alternatively, by selecting a placebo with a negative effect, the trial will appear to show the drug is beneficial. Furthermore, a reader cannot be certain that a placebo was inactive when its actual content is hidden. Not specifying the nature of the "placebo" prevents independent evaluation and delays the scientific process.

Peer review

To be acceptable, a Mantra-trial must be published in a peer reviewed journal. Peer review is a primary stamp of approval in medical research and is the process by which a scientific paper is examined for quality before publication. A scientific journal wants to meet some minimum standards for the information it presents. When a journal receives a paper for publication, the editor sends it out to a number of expert reviewers. The reviewers then recommend publication or rejection, based on its scientific content. We should consider peer review carefully, as it has become a misused benchmark of scientific validity.

Richard Horton, Editor of The Lancet, has explained how peer review was overhyped.

> The mistake, of course, is to have thought that peer review was any more than a crude means of discovering the acceptability—not the validity—of a new finding. Editors and scientists alike insist on the pivotal importance of peer review. We portray peer review to the public as a quasi-sacred process that helps to make science our most objective truth teller. But we know that the system of peer review is biased, unjust, unaccountable, incomplete, easily fixed, often insulting, usually ignorant, occasionally foolish, and frequently wrong.[221]

Peer review is a revered process, which supposedly acts as a quality filter for scientific journals. Unfortunately, in the words of Richard Smith, former editor of the British Medical Journal, peer review is also

> slow, expensive, ineffective, something of a lottery, prone to bias and abuse, and hopeless at spotting errors and fraud.[222]

Similarly, the journal Nature reports

> scientists understand that peer review per se provides only a minimal assurance of quality, and that the public conception of peer review as a stamp of authentication is far from the truth.[223]

The media have assumed that peer review is synonymous with excellence. Reporters often have limited scientific training and need heuristics for checking new research findings. One of the first questions scientists will be asked is whether their results been published in peer-reviewed journals. Indeed, the number of peer-reviewed papers published can determine the future of academic departments and scientific careers. Superiority is estimated further by ranking the journals.

Despite all this, there is no evidence to support the claim that peer review increases the quality of published papers. The Cochrane Foundation "could not identify any methodologically convincing studies assessing the core effects of peer review."[224] Although peer review has an almost mythical status as a quality indicator, there is little or no solid evidence to support its use.

Critics of the system have suggested that peer review is unfavourable to genuine scientific originality.[225] On the plus side, it is a good way of checking for and correcting errors before publication. For example, if a person's weight was stated as 70 grams, rather than 70 kilograms, a reviewer might point out the weight is about 1,000 times too small. The journal, authors, and readers will benefit from such verification.

The decision to publish a paper depends on many factors besides the absence of errors. An editor might reject a paper as not falling within the bounds of the subject: thus, a scientist would be unwise to send a paper on the physics of black holes to the British Journal of Nutrition, if he wanted it to be accepted. Editors can easily reject papers they do not like, by stating that the paper falls outside perceived criteria of acceptability, relevance to the subject, or reader interest. This approach is common and may be used to reject papers that disagree with the status quo. Many papers are rejected at an early stage, even before being sent to referees.

One problem with most peer review is that the reviewers are anonymous. Their names are hidden, so they do not need to defend their comments. Furthermore, the reviewer's comments are not revealed to the readers. Open peer review may be more effective.[222] It is sometimes possible to respond to published papers with a letter. Similarly, it would be appropriate for peer reviewers to submit a signed letter of response, to be published alongside a paper that they deemed lacking, rather than censor publication altogether. Readers could then come to their own conclusions and the information would not be censored. Peer reviewers could provide a private response to the authors on any errors they found, allowing correction, and, if the mistakes were gross, they could suggest the authors might like to reconsider publication. To avoid censorship, in an ideal world, the author should have the ultimate say on whether or not the paper would be published.

One of the original reasons for peer review was the cost of publication. A journal only had so many issues each year and there was a limit to the number of pages. Each additional page had an associated cost. Peer review gave the journal a mechanism to select submitted papers, honing the number down to the limitations of the medium. In recent times, this restriction has been overcome. The marginal cost of an electronically published paper is insignificant. In physics, for example, papers are published, without peer review, online at *arXiv.org*. Indeed, in many arenas of mathematics and physics, essentially all scientific papers are placed on the arXiv (pronounced archive). The size of the repository is increasing by thousands of papers every month. Physicists can withdraw papers that are wrong or refuted. Lack of peer review does not seem to be an issue. Nonsensical papers are rare and are placed in a general category but not usually deleted. However, while arXiv avoids peer review, it has received criticism for censorship and blacklisting of individual scientists.[226]

Unfortunately, peer review has sometimes been used to steal scientific ideas and claim the credit for someone else's work.[227] A dishonest reviewer might give a harsh review to prevent a competitor from publishing. Moreover, if the paper contains a fundamental breakthrough or ideas of similar high value, a reviewer could reject it and then appropriate the concepts, to publish in another journal.

In a well-known case, Drummond Rennie, acting in his capacity as Editor of the New England Journal of Medicine, reportedly sent a paper for review to Philip Felig, Professor and Chief of Endocrinology Research at Yale School of Medicine, who delegated the task to a junior researcher, called Vijay Soman. Soman allegedly rejected the paper, then copied parts of it and submitted them to the American Journal of Medicine, as his own work.[228] Felig co-authored this paper, a common practice within science. Fortunately, the fraudulent paper was sent for review to the department of the original author, who objected vigorously. Despite this, the issue was covered up and not made public until later. The author of the original paper, probably feeling she had not been appropriately supported, resigned her research post in favour of a clinical career.

Tarnished Gold

Sadly, scientific whistle blowing is as likely to destroy a whistleblower's career as that of the offenders.

Peer reviewers are people, with all the normal strangeness, bias, and self-interest that being human implies. Reviewers can always find a reason to recommend rejection and their comments are not necessarily fair or reasonable. Peer review can be used as a mechanism to prevent, or at least slow down, the publication of data by a rival scientist. Authors may have an opportunity to disagree with the reviewers, but this may not be sufficient to convince the editor to publish.

A recent experience illustrates the potential for censorship. The authors of this book are known for having challenged the US National Institutes of Health (NIH) and Institute of Medicine on their assumptions concerning the recommended dietary allowance (RDA) of vitamin C. As far as we could see, their RDA recommendations were unjustified. The recommended intakes were not based on science, and there was evidence to suggest that an appropriate intake for good health could be much larger. As a result of these objections, many people questioned the competence of the official recommendation.

Sometime after our spat with the NIH, we worked with some international colleagues to prepare a collaborative research paper on vitamin C. We helped write the paper and added original experimental results. The paper was submitted to a journal and successfully passed through the peer reviewing and editing process. However, after it had been accepted and was going into print, another co-author (who had little involvement in the work) objected to our names being on the paper. We realised that the NIH funds much of the medical research in the US. Scientists and doctors do not want to criticize the NIH, otherwise future grant applications might not be so favourably received. (Only the naïve would question this assumption.) Since the funding of other co-authors might be compromised, we agreed to have our names dropped.

Having your name removed from a paper you helped to write, and which contains your own original scientific data, is unusual. It never happened to us before or since. However, since challenging the NIH on their science, we have found it far more difficult to publish research papers in the area of nutrition. When giving an invited talk at a scientific conference, one of us (SH) was asked specifically to "be nice to the NIH." (The invitation was from an eminent founding member of the sponsoring organization, but the administrators were concerned that representatives from the NIH would be present.) We regarded this bizarre and strange situation with some humour, considering the size, income, and reputation of the NIH. The worrying aspect is that political and financial considerations often carry more weight than scientific ones.

Peer review and prejudice

Many influential findings have either failed peer review or been published in non-refereed journals. In 1797, the Royal Society rejected Edward Jenner's short paper describing vaccination with cowpox to protect against smallpox.[229] The Royal Society was incredulous at the idea that one disease could prevent another. The following year, Jenner published his experiments privately, in a small booklet. In fact, Jenner was not the first to suggest you could prevent smallpox with cowpox. It was common knowledge amongst dairymaids, who were famous for having clear fresh skin with no pockmarks and were thus favourite subjects with artists. Jenner had known the old wives' tale for perhaps 30 years before his experiments. Vaccination remains controversial, partly because the methods currently used for evaluation are those of EBM; robust methods could have resolved the issues long ago.

Many major scientific and medical works were not peer reviewed. Isaac Newton hated the idea of peer review. Notably, Newton's historic paper on the physics of light in *The Philosophical Transactions* was reviewed by his archenemy, Robert Hooke, who recommended rejection![230] As described earlier, Newton believed light was made of particles, while Hooke considered it was composed of waves. Both were correct, in that light may be validly considered either as waves or as particles.

The Editor decided to publish Newton's paper, alongside critical comments. Unsurprisingly, the paper was of great interest to scientists. Poor Newton had to respond to twelve letters to the editor: his reward for producing one of the most famous and influential papers in physics. This annoyed him so much he that he was discouraged from submitting another paper to the journal. To quote:

It had sacrificed my peace [of mind], a matter of real substance.[230,231]

Later, Newton would issue his famous quotation: "If I have seen further, it is only by standing on the shoulders of giants." It has been suggested that this may have been less a suggestion of his debt to earlier scientists than a cruel dig at Hooke—a short hunchback, who suffered from scoliosis. Peer review of Newton's work was counterproductive, and history has shown that his work stands on its own merits.

One reason often given for peer review—particularly in the field of medicine—is to make sure that readers are not duped by quacks. However, scientists, by definition, ought to be able to evaluate evidence. The fact that a paper has been subject to peer review should have little influence on a scientifically trained reader. Just because someone else thinks a paper is without major errors and has given it a peer review stamp of approval is irrelevant. Real scientists think for themselves.

In more modern times, Frances Crick and James Watson's seminal paper on the structure of DNA was not peer reviewed. This classic paper, based on the experimental work and ideas of Rosalind Franklin and Raymond Gosling, was published in the leading scientific journal, Nature. The elegant structure they proposed was widely accepted, as it fit the available experimental data. The scientists of the day did not need someone else to tell them that the double helix model was correct.

To bring us up to date, Grigori Perelman is one of the leading mathematicians of the century. His work was the first in mathematics to be hailed as the scientific breakthrough of the year (2006). He was awarded this honour by the respected journal, Science, for proof of the Poincaré conjecture. (For those who might be interested, Poincaré's hypothesis was that every simply connected closed 3-manifold is homeomorphic to the 3-sphere.[232]) This problem had been unsolved since it was first posed by Henri Poincaré, in 1904. Perelman was also offered the Fields Medal, which is the greatest award for mathematics and is awarded every four years; however, he declined it. (Mathematics does not have a Nobel Prize; the Fields Medal is the nearest equivalent.)

Perelman's work was outstanding and a landmark in the history of mathematics. For his proof of the Poincaré conjecture, it was announced that he would be the first recipient of the Clay

Millennium Prize. He also rejected this award, along with the million-dollar prize money!

Perelman explained:

> It was completely irrelevant for me. . . Everybody understood that if the proof is correct, then no other recognition is needed.

Perelman shunned peer-reviewed journals, as he did prizes. He published his results by posting his papers to arXiv. Perelman's attitude is clear:

> If anybody is interested in my way of solving the problem, it's all there — let them go and read about it. I have published all my calculations. This is what I can offer the public.[233]

Perelman clearly does not work in medical science. Since Perelman's work was not published in a *bona fide* peer-reviewed scientific journal, then, according to the rules of EBM, it could be disregarded. We wonder what Grigori Perelman would make of EBM.

Case reports

In the course of medical practice, doctors come across rare conditions and diseases and may describe them in what is known as a case report. A case report is a way of communicating information about unusual complaints in a medical journal. The well-known story of the greatly disfigured "Elephant Man", Joseph Merrick, is an example of such a report. Case studies provide valuable and sometimes unique knowledge about uncommon disorders. Individual case studies and Bayesian methods can be combined for investigating uncommon diseases that occur, say, once in a population of one billion. The whole world population with the disease would only be seven subjects, so studying them in a standard EBM clinical trial would be impractical.

Occasionally, a patient may unexpectedly recover from a fatal disease, such as terminal cancer. Other times, new diseases arise, such as when an emerging virus jumps the species barrier from animals to humans. These and other events may be of interest to other doctors and medical professionals, and might be described in a case report.

Many people have an irrational fear of sharks when swimming at the seaside, but do not realise they are at greater danger while digging in the sand. Dr Bradley Maron provided a case series of 52 people who experienced collapsing sand holes over a 10-year period.[234] The fatality rate was 60%: 31 died and 21 were rescued. Most were young people (age range 3 to 21 years), digging and tunnelling on beaches. The holes collapsed when the subject was digging, or had jumped or fallen into the hole. The collapse often completely buried the victim leaving little trace on the surface. This risk may be small, but the knowledge may useful if your child is digging tunnels on the beach.

In EBM, a case study such as this is anecdotal evidence, which means it is considered as a story or even hearsay. Anecdotes are viewed as simple observations and unscientific. The advance of "evidence-based" medicine has led to some people suggesting that case studies are irrelevant or even harmful, since they highlight the bizarre.[235] However, within the more general context of medicine, they have their uses. Importantly, a study of a series of case reports can be as rigorous as a clinical trial.

Consider anaesthesia. Most readers would not want to have a tooth removed or major operation performed without pain relief. This pain reduction information emerged from the practical experience of surgeons and others. Although pain is influenced by the placebo effect, the difference between operating with and without anaesthetic is large and obvious. We predict that readers would not need a committee to tell them that anaesthetics are beneficial during surgery. We also speculate that few supporters of EBM would wish to be in the placebo control group of a clinical trial of severe pain relief.

Case reports concerning drug side-effects are a highly cost-effective means of protecting patients. Adverse effects may be infrequent and the initial clinical trials often fail to pick them up. Sometimes, toxicity may only occur after extended use. A side effect that takes five years to develop will not be apparent in a two-year clinical drug trial. Case reports can monitor users of drugs for adverse reactions.

When a problem is linked with a drug, the existence of just a few case reports provides substantial evidence.[236] If a problem is rare, a cluster associated with a drug is unlikely. The stunted limbs of thalidomide victims were just such an unusual birth defect. Thalidomide children, born to women who took the drug during pregnancy, illustrate the power and necessity of case studies. Dr William McBride of Hurstville in New South Wales, Australia, published a brief letter describing his observation that almost one fifth of children born to mothers given thalidomide suffered these rare abnormalities.[237] The number was far greater than the 1.5% expected for all congenital abnormalities. McBride's letter detailing the problem was just over 100 words long and a mere three paragraphs. The Distillers Company voluntarily withdrew the drug from the market, based on two such overseas reports.

The importance of McBride's thalidomide letter is clear: if a woman thought she might become pregnant, knowledge of this simple report might prevent her taking thalidomide. Rationally, taking the drug as an option to prevent morning sickness would appear to leave the child at high risk of major deformity. To suggest the case reports did not clinically prove the drug had this side-effect, and that it therefore remained suitable for pregnant women, would have been irresponsible.

McBride's thalidomide report came nearly five years after the first child was born with the unusual abnormalities. This illustrates the limitation of case reports. Far less harm would have occurred if the problem had been found earlier. The weakness of case reports is not that they provide scant evidence, but that they have a limited capability for discovering side effects.

As in the thalidomide situation, a number of case reports can combine to form a case series. A case series led ultimately to the recognition of an epidemic of West Nile virus in the United States.[238] Doctors noticed individual cases in both humans and birds, which led to investigation and later identification of the virus. However, there have been few formal studies of the accuracy and utility of case reports.[235] In one investigation of forty-seven case reports of drug side-effects, thirty-five (74%) were claimed to be "clearly correct".[239] The predictive potential of such case reports therefore appears reasonable.

Even finding a new risk of a drug using case studies requires a strong association between the drug treatment and the problem.[240] A problem is only likely to be found if the drug causes a rather obvious side effect with high frequency. Many more side-effects may be present but unnoticed. Despite these limitations, case reports are more likely to pick up rare side effects than are clinical trials. They identify new diseases, and can provide definitive results.

Science or marketing?

It is becoming difficult to separate science from marketing in the medical literature. For a new drug or treatment to be accepted, it has to be shown to provide significant benefits over placebo in a clinical trial. We will show later that this is easy to arrange. Results can simply be inflated during the study design and implementation.[241] Such manipulation is apparent in various areas of medicine. One way would be to terminate a drug trial early, because the treatment seems beneficial. As we have shown, conventional trials are valid for a fixed period and specific number of patients. However, if a treatment is helpful, the rules may be broken to enable all the patients to receive the drug's benefits. Shortening a study offers the company the additional "benefits" of restricting the appearance of longer-term non-responsive patients and giving less time for side effects to develop. It is also good advertising copy, as in "... the drug was so effective it was unethical not to give it to all the patients."

Such flexible approaches to studies are statistically invalid but nevertheless may help guarantee success and thereby enhance future marketing. This is particularly easy when selective reporting of results is employed. One approach is to provide marketing in the form of ghost written medical reviews.[242,243,244] Ghost-written research papers and associated press releases from pharmaceutical companies guide readers to the required interpretation of the data, and sell more drugs.

Cargo cults

EBM is well described using physicist Richard Feynman's term "cargo cult science". This is defined as a futile exercise, with the appearance of a science but lacking in substance.[245,246] Cargo cult science refers to an analogy between certain fields of research and cargo cults. These are religious practices in some traditional tribal societies in the wake of interaction with technologically advanced cultures. The cults focus on obtaining the material wealth (cargo) of the advanced culture through magic and religious practices.[247]

These practices were first described for islands in the Pacific Ocean, in the 19th century following the arrival of Western visitors. The cults were also a feature of World War 2, when islands became the focus of Japanese and American armed forces. Rituals, for example building an imitation landing strip and copying the behaviour of airport staff, were used in an attempt to attract the cargo-bearing planes. Perhaps a rare aircraft would arrive, confirming the validity of the ritual. This process set up a variable reinforcement schedule in which the followers' devotion was occasionally rewarded. Psychologists have found that such reinforcement provides a powerful incentive to continue the supported behaviour.

Feynman noticed the similarity between some forms of research and a cargo cult.[248] Richard Feynman's description fits EBM perfectly. Cargo cult science has ritual methods, designed to produce the "cargo" or results, by way of ritual. Although it has the superficial appearance of science, EBM is based on specific ritual methods that practitioners assert provide the "best" evidence. The rituals of EBM are claimed to increase scientific knowledge in medicine. EBM's rituals are validated by authorities, tradition, and organisational approval, rather than by decision science and the scientific method. As with sacred practice elsewhere, competing belief systems are actively discouraged. The practitioners or high priests anoint reports with scientific "proof" for the benefit of the media. Heretics and their unproven remedies are not tolerated.

At best, EBM generates minor incremental increases to knowledge. For example, over several years a large-scale mantra-consistent clinical trial may suggest a new drug is ineffective. The initial positive trials that introduced the drug may be followed by a series of other trials, over a further period of years. After perhaps a decade, one or more meta-analyses will be performed, to confirm the "proof".[249] There are no earth-shattering breakthroughs, though the expenditure of time, effort, and misallocation of funds may be enormous.

Feynman has provided another example of how conformity and cargo cult science do not make breakthroughs. He uses Millikan's famous oil drop experiment to illustrate the problem. Robert Millikan received the Nobel Prize in Physics in 1923, for this work on the elementary charge of electricity and for research on the photoelectric effect.[250]

Starting in 1909, physicists Robert Millikan and Harvey Fletcher measured the electric charge on a single electron. To do this, they balanced a small drop of oil with an electric charge between two electrodes. Since the forces were known, they could estimate the minimum (quantum) charge of about $1.60217646 \times 10^{-19}$ coulombs. However, Feynman explains that there was something awry with the process. Perhaps we should let Feynman describe this himself:

> It's interesting to look at the history of measurements of the charge of the electron, after Millikan. If you plot them as a function of time, you find that one is a little bigger than Millikan's, and the next one's a little bit bigger than that, and the next one's a little bit bigger than that, until finally they settle down to a number which is higher.[248]

This gradual modification is worrying. The physicists could have simply done a careful experiment and obtained an accurate value immediately. Something was going on to mess up the process. The historical record shows that scientists were selecting their "best" evidence, which resulted in bias. Returning to Feynman:

> It's a thing that scientists are ashamed of—this history—because it's apparent that people did things like this: When they got a number that was too high above Millikan's, they thought something must be wrong—and they would look for and find a reason why something might be wrong. When they got a number closer to Millikan's value they didn't look so hard. And so they eliminated the numbers that were too far off, and did other things like that. We've learned those tricks nowadays, and now we don't have that kind of a disease.[248]

Millikan's original result was a little wrong but the physicists followed the authority of the accepted value that tricked them into using their "best" data and not believing their other results, which were correct.

As we shall show, the characteristics of EBM are those of a selective cargo-cult science. EBM has the appearance, statistics, and rituals of science but it fails to produce the cargo.

Main Points

- EBM is a cargo cult; it has the look and feel of a science, without the content.
- EBM's "critical appraisal" asks are you obeying its rules: this is hardly critical.
- EBM supports corporate medicine and its research is used as advertising.
- EBM censors other viewpoints.
- EBM's evidence hierarchy is irrational and misleading.

> Never tell people how to do things. Tell them what to do, and they will surprise you with their ingenuity.
>
> General George Patton

Authority

> The improver of natural science absolutely refuses to acknowledge authority.
>
> Thomas Henry Huxley (Darwin's bulldog)

EBM is based on authority and the legal system, from which it has inherited its own version of the concept "innocent until proven guilty". In EBM, by analogy, "unproven" therapies can be ignored. Similarly, EBM's assertions of "no evidence" against certain therapies does not imply the absence of scientific data or information, rather it means there is no legal evidence of a particular restricted kind. As a result of practising EBM, doctors are protected by the law. Governments gain additional control and corporate medicine profits from the legal framework.

Despite EBM's legalistic approach, a rational individual would not accept its claim to authority. Legal protection for the doctor and associated organisations can act against the patient's interests. People expect scientific medicine, not treatment based on legal principles. For this reason, practitioners promote EBM as highly scientific. Indeed, if it is to be accepted in an advanced society, EBM cannot avoid claiming a scientific basis. Without a foundation in science, EBM's claims to authority are of little value.

To take an example from another profession, most people would expect a bridge or an aircraft to be constructed according to engineering principles. They might be worried if lawyers or managers started to specify the design. In the event of something going wrong during a flight, concerned airline passengers may not be greatly reassured to know that their aircraft meets minimum legal requirements. Famously, when NASA allowed management authority to overrule its engineers, the Challenger space shuttle exploded on take-off.[251] Richard Feynman was an expert witness to the enquiry and described the cause of the disaster. As he explained,

"For a successful technology, reality must take precedence over public relations, for Nature cannot be fooled."[252]

Medicine and science

Although medicine borrows much of its authority from science, there are cultural differences between the two disciplines. Students wishing to become medical doctors face a long and arduous training, during which they learn a large amount of information. In addition to academic study, they acquire practical skills, gained through treating patients in teaching hospitals. Medical training tends to be authoritarian and the consultant physician or surgeon is the immediate authority.[253] Although the scientific basis of medicine is uncertain and there can be several valid viewpoints, dissent is not always encouraged. When a specialist holds a strong opinion and others in the group agree, it would take a brave medical student to express a heretical viewpoint.

By contrast, young scientists must learn to doubt, questioning everything and tolerating a state of perpetual uncertainty. The aim of science is to discover new ways of understanding. Long-accepted ideas can and should become obsolete: this is how science progresses. Many PhD students, who may have been skilled at learning to regurgitate text books, struggle with the loss of certainty when they start their doctoral work and have to think for themselves. How much more difficult this would be if the result could mean life or death for their patients!

Typical doctors may not have the luxury of experimenting with original or creative ideas, they have to conform to accepted methods. Furthermore, patients might request their doctor to provide them with established and tested treatments. Both doctor and patient are trying to arrive at an optimal strategy in a world of uncertainty. Physicians and surgeons usually try to be appropriately cautious, both in diagnosis and in claims for the effectiveness of an offered treatment. Nevertheless, a confident medical practitioner can recommend a suitable course of action, helping patients make decisions at difficult times in their lives.

Unfortunately, medical training, lawyers, and the expectations of some patients tend to demand conformity to "best practice". By this, we mean the set of procedures that the medical authorities view as most appropriate *on average*. Though this may sound good to an uninformed patient, by now readers will probably realise that this is the medical equivalent of going to a shoe shop and buying a pair of average-sized shoes. If you are lucky, they may not fit too badly but for most people, they will be useless or damaging. A set of generic instructions cannot be successful, no matter how exalted the authority from which they stem. The suggestion that "best practice" can be modified according to current conditions is insufficient to overcome this problem; the variety of patients and their illnesses is much greater than that of the rules of best practice.

Stafford Beer, in introducing cybernetics to management science,[254] explained how information flow needs to be bottom up (starting from the patient's condition and circumstances) rather than top down (starting with medical dogma). We can appreciate that medical bureaucrats will find it disconcerting, but attempts to impose autocratic medicine are doomed to be harmful to patients.

Nevertheless, doctors who do not use the approved "clinically-proven" treatments may find themselves out on a limb or regarded as heretics, despite acting in the patients' interest. A doctor practicing nutritional medicine for a conventionally untreatable cancer, for example, is likely to be accused of using unproven treatments and of putting patients at risk. The EBM faithful think they are avoiding medical risks by following the rules, but they are wrong. What they are doing does not help their patients, it simply allows less competent doctors to cover their backs and avoid a lawsuit.

Doctors conform to the rules of EBM because authority figures tell them that it is the best, safest, and proven form of medicine. We can find no convincing argument that any decision-making authority should overrule the combination of an up-to-date physician and a rational, well-informed patient. However, proponents of EBM implicitly use group conformity and the threat of disciplinary or legal action to enforce their policies.

Unthinking respect for authority is the greatest enemy of truth.

Albert Einstein

Recognising excellence

A defining characteristic of doctors is that they are highly educated. Unfortunately, a certain kind of education can sometimes stifle productive thought. Most postgraduate supervisors will have come across conscientious students, brought up in countries where rote learning is heavily practised. Such students have excellent undergraduate degrees and know their textbooks off by heart. However, they may struggle when asked to think for themselves, seeming to feel they have no right to suggest an idea of their own. This attitude can be as much of a problem as its equally common opposite: the student with lots of ideas who knows little about the subject, so cannot discriminate between worthwhile suggestions and rubbish.

In school, a simple rule for success is to follow what authority figures say and to repeat what the teacher tells you; this is the *authority heuristic*. Repeating information from lectures and textbooks guarantees good marks, even in college. The main drawback is a lack of originality and creativity. Furthermore, in order to use this heuristic, you need to be able to recognise a suitable authority.

If you have missed a lecture, a moderately effective remedy might be to copy the notes from a neighbouring student. However, the nearby student may not be very good, so this might not give the desired results. We could improve the odds of a high mark by using an alternative rule: to copy the notes of an excellent student. This is more difficult, as we need to be able to distinguish exceptional students from average or poor ones. With this modified approach, we need a rule for finding an outstanding student; we might decide to pick one who other people say is good or to check our fellow students' grades. More broadly, when following an authority heuristic, the choice of authority is crucial. In medicine, it could be a matter of life or death, so doctors owe it to patients and themselves to give the matter serious thought.

Copying the consultant is an example of a simple heuristic that can be effective for medical students. Since our knowledge is limited, accepting the word of an authority is an understandable human trait. People often apply the heuristic that something is good if others, especially authorities, say it is. However, if they are left to make their own decision, people may fail to spot excellence, even if it is right under their noses—as when a famous musician went busking in a metro station.

But nobody told me it was good

Joshua Bell is an internationally acclaimed violinist, a Grammy award-winner, and was a soloist with the Philadelphia Orchestra by the time he was fourteen years old. Since that time, he has appeared as a soloist with orchestras worldwide. Joshua Bell also has a sense of humour. When the Washington Post asked if he would busk incognito in a subway, he agreed, saying "sounds like fun."[255] Gene Weingarten, the journalist who arranged this informative experiment, was awarded the 2008 Pulitzer Prize for his article about Bell and the subway.

Wearing jeans and a baseball cap, Bell positioned himself alongside a trash basket at the L'Enfant Plaza Metro Station, in Washington DC. It was the morning rush hour. Passers-by could stop and hear "one of the best musicians on Earth play some of the best music ever written" for free.[255] For three-quarters of an hour, Bell played superlative classical music to over 1,000 pedestrians. The acoustics of the subway were unexpectedly good. Each person who went by had the choice of how to respond: to stop and listen, to drop a coin in the hat, or avoid eye contact and keep going.

Before the experiment and without knowing that the musician would be Joshua Bell playing his $3.5 million Stradivarius violin, Leonard Slatkin, music director of the National Symphony Orchestra, was asked to predict what would happen. He thought that out of 1,000 people, perhaps 100 would stop and listen, and suggested that an excellent violinist might collect up to $150 in donations. This would normally be about the price of a single ticket for one of Bell's concerts.

In the event, Bell took about $32, from just 27 benefactors. Bell was happy with that, joking that he could make a living if Carnegie Hall ever let him down. The remaining pedestrians simply disregarded him. In Bells' words "It was a strange feeling, that people were actually, ah, ignoring me." Several children tried to stop and listen, but their parents were seemingly too busy and dragged them away. The manager of the station apparently enjoyed the music, saying: "He was pretty good, that guy. It was the first time I didn't call the police." So, at least, Bell was not arrested.

One or two people did take the time to listen, including Janice Olu, who had played violin herself. John Picarello also noticed the violinist and was baffled. "This was a superb violinist. I've never heard anyone of that calibre. He was technically proficient, with very good phrasing. He had a good fiddle, too, with a big, lush sound." Only one person realized it was Joshua Bell: Stacy Furukawa, who had been to a free concert by Bell three weeks earlier, at the Library of Congress. Here was the great Joshua Bell playing in a subway, begging for money. She listened with a big smile and thanked him at the end. But most people missed the opportunity to listen to Bell's free concert because they had no context; musicians of international acclaim do not busk for change in the subway.

When you don't know about a subject, having an expert to explain things can be useful. In another example of the appreciation of expertise, an Australian sculptor called Barbara Tribe, an old friend of ours, loved to talk about her work and that of others. On one occasion, she took two similar tankards by craftsmen from the Leach Pottery in St Ives, Cornwall, and described how they differed. She praised the well-turned curve of a handle on one item, and showed how the other tankard was competent but nothing special. As she explained it, we could see the difference—the cups were not at all identical. Barbara's ability to understand and explain the difference had taken years of work and dedication. In a single lifetime, it is not practical or even possible to give such commitment to every subject.[96] When seeking advice, we often need an expert to provide an explanation.

The authority heuristic

Doctors often use the authority heuristic to save time. Used properly, it can be simple and powerful but if it is abused it can be stultifying. Part of a doctor's job as a medical expert is to distinguish accurately between different sources of information. This is not always easy. A classic study showed that a leading medical journal presenting health data is more likely to be believed than when the same information is read in a magazine.

In this experiment, people presented with information that was purportedly from the New England Journal of Medicine found it more credible than when they were told it came from a magazine (in both cases, identical information was given).[256] They apparently assumed that a leading medical journal is reputable and more likely to be correct than a magazine. This suggests they were using an authority heuristic. It seems like a useful rule of thumb and, for most people, it is. However—and this is important—scientists should be able to interpret data themselves, without reference to the authority of the medium.

The fact that a paper is in a top journal does not guarantee its quality. Research papers may be accepted for publication simply because they come from prestigious institutions. In an interesting study, Peters and Ceci took twelve published psychology papers, from first class institutions.[257] They changed the author's names and institutions, made minor changes to the titles, and so on. They invented fictitious institutions that could not be known to the journal editors or reviewers. Amusingly, they resubmitted the papers to the journals in which they had already been published. The editors recognised three papers, but nine entered the reviewing process and were rejected as being of poor quality, despite having previously been accepted by the very same journals. Apparently, the papers had miraculously developed serious flaws!

Unknown authors from less prestigious institutions may have great difficulty getting their research published. It also implies that the quality of a paper is not a major determinant in whether or not it will be published, as these journals accepted poor quality papers from leading institutions, or rejected good quality ones from lesser-known sources, or a mixture of both. With this in mind, we can see how important it is for doctors and scientists to learn to read and understand papers in an unprejudiced way.

Scientists should be able to evaluate research publications, without being told what to think. In the same way, doctors, engineers, musicians, and other professionals are expected to have the skills to assess the value of work in their own fields, regardless of where it is published. If they are too busy to do this, then they risk being misled.

For most people, the use of experts is a simple rule. Not being qualified themselves, they ask a professional what they are supposed to think. For example, it is easier to accept the experts' claim that Leonardo da Vinci was a truly great artist than to study art and art history yourself. Clearly, one person cannot study every subject, as the sum of human knowledge is now too great for a single lifetime. People have to be practical.

Gerd Gigerenzer has described the simple rules that people use as "fast and frugal" heuristics.[258] Fast and frugal is often translated as quick and dirty. These heuristics can be thought of as time-saving ways of coping with a complex world. For such simple rules to be effective, they need to do the following:

- Exploit information in the local environment
- Use regular psychology, such as perception and memory
- Be fast, frugal, and simple enough to be useful when time, knowledge, and computation is limited
- Be powerful enough.

Medical education is long and arduous, so techniques that might help the student to progress more easily would surely be welcomed. The heuristics that serve doctors during their education and training tend to be based on regurgitating information to lecturers and senior doctors. Medical students learn to follow clinical procedures and to accept authority. A student cannot learn the whole of medicine in five years of medical school; even after a long and focused training, they can only expect to be reasonably proficient in one or two specialties. Successful students need to be selective and to learn the core knowledge. A workable heuristic for a medical student might be: learn as much as possible and don't get left behind.

Students are also expected to learn to copy surgical procedures, as in the old medical heuristic "see one, do one, teach one."[259] However, a monkey-see monkey-do approach is not sufficient for creativity or scientific research. Competent musicians play as they were taught, whereas brilliant musicians make their own rules. We suspect that most patients, like the authors, would prefer an outstanding physician to one who is just about competent. Unfortunately, the medical education system is not usually set up to nurture brilliance.

The effect of years of medical training, like those of many other disciplines, can instil recipients with a stultifying respect for the status quo. A student may be highly intelligent, but all the students are bright. The professors are leaders in their field, and are imparting knowledge that has taken centuries to accumulate. The volume of information and medical technology that a student has to grasp is overwhelming. In this context, it might require the confidence of an egotistical narcissist to question the combined wisdom of centuries. However, a scientist should question everything.

Conformity?

A family doctor tries to achieve the best individual treatment for his patient, while being expected to conform to EBM, best practice, and peer pressure. Whether they know it or not, most people are subservient to authority, to an extent that is most unwelcome. American social psychologist Stanley Milgram's now well-known results on this topic shocked the world and changed our view of humanity.[260]

In the early 1960s, Milgram performed a series of psychology experiments that demonstrated the power authorities exert over people.[261] In the experiment, a white-coated scientist instructed an experimental subject to give a series of increasing electric shocks to another subject when he or she answered a question incorrectly. Before the experiment, it was thought that few people would be willing to give a powerful electric shock to another, even when instructed by an authority figure. Milgram showed that even though they might feel uncomfortable in carrying out the order, about two thirds of people complied and some even gave a potentially deadly 450-volt shock to their fellow subject. Most administered large shocks before refusing. Only one subject refused before the 300-volt level. (The subjects administering the shocks did not know that the electricity was not connected or that the screaming victim was, in fact, an actor.) The experiment suggests that people have a tendency to give up responsibility for their actions when asked to do so by an authority figure.

Milgram's experiments caused great controversy because some critics thought it unethical to deceive people into thinking they were giving another person a strong electric shock. Not surprisingly, the experience stressed and upset the subjects. However, other researchers thought that Milgram had been justified, because of the experiment's implications for understanding war criminals and others who claim they are just obeying orders.

Related studies throw further light on the capacity of people to defer to authorities. In the Stanford Prison experiment, Phillip Zimbardo showed the difference between the behaviour of two groups of people, who were classified as "prisoners" or "guards".

The chosen subjects, who appeared to be psychologically stable and of good character, were randomly assigned to their roles. Despite this, the experiment had to be terminated early; about one third of the guards were displaying sadistic and psychotic tendencies, and the prisoners were being traumatized.

Milgram's experiment and similar studies have been repeated many times and the results are consistent: almost two thirds of people demonstrate extreme subservience to authority.[262] Over time, there is a suggestion that people are less likely to display blind obedience to authority, because of increasing nonconformity, narcissism, and self-esteem.[263] However, these interpretations are highly optimistic.[264] Humans evolved as social animals and may require a level of obedience, conformity, and peer pressure to enable group functioning and cohesion. The recent inhumane treatment and torture of prisoners at Abu Ghraib prison in Iraq demonstrates that the findings of Milgram and the Stanford Prison experiments should remain a warning to us all.

Each of us would like to believe that we are one of the few individuals who are immune to such obvious subservience. This may be especially the case with those of us who are highly educated and think we have a substantial intellect and highly tuned critical faculties. We can make up our own minds about a topic and reach our own conclusions. We all want to believe that we are one of the people who would refuse an instruction to torture a fellow human. Unfortunately, in most cases, the experiments suggest that this is wishful thinking.

It would be going a bit far to suggest that a medical training is equivalent to being in a prison camp, although there are similarities—sleep deprivation being an obvious one,[265] and bullying another.[266] Both these factors are likely to result in medical errors. However, the application of authority in medicine is generally more subtle than that in the Milgram and related experiments. The medical establishment espouses a legitimizing ideology and an apparently ethical philosophy, to which it gives social and institutional support. Unfortunately, this arrangement provides an ideal environment for the potential abuse of authority. In medicine, those in authority are selected partly for their ability to manage others. Medical authorities have other control methods in their efforts to preserve orthodoxy. Few doctors are willing to risk a decade or more of training and an investment of tens of thousands of dollars to challenge the authorities by treating a patient using an "unproven" or unapproved therapy.

The pressure to conform in medicine deters many doctors from expressing independent views. Some naïve medical researchers may doubt this statement, so we will discuss an example. The power of conformity to hold back medical progress is illustrated by Dr Devra Davis, in the preface of her book *The Secret History of the War on Cancer*.[267] Davis has made a solid contribution to cancer research and is a highly intelligent and independent-minded expert in the field.

Dr Davis's book is a fine account of the recent history of cancer research and blows the whistle on the tragedy of opportunities lost through special interests. She published the book in 2007, after some twenty years delay. In 1986, Davis was offered an advance equal to half her annual salary for what would be her first book. At that time, she was working at the prestigious US National Academy of Sciences and told her boss, MIT Professor Frank Press, about the book. Press, a diplomat and former advisor to President Jimmy Carter, responded with the following warnings:

> It had better be a really, really good book. ... because you won't be able to work here after you write it.

> You can't write a book critical of the cancer enterprise and hold a senior position at this institution.

Professor Press was not threatening Dr Davis; he was trying to let her know that publishing the book would destroy her career. This was not intimidation or blackmail, but helpful advice. She would not be promoted, she would not be given research funding, her colleagues would shun her, and her research papers would be rejected. Publishing the book would probably result in the end of her research career.

The question for the reader is as follows: what would you do, if you were faced with this decision? If you had the intellectual courage to ignore the advice, it might be the last scientific contribution you ever made. Years of study would be wasted. As a trained scientist, you might make many discoveries to help cancer patients over the course of your career. Those contributions may be thwarted by the publication. If you publish the book, your career may be over. It may also cost you a fortune in lost salary.

In view of all this, you could delay publishing the book and work from the inside, trying to change the system. You would keep your career, salary, and may make an outstanding contribution to cancer research in the future. You would not waste your education, effort, and expense. Working on the inside appears practical. However, if you buckle under the pressure of this decision, it is unlikely that you will remain an iconoclast. You may become just another conformist researcher, independent at heart but conventional in practice. Dr Davis describes the choice well—there is no correct answer. Doctors are faced with decisions like this throughout their training and medical practice. The individual issues may be smaller and less explicit but the balance between scientific integrity and conformity is ever present.

In this case, Davis published her book years later. Publication became a safer proposition when sufficient time had elapsed. Davis had gained more experience and moved on to more supportive organisations. Devra Davis should be applauded for the book she eventually produced. Unfortunately, because of the demands of conformity, the public had to wait 20 years for the information.

Professional pressure

> I am compelled to fear that science will be used to promote the power of dominant groups rather than to make men happy.
>
> Bertrand Russell

In addition to the requirement to conform to expected standards, doctors face peer pressure. Medicine, like every other social activity, is subject to group behaviour. This is more apparent in nursing, where a lack of leaders has been attributed to the profession being a repressed group.[268] Societal pressures on nurses have inhibited people with leadership potential from entering the profession. However, peer pressure has beset medicine throughout history.

A classic example occurred in the 1840s, when Dr Ignaz Semmelweis was able to show that if physicians washed their hands, hospital childbirth death rates were greatly reduced. Unfortunately, his idea went against current medical practice and was rejected.[269] Semmelweis' finding is normally considered part of the history of medicine, which ultimately led to saving many women's lives. However, in 2003, Mary Lankford and colleagues showed that group pressures were still active in this arena.[270] Compliance with hand washing is influenced by the behaviour of other staff. Healthcare workers, including doctors, were far less likely to wash their hands if a peer or higher-ranking person in the room did not.

Throughout their long training and professional practice, doctors are subject to groupthink. This is the pressure in a cohesive group to resolve differences and reach consensus, by repressing the ideas of individuals.[271] The power of groupthink is sufficiently strong to produce an effect called the *Abilene Paradox*.[272] This suggests that the pressure to "not rock the boat" can lead to a group decision that none of the individual members prefers. Jerry Harvey realized this paradox during a discussion with his bored family, after a long day trip to Abilene. When they returned, it became apparent that not one of them had actually wanted to go. They each went along with the idea for the benefit of the others, who they had assumed were enthusiastic for the trip.

EBM is also supported by the related bandwagon effect.[273] So many medical professionals believe in it and support it, that individuals assume it must be valid. Bandwagons are contagious. Part of medical training involves conformity to the rules and learning the expectations of the profession. A doctor may be properly influenced by the fact that thousands of doctors and the medical authorities believe an idea which is claimed to be based on centuries of progress. The aim and effect of EBM is to influence the decision making of individual doctors. Unfortunately, a direct effect of doctors conforming to EBM is to reduce the variety of treatments available to patients.

Nice?

>Science commits suicide when it adopts a creed.
>
>Thomas Henry Huxley

The UK National Institute for Health and Clinical Excellence (NICE) provides guidance, sets quality standards and manages a national database to improve people's health and to prevent and treat ill health. NICE employs an "evidence-based" approach, using randomized clinical trials and cost-benefit analyses, to determine whether a particular drug should be available for physicians to prescribe. It also provides accreditation and a seal of approval for other information providing organizations. Health professionals and the organizations that employ them are expected to take

NICE's recommendations into account when deciding what treatments to give people.[274]

The idea behind NICE, to help prevent illness and treat it effectively, is like motherhood and apple pie: no-one could object to it.[275] The problem is the implementation. Putting EBM into practice is likely to impose control, rather than improve patient health.[276] Despite its name, NICE is not so nice.

Professor Bruce Charlton, of St Bartholomew's Hospital, London and the University of Newcastle upon Tyne, explains the issues.[277] In 1993, the National Health Service started using contracts that controlled details of clinical practice.[278] Specific treatments or drugs were approved, for example, beta-blockers and aspirin following heart attack. The controversial explanation was that the treatment was proven. This was the start of a continuing process. State organization is taking control of medicine and is devaluing the doctor's expertise. Unless government recommendations are based on rational decision making, rather than EBM, and are implemented voluntarily, Charlton claims that:

> NICE guidelines will amount to little more than government propaganda backed up with a big stick.[277]

NICE and similar organizations do not have unique access to data. Their decision-making is the kind of run-of-the-mill statistical analysis that could be performed by any student of a quantitative subject with a computer. In other words, their analysis is rather rudimentary. When Dr Hickey was teaching computer science at Staffordshire University, he had the opportunity of visiting a group performing statistical analysis for NICE. His first surprising observation was that the analysts typically had a background in accountancy, rather than science. The analysis was being performed on Microsoft Excel spreadsheets.

At first, Hickey thought they were using the spreadsheet as an interface to more advanced software, so he asked an analyst, who replied as follows:

> Analyst: No, we do all our calculations on the spreadsheet.
>
> Hickey: But your Monte-Carlo simulations and Bayesian analysis, that's done elsewhere? You are very limited with what the spreadsheet can do.
>
> Analyst: We don't do any Monte-Carlo analysis or anything like that.

Hickey (while looking at the spreadsheet and diagrams that appeared similar to a first year undergraduate computing exercise): This is one of your smaller calculations?

Analyst: No, this is one of the big jobs. But with some of our big projects like this one, we are finding it difficult to fit it all into the spreadsheet. I keep having to simplify the VBA [a limited computer language] code.

Hickey: You do know that you can plug in software extensions to the spreadsheet and effectively have unlimited computing power?

Analyst: No, I didn't know that. We just use the spreadsheets. None of us are proper programmers.

The conversation continued, becoming ever more bizarre. The analysts had little, if any, scientific training and used elementary computing methods. Their decisions involved simple statistics, based on data typically provided by the drug companies. The process was an extension of accounting methods—their real interest was cost effectiveness, or just reducing costs. Do we really want treatments for cancer and heart disease to be determined by accountants?

As Professor Charlton points out, NICE has no unique advanced techniques for its analysis. There is no reason to suppose that organizations such as NICE can provide improved guidance to doctors. NICE is unlikely to perform with greater success than any other government bureaucracy. Despite this limitation, the statutory powers of NICE and other such organizations imply that their guidelines carry the certainty of law. We are expected to believe that these accountants and their simple spreadsheets can achieve what scientists and doctors cannot: remove uncertainty to give definitive medical guidelines. They cannot.

As we write this, the UK government has explained that it does not want scientific experts on its "independent" drugs advisory group, the Advisory Council on the Misuse of Drugs (ACMD). This comes after Dr David Nutt, chairman of the committee, was a little too independent and gave his interpretation of the data on drug abuse and regulations publically. The Director of the Campaign for Science and Engineering, Imran Khan, put it eloquently, saying, "It's incredible that the government are trying to take us back to the time of 'Minister knows best'."[279]

Top down?

Governments use EBM to control medicine. EBM allows governments to generate executive organizations such as NICE in the UK, the FDA in the US, and the international Codex Alimentarius Commission for nutrition. These organizations initiate a top-down managerial hierarchy that allows governmental and legislative control. Often, the result is that the people making the decisions are not fully independent doctors or scientists. Managers and accountants specify medical treatments that determine whether you live or die. Scientists, by contrast, are seen as mere technicians, selected to rubber stamp the political and commercial requirements.

There is no scientific support for NICE and similar governmental organizations. They are justified by political needs, balanced by those of corporate medicine. Once these organizations are formed, the agency problem comes into play. Each agency or organisation starts to act to enhance its own power, funding, and influence. Independent academics, doctors, and scientists have little say in the process. By contrast, in an ideal world at least, science is a collaborative, open process.

Professor Charlton has provided an excellent description of the deficits of such bureaucracies.[277] Managers in NICE and others implementing health decisions have their own agendas, which may conflict with individual health needs. Governments promote basic nutrient requirements, such as the RDA (Recommended Dietary Allowance), which have been highly criticized.[280] Recently, they have gone further, aiming to restrict the availability of vitamins and other nutrients, based on standardizing trade laws. According to this approach, health is supposed to be secondary to rules of trade and commerce (though few individuals would support this notion with respect to their own health). The apparatchiks have the same personal motivation as other officials: they are interested in furthering their own careers. Promotion does not depend on the accuracy of their decisions, but on meeting the internal demands of the system.

Safety or authority?

If EBM were effective, medicine would be gradually becoming safer. However, in the US, adverse drug reactions in hospitals kill more than 100,000 people a year.[281] Estimates for the effects of medical error vary but it is clear that medicine is a leading cause of death. As the US Institute of Health put it, more people die each year because of medical errors than from motor vehicle accidents, breast cancer, or AIDS.[282]

As the number of people who are dying as a result of bad medicine becomes more widely known, EBM has responded.[283] In 2004, the US Institute for Healthcare Improvement (IHI) started the "100,000 Lives" Campaign.[284] The Institute approached over 3,000 US hospitals, with the aim of preventing 100,000 unnecessary deaths over 18 months. They wanted the hospitals to try six initiatives that might help save lives:

- Rapid Response Teams
- Medication Reconciliation
- Prevent Central Line Infections
- Prevent Surgical Site Infections
- Prevent Ventilator-Associated Pneumonia
- Evidence-Based Care for Heart Attack.

By setting a number of lives to be saved, it was hoped that the objective would be clear and results measurable.[285,286] Eighteen months later the IHI proudly announced that the campaign had exceeded its initial aims and 122,342 lives had been saved.[287] Hospitals had responded successfully to the campaign.[288] The self-congratulation was apparent.

Without irony, one paper suggested a new target: "Can hospitals save 5 million lives over the next two years?"[289] They wanted a "Save 5 Million Lives" campaign. Declaring that 15 million adverse events occurred in hospitals each year, it was suggested that there were 40-50 incidents for each 100-hospital admissions.[290] The aim of the new campaign was to lower the number of adverse events by 5 million a year. Understand what the advocates of this campaign are admitting: in US hospitals, medical mistakes are killing 2.5 million patients every year!

Unfortunately, the estimates for the number of deaths prevented in the 100,000 lives campaign were optimistic.[291] There is no solid data to support the number of lives saved. In 2009, the Agency for Healthcare Research and Quality checked the figures. They reported a decrease of 23,623 deaths between 2004 and 2006. Using the dates of the Campaign, they suggested, only 12,342 lives were saved.[292] At least some people did not lose their lives because of the effort, which is a positive outcome. However, the whole saga raises a question mark over medical safety. We hope that the aim of preventing five million deaths from bad medicine was an overstatement, but fear it may not be.

Authoritarian management does not prevent bad medicine. Preventive medicine, which enables people to avoid treatment, would be an obvious place to start. Despite EBM, or maybe even because of it, being a patient remains a hazardous activity. Bizarrely, someone engaging in a dangerous or extreme sport may be at less risk of accidental injury than a hospital patient.

Confirmation bias

Once EBM became established, it was logically self-supporting. While it may be irrational, people engaging in EBM are rewarded, as their prejudices are confirmed. A *confirmation bias* means that people are predisposed to focus on evidence that supports their beliefs; evidence that disagrees with current ideas tends to be neglected or ignored. To a first approximation, this confirmation bias is built into the EBM evidence hierarchy.

Throughout the history of medicine, selective evidence has been the bane of progress. For 1,500 years, knowledge provided by Claudius Galen—surgeon to the Roman gladiators—was believed to outweigh observation and experiment. While Galen himself was an experimentalist, his ideas were regarded as established fact in the years that followed. In today's language, they were regarded as "proven", having stood the test of time and attracted a "consensus of medical opinion". Once Galen's models were established in this way, other evidence was either fitted to the idea or ignored. Reliance on authority, certainty, and proof produced a confirmation bias.

Confirmation bias refers to "unwitting selectivity in the acquisition and use of evidence."[293] Dr Raymond Nickerson, an American experimental psychologist with substantial industrial research experience, gave an interesting description of confirmation bias.[293] Nickerson's account complements some of our arguments about the irrationality of EBM. He describes the following features:

Restriction of attention to a favoured hypothesis

Since EBM is dominated by the concepts of risk factors and multivariate explanations, its supporters do not look for direct interpretations of the data or for simple cures.

Preferential treatment of evidence supporting existing beliefs

This is related to the selection of data. EBM places inordinate emphasis on social and statistical studies and thus avoids information that might refute its core ideas and findings.

Looking only, or primarily, for positive cases

There is a bias in the medical and scientific literature, such that clinical trials reporting positive or significant outcomes are more likely to be published than those showing negative or non-significant results.[294,295] However, EBM restricts its evidence-base even further—to those studies that meet its specific methodological requirements. It thus filters out different scientific viewpoints. By way of analogy, Nickerson asks people to consider trying to find a small circle, beginning with a hypothesis of "a small red circle". By selecting only circles that are small and red, one will never discover other small circular things, such as those that are yellow, blue, or any other colour apart from red.

Overweighting positive confirmatory instances

By giving large-scale trials and meta-analyses a high profile, EBM reinforces their relative importance. The reputation of the EBM approach is thus confirmed with every significant result reported by the media.

Seeing what one is looking for

The method of searching for associations using large multi-variable trials inevitably finds correlations with a variety of things, which are then called "risk factors". There are always associations and some of them, by chance, will be "statistically significant". Such approaches find what they are looking for, in the way that a person looking through a telescope will find stars, but would need a microscope to see bacteria.

Revenge of the daisies

> The sciences do not try to explain, they hardly even try to interpret, they mainly make models.
>
> John von Neumann

Scientists view the world at different levels of size and organisation. While most people understand that systems exist, some specialist scientists have difficulties in understanding the role of systems theory and models. Self-organising systems are commonplace in science. The sun, for example, is stable because of numerous nuclear processes, heat diffusion, rotation, gravity, and so on, which maintain a more or less constant structure. Although it is an inanimate object, a balance between the mechanisms has kept it stable over millions of years.

The Gaia hypothesis,[296] which proposes that the world is regulated by living organisms, is also a standard cybernetic idea. Dr James Lovelock, a multi-talented British scientist, developed the initially vague notion that plants, animals and microorganisms collaborate in regulating the atmosphere, keeping the environment suitable for life. On earth, plants take in carbon dioxide and release the oxygen that animals need to exist. In turn, animals take in oxygen and release carbon dioxide. The oxygen in our atmosphere is the result of plants that have released it as a waste product, over millions of years.

When Lovelock published his intriguing Gaia theory, religious groups and new age followers soon took it up. One problem was that Lovelock adopted *Lord of the Flies* author William Golding's suggestion to call the theory Gaia, after the Greek earth goddess. To Lovelock's chagrin, this fuelled an over-literal new age pagan interpretation, based on Lovelock's metaphor of the earth as a living organism. Lovelock's approach was an excellent marketing ploy but was unlikely to be welcomed by mainstream science.

Scientists such as Richard Dawkins objected strongly, saying there was no way that plants and animals could cooperate in this way. It seemed to require long-term intelligent behaviour, and cooperation apparently goes against Dawkins' particular view of biology. Lovelock might have found this somewhat hypocritical, given that Dawkins was the originator of what Lovelock described as the "wonderful metaphor" of the selfish gene. As Lovelock pointed out, few say: "How absurd—how could a gene take thought and be selfish?" Correspondingly, the name Gaia was a metaphor for Lovelock's theory of the earth as a self-regulating system; it was not intended in a literal or religious sense.

As is often the case, the controversy forced Lovelock to study his ideas in relative isolation, while scientific journals refused to publish his work. Lovelock described this as the usual scientific censorship of new ideas by the establishment. He was not one to give up easily, however, and his ultimate response was brilliant: he produced a model that showed his idea could work.

Together with PhD student Andrew Watson, Lovelock simulated a planet called Daisyworld, which contained only two types of plant: black and white daisies.[297] According to the model, sunlight on the planet varied but the plants controlled the temperature, acting effectively as a thermostat. When the sun was dim, the white daisies did not absorb enough light and tended to die out, whereas the dark daisies absorbed light and flourished. By absorbing heat and light, the dark daisies caused their surroundings to warm up; the planet thus absorbed more heat when the sun was less active. When the sun became brighter, the dark daisies overheated and lost out to the white daisies, which spread rapidly. Large colonies of white daisies reflected light and heat away from the planet, cooling it down. Watson and Lovelock's Daisyworld model demonstrated that the two kinds of daisies could regulate the planet's temperature to a point that was more or less optimal for the overall daisy population.

The Gaia hypothesis describes the earth as a cybernetic system. Lovelock's daisies were not intelligent, their temperature control feature arose as a result of simple rules—a mechanism known as emergence. Although the descriptive term emergence may also seem to have a new age flavour, all it means is the logical appearance of order out of chaos, according to simple rules. The synchronised patterns in a flock of birds, or the behaviour of water molecules forming ordered lines of waves crashing onto a beach, are two examples of emergence.

Self-regulation provides controls that stabilise complex systems and without such regulation there would be no system. The earth and other large celestial bodies are often almost spherical because of the action of gravity—there is no need to invoke mystical forces to shape a planet. Similarly, as the moon revolves about the earth, a balance between the forces affecting both bodies produces a regular orbit.

The most complex systems are biological. In cybernetic terms, the idea that biological organisms control and influence their environment is inevitable, rather than fanciful. It is standard systems science and should be evident to anyone who has ever taken an intelligent walk in the woods. Had the Gaia theory been named otherwise or presented less poetically, it might have been more acceptable to scientists—but far less influential.

By now, some readers might be asking what all this has to do with medicine. Surprisingly, Daisyworld turned out to have potentially important medical applications. Mathematician Peter Saunders, working with physiologists Johan Koeslag and Jabus Wessels, produced a theory of Daisyworld control in medicine. The mechanism is a possible control process whenever two factors pull in opposite directions; for example, the control of blood sugar in the treatment of diabetics, based on the interaction between insulin and glucagon.[298] Blood sugar levels depend on the balance between these two hormones, in a similar process to the temperature control by black and white daisies on Daisyworld.[299] The interaction may partly explain why late onset diabetes is easier to treat than the juvenile form. A second example concerns the hormonal control of calcium by the interactions between parathyroid hormone and calcitonin.

The Gaia story shows how new ideas are fragile and need nurturing. As initially presented by Lovelock, Gaia was an easy target for sceptics, although it contained an important concept. However, Lovelock did not deserve to be censored: he had every right to express a novel opinion. Authorities are often too quick to use peer review and editorial muscle to prevent or delay publication. Daisyworld provides an example of how a development in an apparently unrelated area can inspire new medical understanding. This cross-fertilisation is particularly important when it involves new theory or information flow.

The primary problem in medical science is to understand the mechanisms our bodies use to stay healthy and to discover ways to control disease. Such understanding requires real science, rather than amalgamations of statistics on the behaviour of groups in clinical trials. Whether in medicine or science, authorities unfortunately depend on a form of simple-minded rationalisation, which all too often results in censorship of new ideas.

Delusions?

Supporters sometimes argue that EBM is not authoritarian and that it increases choice, rather than decreasing it. A recent example by Professor Kay Dickersin and colleagues included the following statement:[300]

> Critics of evidence based medicine worry that it dictates a single 'right' way to practise, despite differences among patients; that some self appointed group of 'experts' will declare only one type of study to be useful; or that healthcare decisions will be made solely on the basis of costs and cost savings.

This seems to us to be a reasonable and accurate summary of some aspects of EBM's authoritarian approach. Shortly afterwards, Dickersin made the following contradictory statement on the reason why EBM is necessary:

> Undesirable gaps and variation in practice exist.

The suggestion that, under EBM, medical choice will be increased but undesirable variation in practice will be reduced, is inconsistent. Variation is a result of the different decisions people make when given choice, and who is to say when such differences are "undesirable"?

Dickersin imagines a world without EBM, in which, apparently:

> Most women with early breast cancer would still be undergoing mastectomy instead of lumpectomy and radiation. Now they can choose.

EBM does not provide such choice: it is a matter for the individual patient. The patient should always have had the choice; surgery and medical physics provide the options, not EBM. What the patient needs in order to make a rational choice is for the doctor to provide the likely (Bayesian) outcomes for the individual patient. Without this information, the patient is unable to make a properly informed decision. Moreover, EBM generally avoids the (Bayesian) trials and explanation that would provide the patient with direct and useful data.

A history of failure

> We doctors have always been a simple trusting folk. Did we not believe Galen implicitly for 1500 years and Hippocrates for more than 2000?
>
> William Osler

To conclude, we may consider a long quote from Dr Lewis Thomas, on the failures of medical science throughout history. Thomas is warning about trial and error experimentation that, like EBM, lacks both guiding theory and the risk of refutation.

> Virtually anything that could be thought up for the treatment of disease was tried out at one time or another, and, once tried, lasted decades or even centuries before being given up. It was, in retrospect, the most frivolous and irresponsible kind of human experimentation, based on nothing but trial and error and usually resulting in precisely that sequence. Bleeding, purging, cupping, the administration of infusions of every known plant, solutions of every known metal, every conceivable diet including total fasting, most of these based on the weirdest imaginings about the cause of disease, concocted out of nothing but thin air—this was the heritage of medicine up until a little over a century ago. It is astounding that the profession survived so long, and got away with so much with so little outcry. Almost everyone seems to have been taken in.[301]

In our view, EBM has codified this scientific-theory-depleted form of trial and error into a new authoritarian medical philosophy and, once again, almost everyone has been taken in.

Main Points

- Science has no respect for authority.
- People and doctors use the authority heuristic to decide quality.
- Doctors are trained to conform, scientists to be iconoclastic.
- Medical whistle-blowers tend to be ostracized and excluded.
- EBM sees only large group statistics, which confirm its flawed ideas.
- New ideas are fragile: distrust them, but do not censor them.
- The history of medical authority is full of unnecessary harm.

> Have no respect whatsoever for authority; forget who said it and instead look at what he starts with, where he ends up, and ask yourself, "is it reasonable?"
>
> Richard Feynman

Powerfully Deceptive Trials

> Mounds of data are collected, which are statistically decorous and methodologically unimpeachable, but conclusions are often trivial and rarely useful in decision making. This results from an overly rigorous control of an insignificant variable and a widespread deficiency in the framing of pertinent questions. Investigators seem to have settled for what is measurable instead of measuring what they would really like to know.
>
> Edmund Pellegrino

EBM's clinical trials have no special position in science. In this part of the book, we deal with some myths about the power of large-scale trials. Such trials are useful as a crude, if expensive, test for finding drug side-effects and uncovering rare events. However, rather than being a gold standard, a clinical trial is merely a rather mundane practical test. Indeed, we suggest that the clinical trial as practiced by EBM is fool's gold. Like iron pyrite, it has the look and lustre of gold, but without the weight.

No gold standard

We need to reassess clinical trials. Most good scientists and research oriented doctors know that randomized clinical trials do not provide an unequivocal guide to clinical practice.[302,303,304,305] Randomized clinical trials are as unreliable as other forms of evidence. Clinical trials are often performed with inadequate controls, limited and inappropriate statistical analysis, and unrepresentative groups of patients. In addition, rational interpretation of clinical trials is extremely difficult.[306]

EBM is obsessed with mega-trials. The larger and more expensive the trial, the more prestigious is the resulting publication. Supporters claim that a trial becomes more valid as it grows larger. Still greater admiration is reserved for those so large that they require multiple clinical centres. However, as a trial grows, any advantage gained from size is overwhelmed by problems in experimental control and by loss of detail. Earlier, we showed how difficult it is to understand a simple probability problem. Correspondingly, large trials often confuse rather than illuminate.

A PhD student doing a three-year trial on, say, 25 subjects and 25 controls, will spend about three weeks on each subject. Time is spent ensuring the subjects are suitable for the experiment. The controls are carefully matched to the patients. There is time to evaluate each subject, their background, their response to the treatment, and so on. The aim is to avoid bias and systematic error. However, if the student were to investigate 1,000 subjects and 1,000 controls, he or she would have only a few hours for each subject. In this large study, the student would not have sufficient time to validate individual subjects, or their results, with the same rigor as in the small study. The student would need to take shortcuts, in order to complete the study in the time available.

Large clinical trials do not exercise the same level of control as our PhD student with a small-scale trial. Taking three weeks over each subject, it would take about a year to study sixteen subjects properly. A similar but massive study of, say, 10,000 subjects and controls, would take over 600 person-years of effort, not counting the communication and management overheads. The drug companies have a stake in keeping the cost of trials high and the introduction of new drugs expensive. It provides a monopoly for a small number of huge companies that are able to cover the entrance fee.

Writer Timothy Noah describes how it suits drug companies to claim costs of approximately a billion dollars to research and develop a new drug.[307] These huge costs mean that even large universities may be forced to team up with drug companies to introduce new drugs. Pharmaceutical companies have high profit margins, which they claim are necessary to cover their massive R&D risks.[308] Investing a billion dollars in a new drug that might never be released is a big financial risk. However, according to an independent assessment by Donald Light and Rebecca Warburton, the real cost of introducing a new drug is about $50 million.[309,310] This is a lot of money, but far less than a billion dollars. As Timothy Noah amusingly put it:

> So the drug companies' $1.32 billion estimate was off, according to Light and Warburton, by only $1.265 billion. Let's call it a rounding error.

Tarnished Gold

It would appear that, expensive as EBM style trials are, they do not cost enough for big drug companies trying to create a monopoly market for themselves. It is easy to see why large studies often cost millions of dollars, take years to complete, and consume resources. In addition to helping create a monopoly, they also appear impressive. However, large studies become increasingly inadequate in terms of the quality of their results. In some cases, the data in large studies is obtained from simple questionnaires. Increasing the size of the study does not compensate for this loss of care in the experimental method.

Large trials are not simply bigger versions of smaller, precise experiments. They are different in their objectives, methodology, and results. Larger trials are less rigorous in collecting, processing, and analysing data. Professor Bruce Charlton puts the issue well. To insist that large-scale studies are better, he says, "is absurd, rather like asserting that microscopy is the 'gold standard' of biology, without regard to the question being asked or the quality of the instrument."[303]

Obsessed with size

> In the physical world, one cannot increase the size or quantity of anything without changing its quality. Similar figures exist only in pure geometry.
>
> Paul Valéry

The recent change in the size of clinical trials is dramatic. Martin Bland, a statistician from the University of York, has described how the size of trials has increased. In 1972, he found that the average (median) sizes of trials in the Lancet and British Medical Journal (BMJ) were 33 and 37 subjects respectively.[311] For the same month in 2007, 35 years later, the average figures for the Lancet and BMJ were 3,116 and 3,104 subjects. This increase is about two orders of magnitude: the later studies were almost 100 times larger.

To put this in perspective, an elephant is of the order of 100 times longer than a mouse. Differences in orders of magnitude suggest different properties. So, for example, if you cruelly dropped an elephant from a skyscraper, it might disintegrate on impact with the ground. Drop a mouse, on the other hand, and it may simply walk away, as its relative surface area is large and its terminal velocity is low. Similarly, large experiments have different properties to those of small trials.

For experiments, small is beautiful. A small, simple, cheap experiment is ideal. Almost anyone can check the result. Small clinical trials are more likely to advance scientific knowledge. You do not need to believe the report from Isaac Newton that unsupported apples fall to the floor. If Newton's claim had been wrong, it could be quickly refuted. Small-scale experiments are particularly appropriate in medicine, because doctors work with individual patients and their illnesses.

As mentioned, a useful heuristic is to *trust but verify* the research of others. We should be sceptical of any medical claim that cannot be replicated easily by other scientists. Scientists are no more honest than other groups of people. However, they tend to stick to the truth because they know their findings will be replicated and fraud will eventually be detected. The ability to copy and repeat experiments is at the heart of the scientific method. In large-scale experimental science, such as high-energy particle physics, replication is necessarily difficult and expensive: a particle accelerator could cost billions and require international cooperation. Unfortunately, researchers may feel less need to be truthful when conducting large expensive clinical trials, which are almost impossible to repeat without being a member of the EBM establishment.

Simple observation and replication has advanced medical knowledge throughout history. In 1673, the Royal Society published microscopic observations by Antonie van Leeuwenhoek. Leeuwenhoek had developed a powerful new microscope, and was using it with success. Three years later, Leeuwenhoek reported the first observations of microorganisms.[312] He reported numerous single-celled organisms that no one had seen before, living in a drop of apparently clean water. Not surprisingly, these reports were met with healthy scepticism. It was difficult for people in those days to accept that a drop of clear pond water was teaming with tiny creatures, too small to be visible to the naked eye.

With some effort, Robert Hooke of the Royal Society was able to improve the resolution of his own microscopes. Having done this, he reported that the tiny organisms did indeed exist. Hooke had replicated Leeuenhoek's observations and they had taken the initial step in generating a new scientific field: microbiology. Without Hooke's replication, the microscopic entities might be considered fantasy; his confirmation helped the research to progress forward.

Most breakthroughs in medical and biological science have come from small experiments and observations that were repeated and checked.

Many people assume that larger trials are more reliable. This is a statistical fallacy: there is no difference between the reliability of a comparable result from a large and a small clinical trial. By comparable, we mean a result that has the same probability of having occurred by chance.

Consider two clinical trials, to test a fictitious drug, called Obecalpine. Apart from their size, the design of the trials is identical.

Trial A showed that Obecalpine helped prevent heart disease in a group of 20 patients, compared with 20 control subjects, 40 subjects in total. The statistical analysis showed that the result was significant (p=0.05). The study was described as a preliminary investigation and the authors suggested a large-scale clinical trial was needed to verify this finding.

Trial B was massive and showed that Obecalpine helped prevent heart disease in a group of a million patients compared to a million controls, a total of two million subjects. The statistical analysis showed that the result was significant (p=0.05). This study was described as a definitive large-scale trial, which proved the benefits of the drug Obecalpine.

Question: Which of these trials is more important?

Most people might respond that Trial B is more reliable and important. It is, after all, a huge study, involving two million people, whereas trial A involves a small study of only 40 individuals. This appears to be common sense. The conclusion is supported by the description of it as a large-scale "definitive" trial that "proved" the drug's benefits.

In fact, neither of these trials provides any indication of greater merit than the other. The probability of both trials (p=0.05) is identical. The meaning of this probability is that, if the drug had no effect at all, the result might be expected to have arisen by chance 5 times in every 100 experiments. (For the benefit of pedantic statisticians, we will point out that the trial data in these experiments were randomly selected from the same population.) If the larger study were actually more reliable, its probability would be lower. In other words, *the chance of either result occurring by chance is the same!* This means that if you repeated the experiment and the drug was completely ineffective, either result would occur with equal frequency.

If a medical researcher report results from a small and relatively inexpensive trial, using 40 patients as in Trial A, it will not carry much weight in EBM. Ideally, however, the smaller trial should be preferred, if only because it is easy to repeat.[313] This is not the end of the story. A rational patient with heart disease would be interested in the smaller study rather than the large one, as it is more likely to be of benefit to him. This is because, in order to get the same level of significance as the large trial, the small Obecalpine study (Trial A) will have estimated a much larger potential benefit than the large one (Trial B). A small study requires a larger difference to produce the same probability value. As the number of patients in the sample increases, the importance of the difference is reduced.

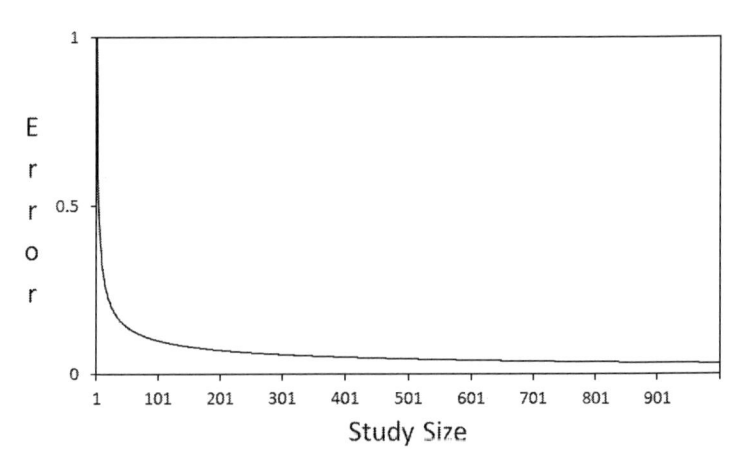

Decrease in standard error with sample size

The reason people assume that the large study is more reliable comes from the improvement in precision. In estimating an average (mean) value from a set of values, there is always some error. This error is called the *standard error of the mean*. The standard error decreases as the number of samples increases. However, the rate of change tails off as the number of values increases.

The reduction in error with sample size decreases rapidly for low numbers. For higher numbers, above about 100, the decay in error is small. The reduction in error size for ever larger numbers is increasingly tiny.

Suppose we are testing a drug to reduce pain. Once again, we have a small trial and a large trial, and both have the same 1 in 20 level of significance (P≤0.05). All groups have a spread, or standard deviation, of 50% of the average value of 100 pain units. This standard deviation indicates that about two thirds of the people in the control group have between 50 and 150 units of pain. That is the population and probabilities are statistically identical for both the small and the large trial.

Small Significant Study

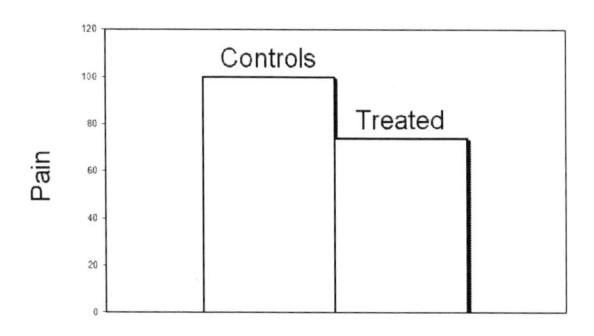

Large Significant Study

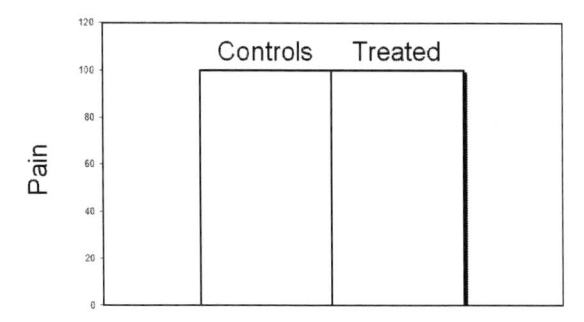

Large clinical trials find small benefits that may be irrelevant to a patient

In our small experiment, there are 30 subjects in each group. For this little trial, the treatment shows a significant result (at p=0.05), with a 26% improvement in the pain score. The average pain score drops from 100 to 74. This corresponds to a substantial benefit and the majority of patients report feeling substantially better. The drug works.

The group in a corresponding but massive trial contains 1,000,000 subjects and controls. This is clearly a large and impressive clinical trial. The same significant result (at p=0.05) now occurs with a benefit of only 0.14%. For example, the average pain score drops from 100 to 99.86 pain units. This average reduction in pain is so slight that not one patient even notices a benefit. Despite the significant result, the drug is useless.

Results in the large trial are far less relevant to patients than are those from the small experiment. Dr David Horrobin, after 40 years of medical research, found himself with terminal cancer. When he looked at the problem from the patient's viewpoint, he was aghast. He wanted a treatment that would save his life, or at least give him a year or two longer. What he found was large studies and EBM research, which highlighted statistically significant minor benefits, or, in other words, ineffective treatments. Horrobin put it well:

> If a trial has to be large, say more than 100 patients, it is large only because the expected effect size is very small.[314]

David Horrobin was well aware of the points explained above. Archie Cochrane was also mindful of this issue and related that "with large numbers it is often possible to achieve a result that is statistically significant but may be clinically unimportant."[179] We agree. By concentrating on these large-scale trials, EBM has lost its way.

> No effect that requires more than 10% accuracy in measurement is worth investigating.
>
> Walther Nernst

At equal levels of significance, a large-scale trial measures a smaller effect than a small trial. The fact that a trial is large makes people think that the result is more impressive. So, a drug company wanting to promote a treatment that provides only a tiny advantage to the patient might use a large trial. The new drug that is only slightly effective will then give a significant result. The company gets multiple advantage. Firstly, the minuscule benefit is statistically significant. Most people, including doctors, do not realize that the trial *had* to be large, because the drug effect was so small. Furthermore, anyone wanting to repeat the experiment will need lots of funding and time, leaving the company free to get on with making money. The drug can be on the market for years before the study is refuted.

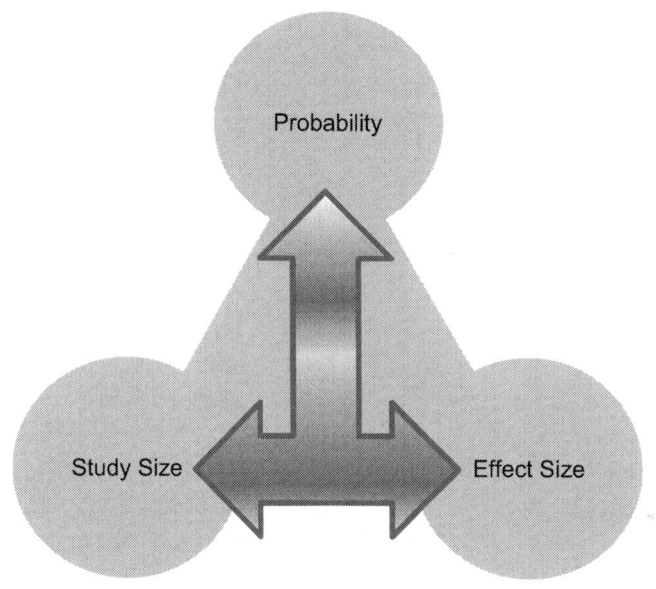

There is a balance between the size of a study, the p-value, and the size of any effect.

These three things vary together: they are not independent.

For the same probability, if we increase the study size then the size of the effect goes down (and vice-versa).

By comparison, researchers using small trials will find it more difficult to obtain a significant result, unless the effect they are investigating is large. Independent replication of results from such small trials suggests a substantial therapeutic effect—one that would be useful to patients. As Cochrane himself said of small trials:

With small numbers, it is easy to give the impression that a treatment is no more effective than a placebo, whereas in reality it is very difficult indeed to exclude the possibility of a small effect. [179]

So, it is hard to detect minor benefits using small trials—but then, who wants tiny benefits? Patients want their treatments to work, they want large effects. They want to be cured or, at least, to be free of symptoms. You will see where we are heading: the way to find treatments that stand a chance of benefiting an individual patient is to use small trials.

Will the treatment help the patient?

If a small trial does not find a significant benefit, then the drug is most likely irrelevant to an individual patient. Both doctor and patient are interested in the number needed to treat (NNT). As explained previously, this is a measure of how many people will need to take the drug in order for one person to benefit. The NNT is thus an easy to understand indicator of the likelihood of a patient gaining benefit. If the NNT is one, every patient taking the drug will benefit. This is presumably close to what patients are expecting! However, if the number needed to treat is 100, then a hundred people must take the drug for just one to benefit, though all will risk its side-effects. Large trials can find significant results, even when few patients will benefit.

Consider statins, the new wonder drug of EBM. Some doctors have joked that statins are so good they should be added to the water supply. Depending on the outcome of interest, the number needed to treat for a typical statin drug is somewhere between 30 and 300; the actual value remains controversial. Let us assume a value of 100. If 100 or more people take the drug for a year, perhaps one fewer person in the group will have a heart attack than if they had not taken the drug.[315] (In EBM, such a result may be a statistically significant improvement, used to justify mass prescription.) Such results mean that an individual prescribed the drug may pay in the region of $1,000 to lower their risk of having a heart attack by, at most, 1% over the year. Furthermore, the patient should not expect a reduction in his risk of death, as the side effects may balance out the benefits.

One company claimed that their statin drug "Lipitor reduces the risk of heart attack by 36%...in patients with multiple risk factors for heart disease."[316] What this meant was that, in a large clinical study, 3 in 100 patients taking a placebo had a heart attack, compared to 2 in 100 patients taking Lipitor. Notably, this re-evaluation came from

John Cary in a Business Week article, not a medical paper. The drug company's original claim was correct but misleading. The patient would actually benefit from a 1% lower risk, as the percentage of heart attacks deceased from 3% to 2%. This inflation of drug benefits is conventional in EBM.

The problem with drugs—such as statins—that have a high number needed to treat is that an individual patient is unlikely to receive any benefit from taking the drug. Indeed, the longer the patient takes the drug, the greater is their risk of side effects. There are further hidden problems with these drugs. A recent systematic review of EBM studies of statins concluded that "there was evidence of selective reporting of outcomes, failure to report adverse events and inclusion of people with cardiovascular disease. Only limited evidence showed that primary prevention with statins may be cost effective and improve patient quality of life."[317]

Large trials do have value in estimating safety. For example, if a drug kills an average of one person in 100 users, a small trial of 30 people would be unlikely to record a death. In a larger trial, say 1,000 patients, the expectation would be 10 deaths. So, large trials can help uncover relatively rare events. But remember that clinical trials are not as effective as case reports for determining rare side effects, as the sample size would need to be prohibitively large.

Using Stafford Beer's POSIWID heuristic (*the purpose of a system is what it does*), we can determine why clinical trials have increased in size, from about 30 to 3,000 patients, since the 1970s. We begin by estimating the number needed to treat (NNT) in a 1970s style study, with 30 subjects and 30 controls. To do this, we assume that 15 of the controls will improve naturally during the trial; these assumptions are not critical, we just need a control group for comparison. In order to reach standard significance, we need 5 extra treated patients to recover in our small trial. That means the NNT is about 6 and our drug would need to help about one patient in every 6 treated. Clearly, our 1970s drug does not need to be particularly effective to get a significant result in a small trial. However, in the corresponding EBM trial, with 3,000 subjects in each group, an average patient would receive a 1 in 67 chance of benefiting from the treatment! Applying Beer's POSIWID heuristic: the purpose of large trials is to promote ineffective treatments.

Accurate trials?

One of the reasons for large-scale trials is purported to be to make the results more accurate. However, this may not happen. To see why not, we need to understand the difference between two apparently similar concepts: accuracy and precision.

The term *accurate* applies to a measurement that is close to an objective or true result. If you take a number of measurements they might not be close to each other, but on average they indicate the true result. Weighing a person requires accurate scales that give the true reading. If a person is weighed every day, the reading may vary slightly but, on average, well-calibrated scales will give an accurate indication of the person's weight.

A *precise* result means that the measurements from a particular instrument are all very similar, though they may all be quite wrong. So each time you find a person's weight, the scales would give the same or a similar value; the measurement is reproducible. However, if someone has left a 30 lbs. weight on the other side of the scales, the results will still be as reproducible, though of course they will be biased. Although the person's real weight is 170 lbs., the scales report 140 lbs., with little variation. While we know of people who might find this particular deviation more than acceptable, it is a result of bias, rather than of diet.

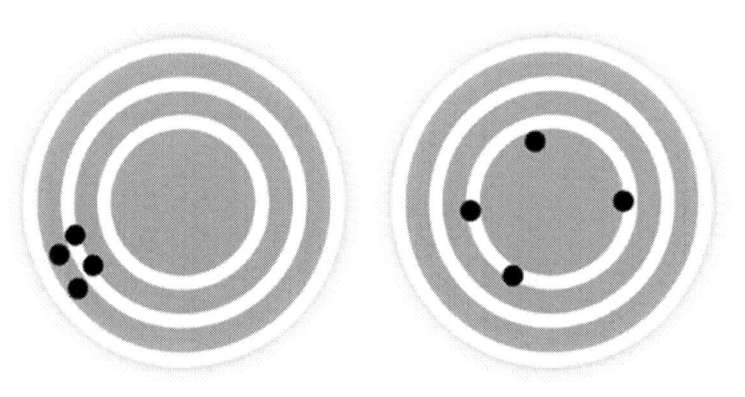

Precise not Accurate   Accurate not Precise

In the diagram of targets, one shows a result that is precise (all points close together near the outer edge of the target), the other a result that is more accurate, though less precise (points spread out, but surrounding the bull's eye).

Tarnished Gold

A large trial may be precise, without being accurate. The number of people investigated in large-scale studies is no indication of lack of bias. A huge study that used a biased questionnaire would give an inaccurate result. However, a series of small trials by independent researchers, using different methods, in diverse environments will average out such bias. Repeated small studies are less expensive to perform, robust, and generally more accurate.

No more breakthroughs?

The increasing size of clinical trials reflects a loss of confidence in medicine. It suggests that scientific breakthroughs are no longer sought. Consequently, researchers are not funded for the kind of work that might provide real help to patients. When patients are treated, they want a therapy to help them get well again. Perhaps a desperate or terminal patient might agree to an expensive or onerous treatment that offered only a small probability of saving his or her life. However, such patients would still expect scientists to be looking for cures or, at least, highly effective and safe treatments.

Although it may sound an outrageous suggestion, a scientist wanting to perform a trial on a possible cure for a serious condition is unlikely to be funded. Surely, you may think, many organizations are funding research designed to help patients, to extend their lives, and return them to health? Fundraising charities certainly make claims along these lines. Martin Bland, Professor of Health Statistics at the University of York, UK, and a member of many a grant-giving committee, describes the problem well, saying,

> funding committees often shake their heads over the implausibility of treatment changes reducing mortality by 50% or more.[311]

Bland's statement was intended to show that researchers were "widely optimistic" in their assessment of the possible benefit their treatment would produce. (We note however that this 50% reduction might be from just two deaths in a thousand to one.) The statement illustrates our point: a treatment that saved the lives of only half the patients was considered unrealistically hopeful! Modern medicine does not expect to find or even fund research into the possibility of treatments that might be of exceptional benefit to patients.

Consider an example from the history of medicine: Louis Pasteur and anthrax.[318,319] Pasteur had a little success with cholera vaccination, so, inspired by the germ theory of disease, he set about finding a vaccine for anthrax. Nowadays, anthrax is in the news because of its potential use in germ warfare. In Pasteur's day, anthrax was laying waste to the farming areas of France. Sheep were succumbing to the disease and fresh outbreaks were occurring in fields that had held infected sheep, even if they had been empty for months or years. After some work attenuating anthrax samples and using the results of Charles Chamberland, another French bacteriologist, Pasteur announced a trial.[320] Fifty sheep were separated into two groups of 25. He treated one group twice with the new vaccine, with 12 days between each dose. After two weeks, all the sheep were injected with anthrax. Pasteur publically announced that the vaccinated sheep would survive; this was either a brave or a foolhardy thing to do, as he could not be sure that the vaccine would work.

A couple of days later, a crowd gathered to see the results. Out of 25 vaccinated sheep, one pregnant ewe died, though the death was apparently unrelated to anthrax. The other 24 were healthy. All the controls were dead. The number needed to treat was one. This is what we might call a clear and definitive result: statistical analysis would have been spurious in this case.

We did a quick check of the expected risks to the sheep. Though this is hindsight and is not technically valid, we thought it might provide some insight. We can calculate the probability of an untreated sheep dying from anthrax. To keep things simple, we assumed that 24 out of 25 unvaccinated control sheep would die, so the risk of death is 96 out of 100. This is fewer than the observed number, but we are conservatively allowing for occasional survivors. The corresponding result with vaccinated sheep was 1 death from 25 vaccinated. It is exceedingly unlikely that Pasteur's result would occur by chance: if even 9 or more vaccinated sheep had lived, the probability would be less than a million to one against. The probability of 24 or more treated sheep living is astronomically small (about 7×10^{-33})—even less than the chance of throwing a fair coin and getting 99 heads in a row!

With such a low probability of occurring by chance, it is obvious that this was a major breakthrough. The only other explanation would be a major error in Pasteur's experiment, which could easily be checked by repeating it. At least for sheep, here was a clear demonstration that Pasteur's method worked. Pasteur's simple experiments did much to raise medicine from the scientific gutter of quackery.

The large-scale trials endorsed by EBM are only necessary if you no longer believe you can come up with a real benefit and so need to be able to detect small differences. So-called evidence-based medicine would find no place for a genius such as Pasteur. EBM's reliance on super-sensitive techniques implies that current researchers lack confidence and can only tinker around the edges of medical science.

Pasteur used simple experiments to search for major, obvious, solutions. EBM looks for minor incremental effects, using large-scale trials. Pasteur and colleagues were successful because of their genius in developing and testing simple cures. EBM replaces such progress with administrators and expensive mega-trials. Progress is correspondingly slow and incremental.

In recent history, there are many occasions where a simple treatment brought about a large benefit to the patient. These are the famous medical breakthroughs. The discovery of vitamins prevented fatal and incapacitating diseases, such as beriberi, pellagra, and scurvy. Insulin was found to be effective at preventing acute death and disability from diabetes mellitus. Penicillin and other antibiotics were similarly effective against bacterial infections, before their misuse promoted the growth of resistant strains. The connection between these breakthroughs is that they were discovered using small experiments, observation, and basic research.

Surprisingly, using the methods of EBM, researchers can offer a funding body results that are guaranteed, though almost certainly unimportant to patients. The use of language is telling: such larger studies are described as having greater "power".

Power studies and rigged results

Prévoir pour pouvoir. (Foreknowledge is power)

Auguste Comte

Suppose a drug company wanted a guaranteed significant result, to show the benefits of a new drug. Not only is this possible, it is easy—provided you have the time and resources to collect sufficient data. A statistical trick can more or less guarantee a positive result in a clinical trial.

The trick is to determine the experiment's power. The power tells the researcher how many subjects a trial will need, in order to show a significant difference. Determining a study's power allows the researcher to design a trial to ensure a significant result for even negligible drug benefits. The technique can also be used when the drug will help only a small proportion of patients. Calculating the power tells you how many people you need in a trial in order to achieve statistical significance. You can then design the experiment for a positive outcome and the significant result becomes likely; indeed, it is expected.

The question that the trial addresses is changed with a power calculation. Typically, power is used to increase the size of the study until it has an 80% chance of finding an effect significant. Usually, the difference is calculated from the p-value, i.e. significance level. Often the trial is no longer searching for a difference but validating a small treatment effect. Using a power calculation is the same as asking whether we can build a big enough trial to make a tiny effect look acceptable (significant). If you know before the experiment that you have an 80% chance of a significant result, the question arises: what does the reported p-value, of 95% or 99%, mean? Since the p-value has been used to determine the size of the trial, it is not an independent criterion but an expected outcome.

Perhaps there are not sufficient patients to give your study enough power to demonstrate your effect. In this case, you can use the "sample size samba".[321] You calculate the effect size you could find with this many subjects and use this figure as your target for prospective drugs. *Voilà*, your trial now has an acceptable power. Moreover, all is not lost if the drug cannot even meet this level of benefit. The next ploy is to combine the trial with others in a meta-analysis, to give the required significance. In the words of Dr Kenneth Schulz and Dr David Grimes, "All trials have an infinite number of powers, and low power is relative."

Often, power estimates are used to show that small studies are unable to detect small effects. *Underpowered* is a descriptive term for this, which delivers a derogatory emotional effect; we might compare the result to an underpowered car and think that this would not be a good thing for a clinical trial. In reality, EBM trials are *overpowered*: they find tiny effects of little relevance to a doctor treating a patient.

How might you use such techniques in practise? Let us imagine you have a drug that has only a small beneficial effect. To market the drug, you need to show a significant result from a clinical trial. To begin with, you run some animal experiments and a small clinical trial, which show that the drug gives about a 4% improvement in symptoms—the blood pressure might be slightly lower, for example. You can then use this information to calculate how large your study needs to be in order to get a significant result. A statistician can compute the expectations to give a required amount of confidence in the outcome.

Now, suppose you calculate that 200 subjects will give you the p-value you want. In this case, running the trial with 1,000 patients will give you an excellent chance that your clinical trial will be a success. However, if you are working for a rich drug company and want to make a marketing impression, you might use 10,000 subjects. An impressive and highly significant result is almost certain. Furthermore, replication will be expensive and time consuming, in case someone wishes to show the drug is ineffective. In other words, this is a statistical technique for rigging a trial to give the required results.

Surprisingly, some statisticians who support the rigging of clinical trials by calculating the power have suggested that 'underpowered' studies are unethical. They claim that studies where the power calculation is not used do not test the hypothesis and are "scientifically useless".[322] In the words of Douglas Altman,

> A study with an overlarge sample may be deemed unethical through the unnecessary involvement of extra subjects and the correspondingly increased costs. Such studies are probably rare.[323]

However, Altman's comment on rarity was made back in 1980, when studies were typically small and had not grown "unethically" large. Altman would thus have considered most of the modern EBM trials unethical.

Power analyses can be used in many ways. As we have suggested, a pharmaceutical company may view a clinical trial as a form of marketing.[324,325] It is an opportunity to publicise the efficacy of a drug and is a core element in promoting sales. There is nothing wrong with this, the company exists to maximize profits for its shareholders.[326] Drug and tobacco companies have a legal obligation to promote their products and their directors' primary duty is to benefit the company and its shareholders. If they do not put profits before patients, they are not doing their jobs properly. A successful clinical trial is a marketing opportunity, which explains why power calculations are so popular.

Let us see how this might work in practice. Earlier, we saw how large trials provide cover for useless drugs that work on few patients. In such cases, we are talking about a tiny average benefit. For this example, we performed a power calculation for some hypothetical medical trials, using an online calculator.[327] We also did similar calculations from first principles. Suppose that people with bronchitis are sick for an average of 5 days. People vary a little and the spread (standard deviation) of days ill fluctuates from 4 to 6 days. Now, our drug (Obecalpine) does not work particularly well, but we think it might reduce the days of sickness to 4.5 days. So, we asked how big would the trial need to be to show a significant result with a small benefit of around 12 hours shorter illness. For this slight benefit and a standard 1 in 20 probability ($p \leq 0.05$), we computed the power and found we would need a sample size of 22 patients in each group to demonstrate a significant result.

Twenty two patients? Is that all? So where, you may well ask, do the huge EBM-type studies come from? We repeated the calculation to see how many subjects we would need if the drug was even less effective and only reduced the period of illness by one hour. In other words, our patients are in bed for 4 days and 23 hours, instead of 5 days. We feel sure that most patients would prefer a more effective remedy. In this case, we would need a sample size of about 3,068 subjects. That is more the level we have come to expect from EBM's clinical trials.

Now, let us suppose Obecalpine is an altogether hopeless drug. Perhaps we can only expect a few minutes average reduction in illness. If we could get the patients out of bed 15 minutes earlier, we could get a significant result with a sample size of around 50,000. So, we need a very large scale trial for our drug—if we expect the patient to benefit to the extent of reducing 5 days sickness in bed to 4 days 23 hours and 45 minutes. This is evidence-based medicine!

To argue that small studies are underpowered is irrational. The power is the ability to detect an effect with a given statistical significance. However, if you need a large "powerful" study, the treatment is not effective!

One defence of the power study approach is that the effect being elucidated is real. In other words, the power provides an estimate of the validity of the observed drug effect. Moreover, the probability that is calculated in a power study still depends on the underlying reality. This defence is somewhat devious. The experimental question has been transformed and no longer asks whether we can find a cure or effective treatment. Instead, researchers are often asking questions of the form "How big a study is needed to give a significant result with our useless drug?" When they have selected the number of patients needed, there will be a high probability that the drug will give a statistically significant result. The game has changed and the experiment is rigged.

Real world critical appraisal

Earlier, we saw how EBM recommends doctors to appraise a clinical trial. Here we suggest a few alternative heuristics for this purpose.

- If the NNT (number needed to treat) is greater than 10, then the treatment will not help your patient. Patients generally expect more than a 1 in 10 chance that a drug will help them.
- The size of the benefit should be at least 20%. For example, patients are sick for at most 4 days instead of 5.
- The benefit should be a definitive direct measurement.

These requirements represent a minimum expectation from a patient's viewpoint. Most patients would hope for a treatment with a reasonable chance of helping them and for the benefit to be noticeable.

Large-scale confusion

> It is not necessary to change. Survival is not mandatory.
>
> William Deming

As supporters of EBM are disposed to claim, a p-value is not the probability that a result is right or wrong. Nor is it a measure of the clinical significance of the results. The p-value is the probability that a particular result would be expected by chance alone with *that particular sample size!* However, if they have used information from a previous experiment to obtain this result, the significance is misleading. There is a difference between an experiment searching for an effective treatment or cure, and one designed to confirm earlier data with a significant result.

As we saw in the Monty Hall game, information or prior knowledge can change the outcome. Probability is a measure of our uncertainty or lack of knowledge. Calculating the power reduces the uncertainty in the experiment as a whole. In a circular argument, the earlier results are used to control the outcome of the new study. Calculating the power can breach Feynman's Conjecture that, "it doesn't make any sense to calculate [probabilities] after the event",[328] and introduce hindsight bias.[329] Calculating the power changes the question.

Experimenters can remove uncertainty and rig their clinical trials. There is nothing intrinsically wrong with this approach, provided the nature of the experiment is made clear. Large-scale EBM studies might carry a disclaimer, such as

> This study demonstrates that even a miniscule effect can be made significant and the result may have little or no clinical importance.

EBM's trials differ qualitatively from traditional medical research. They address questions unrelated to the treatment of patients. Indeed, did its practitioners but know it, large-scale clinical trials are EBM's declaration of failure.

Main Points

- Large-scale, randomized, placebo-controlled trials are not a gold standard.
- Megatrials provide weak evidence of small effects.
- Power calculations yield over-determined trials.
- Power studies make ineffective drugs appear significant.
- EBM's "proven" treatments rarely benefit patients.
- Numerous small trials can be performed for less cost than a single EBM trial.
- Simple small clinical trials find useful effects.

> If you want a guarantee, buy a toaster.
>
> Clint Eastwood

Beyond Right and Wrong

This isn't right. This isn't even wrong.

Wolfgang Pauli

From its inception, EBM has had its own built-in gremlin, which renders it ineffective. Here we return to the idea of information overload and a phenomenon called the *curse of dimensionality*—a problem that decision scientists often encounter. EBM's approach invokes this curse because it consistently introduces multiple risk factors.

The large-scale studies favoured by EBM generate numerous risk factors. Diseases are described as being *multifactorial*, which means they depend on many environmental, biological, and genetic factors. For example, the causes of heart disease supposedly include risk factors such as saturated fat in the diet, high cholesterol, trans fats, stress, homocysteine, gingivitis, obesity, lack of exercise, high blood pressure, faulty genes, multiple environmental influences, and so on. Since the disease depends on so many different things, it is difficult to suggest an effective form of prevention or treatment. Under EBM, disease is complicated and needs multifaceted solutions.

We have seen that EBM's requirement for complicated explanations breaks the principle of Occam's razor, which favours simple solutions. However, simplicity was not the original aim of Occam's heuristic: there is another way of interpreting the principle of parsimony. Occam suggested "entities must not be multiplied beyond necessity" and modern science is built upon this idea. Isaac Newton explained "we are to admit no more causes of natural things than such as are both true and sufficient to explain their appearances." This means that you should not have more than the minimum number of factors required to explain the disease. A scientist should value a single cause explanation more highly than one that depends on multiple factors.

Finding simple but appropriate models is difficult and has been the aim of centuries of science. By contrast, the process used by practitioners of EBM to generate a new risk factor is straightforward and has launched many a promising career. EBM has steered medicine away from its traditional search for direct explanations. As a result, it consistently fails to find the causes of disease and any associated cures become lost in its confusion of risk factors. The true cause for a disease, such as heart attack, could be a simple and tractable nutritional deficiency that is hidden by EBM's methods.

Multiple risk factors

> To assign what purports to be precise values to such essentially vague quantities is neither useful nor honest. Any pretence of applying formulae to these loosely defined quantities is a sham and a waste of time.
>
> Norbert Wiener

EBM's multifactorial explanations are often difficult to refute and have a low predictive value. Commercially, however, the use of multifactorial risk factors helps corporate medicine maintain a conveniently high level of uncertainty. Tobacco companies led the way. Experts for the companies, collectively known as *Big Tobacco*, avoided admitting that smoking causes lung cancer or heart disease. When asked, they reframed their response from *cause* to *risk factors*.[330] An example of this expert testimony is as follows:

Ms. Sherman: Do you believe that active smoking causes lung cancer?

Dr Raphael Witorsch: I'm going to give you a response that you're not going to be satisfied with because it's going to go back to the old multifactorial.

Judge Vittone: Just give the response, doctor.

Dr Witorsch: Okay. I believe that it is a risk factor for lung cancer.

Ms Sherman: As I said to Dr. LeVois, is this a semantic problem between a layman and a scientist?

Dr Witorsch: No.

In this exchange, Dr Witorsch was giving an accurate and honest response, which conforms to the scientific approach that would later become known as EBM. The problem here is not with the expert, who was providing a partial interpretation of the data, but with the methodology used. EBM grew as a response to the legal requirements for "scientific proof", such as attributing the blame for lung cancer to smoking. In the context of protecting tobacco companies from the lawsuits of dying patients and their relatives, multi-factorial risk factors were just what the doctor ordered.

The EBM explanation for, say, heart disease, is a system of connected risk-factors. There is no real mechanism or explanation, just a bad statistical model. Such a system is irrefutable: almost any experimental result can be incorporated, because the explanation adapts to changing experimental data.

Suppose a study shows that women aged 53 with low cholesterol get heart attacks with alarming frequency; this finding can be accommodated by appealing to one or more of the other variables, so it does not refute the multiple risk factor "explanation". The relationships between the risk factors can be modified slightly, so the system adjusts to the anomalous result. Researchers might claim that women of this age tend to have hormone changes, which can outweigh the effects of low cholesterol. Essentially, there are so many connected factors that a stable state can be found to explain almost any set of clinical trial results. The danger of trying to use an *adaptive system* of correlated risk factors as a theory is that it can "explain" almost anything.

Because the risk factor explanation for heart disease is so broad, the same list could be applied to other diseases, such as schizophrenia. Patients with mental illness may tend to have problems with dental health and gingivitis.[331] Cholesterol may be raised in schizophrenia, as may leptin, a hormone involved in the control of body weight.[332] The mentally ill tend to be obese.[333] Schizophrenics tend to smoke[334] and have raised homocysteine levels.[335] In short, cardiovascular risk-factors are also associated with schizophrenia.[336]

In defence of EBM, its proponents may counter that poor mental health is a risk factor for cardiovascular disease. The evidence suggests that depression, anxiety disorders, bipolar disorder, and schizophrenia are important cardiac risk factors; patients with these illnesses are at higher risk for cardiac disease than the normal population.[337] Of course, this misses the point entirely. We selected schizophrenia as an essentially unrelated condition, to illustrate the weakness of such explanations. We could have chosen any of a number of chronic diseases that share risk factors with heart disease.

A curse on medicine?

EBM researchers apparently think that additional risk factors will result in better explanations. However, increasing the number of risk factors in an explanation is different from increasing the number of measurements of a single parameter. Far from enhancing the precision of the result, excessive risk factors are associated with increased levels of error. The *curse of dimensionality* implies that explanations that rely on multiple risk factors will be overwhelmed by associated errors, to the extent that the explanation rapidly becomes meaningless.

An EBM clinical trial might involve a 90-question survey, together with multiple clinical measurements. Each examination might measure blood pressure, blood-clotting time, the patient's weight, and so on. If a trial lasts five years and costs millions, it makes sense to extract every bit of information. So, measuring more parameters might seem an excellent and prudent idea. It is not. The large number of parameters will guarantee that the study fails to throw genuine light on the problem.

When you add extra factors, there is a high probability that they will be correlated with each other. For example, if the first factor is height and the second is weight, these are likely to be connected, as taller people will tend to be heavier. This means that two factors do not provide twice the information of one; similarly, four factors do not provide twice the information of two, and so on. The more parameters you add, the more likely it is that you are replicating information already represented by earlier factors.

On the other hand, every factor you add has an associated error. If you are measuring height, then your measurement will be plus or minus so many inches, and if you are measuring temperature, it will be plus or minus so many degrees. These errors are random and independent: length and temperature errors are nothing to do with each other. You cannot compare apples with oranges, as the saying goes.

This problem gets worse as the number of factors gets higher: the errors keep increasing, whereas the added information fades to nothing. (For the mathematically inclined, note that the hypervolume of the decision space increases exponentially with the number of parameters.) If you don't follow this, it doesn't really matter; all you need to know is that the more factors you include in a study, the more likely it is that experimental errors will lead you to a false or misleading result.

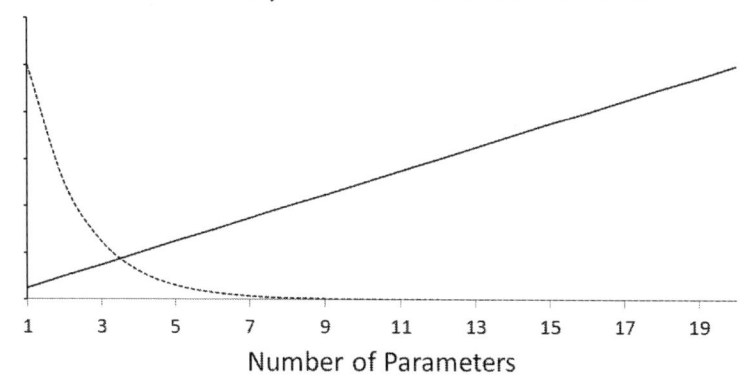

How Multiple Risk Factors Add Error

Number of Parameters

The result of using multiple risk factors in the real world is illustrated. The added information (dotted line) rapidly dies away as the number of risk factors increase. The error (solid line) accumulates with each additional factor.

The curse implies a Goldilocks requirement for successful trials: the number of factors must be "just right". As we increase the number of parameters used, we reach the point where we have captured all the information we can find. At this point, we have achieved our maximum prediction accuracy. Beyond this, each new parameter cannot increase the amount of information; we have already captured all that is available. However, each new parameter contains errors or random noise.[338]

Now, you might think that perhaps a super-computer would be able to make sense of all the extra information. Not so! There are mathematical tricks to help overcome the problem but it is not possible to separate the real information from the error. This random noise is independent and indistinguishable from useful data. The noise simply swamps the useful information and the accuracy of prediction falls.[339] This is yet another reason for the failure of EBM.

Cursed!

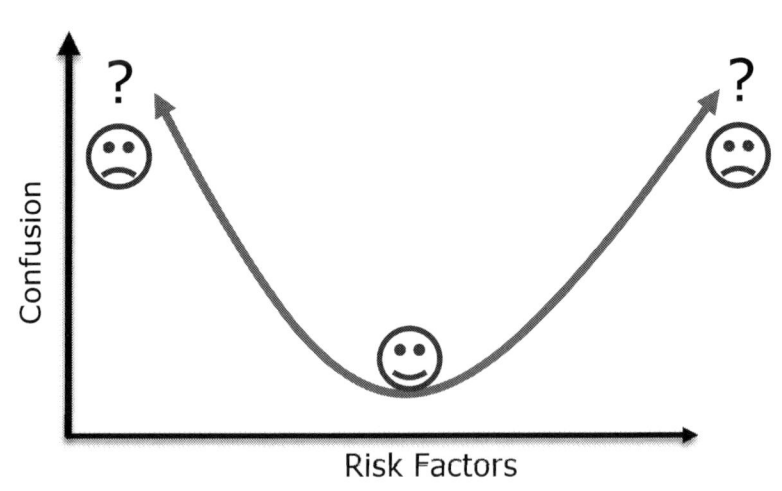

Graph showing Confusion (y-axis) vs Risk Factors (x-axis) as a U-shaped curve, with sad faces with question marks at both ends and a smiley face at the bottom.

In this diagram, a person starts out on the left with only one risk factor and very little information; he has no idea what is going on. As he gathers more risk factors, he begins to understand. However, beyond a certain point, the curse of dimensionality kicks in and he is overwhelmed by errors!

Dimensionality

The use of many different parameters is different from repeating the same measurement. By repeating measurements, we can increase the precision of our result. However, if we increase the number of parameters, or risk factors, we swamp our useful information with noise. The property known as *dimensionality* refers to the number of independent parameters used to describe a problem. When you ask many different questions, you cannot take an average. There is no sensible average of a person's hair colour, foot length, religious belief, and number of teeth, for example. Each parameter asks a different question of the data, and each represents a different dimension.

So, if you ask 100 questions, you have a potential dimensionality of 100. However, because of overlap between the questions, the actual dimensionality is likely to be much smaller. Remember 20Q or the doctor asking questions in order to reach a diagnosis: with a million illnesses, 20 yes-no questions were enough to specify each disease. This smaller number, 20, is the real or intrinsic dimensionality of the million-disease diagnosis problem. Any additional questions (the other 80 in this case) do not add information, just noise.

The *intrinsic dimensionality* is the minimum number of parameters (or risk factors) you need to specify the data and to solve the problem at hand. For an accurate diagnosis of over a million diseases, a brilliant doctor needs only to ask 20 questions at most—provided they are the right ones. However, a less experienced doctor could ask questions all day without reaching the correct answer: thousands of queries and medical tests, nearly all of them irrelevant, redundant, or otherwise unnecessary. These additional questions confuse the issue, making it harder to identify the illness.

Dimensionality in practice

One of the authors (SH) has investigated numerous pattern recognition problems, in fields as diverse as medical imaging, industrial machine vision, security applications, robot control, business applications, stock market prediction, and others. Experts in each of these applications could list hundreds of parameters that might affect the decision they were trying to make. Frequently, they would present so many that it was extremely confusing. Furthermore, they had no idea what form the solution would take. In every case, the first step was to estimate their problem's true dimensionality.[340,341]

Often, the problem seemed difficult and intractable. However, in each application we found something quite interesting: even the most apparently difficult question depended on just a few variables. We never came across a problem that was not adequately represented by a handful of parameters; a typical solution required perhaps three to five. This means the intrinsic dimensionality of these practical problems was quite low. The problems included several medical applications, particularly different forms of imaging. The solutions were generally far less complex than the experts had imagined.

Intrinsic dimensionality is related to requisite variety. We need a minimum amount of information to solve a problem. Since we have established that every good solution is a model of the problem it needs to solve,[44] our solution needs requisite variety—which means enough information—but it should not have too much.

From Ashby's law, we know that asking too few questions in a diagnostic interview will leave confusion between certain diseases. Likewise, the curse of dimensionality states if we ask too many irrelevant questions, we will become confused and not get an accurate diagnosis. In the large clinical trials favoured by EBM, researchers do not know what the important questions are. The tendency is therefore to make as many measurements as is practical, thus inviting the curse of dimensionality to ruin the study.

Risk factors can guarantee a successful trial

One of the tricks used to ensure a statistically significant trial also makes the results untrustworthy. The trick is to measure more risk factors and outcomes. Here, a risk factor is a possible "cause" while an outcome is a result. The more outcomes you measure, the more thorough the study will appear. You will not be wasting scarce research funds on a massive study of a single outcome. This approach can guarantee the trial's success and produce significant positive results for the drug, if not for the patients.

In other words, to ensure an EBM study is well rewarded, it is important to measure lots of risk factors and outcomes. One study reported over 20 outcomes from an average trial, and 10,557 outcomes in 519 trials.[342] One reason for the popularity of multiple outcomes is that they can be sure to provide statistically significant results.[343,344] In any study, significant differences can just happen by chance. If 20 outcomes are collected in an experiment, there is a high chance (about 64%) that one or more will be found to be a significant but misleading result. This means that two out of every three of these trials can be expected to give at least one significant result by chance alone. The result will be unreliable, but may help progress the researcher's career. As well as providing randomly significant results, multiple outcomes make the study appear larger and more thorough, conferring even greater kudos.

Almost any measurement made on two randomly selected groups will show a difference. The average age, height, blood pressure, and blood cholesterol levels in any two random groups are not likely to be identical. A researcher wanting to show that a new drug is beneficial in preventing migraine may make multiple measurements.

Instead of choosing just one measure, the trial includes many: the number of headache free days each month, the level of nausea, number of days off work, the duration of an attack, the number of attacks, intensity of pain, and so on. Many such factors can be included in a simple questionnaire. It is easy to ask a large number of questions in a survey; it might even be expected. The researcher knows that if you make 100 measurements on the two groups, about five will give a significant result by chance. So, by asking 100 questions, researchers can expect to have five significant results for their research paper—and significant results are more likely to be published.

A new dodge

Increasing the number of outcomes in a trial may make it easy to get a significant result but there are several more tricks that can help ensure an apparently successful clinical trial. Even if a clinical trial produced no significant results, all is not lost; there are ways to get the all-important statistical significance. One technique is to split the groups and run the tests again. For example, if you find no publishable result, split your subjects into age groups and retest. Each test gives you another dip in the lucky bag and the chance of an apparently significant result. The drug might appear to be effective in adults between 60 and 70 years, by chance alone. Problem solved. The paper will be published with an unfortunate and misleading result, but the drug has been "proven" to be beneficial using a large-scale clinical trial, and the research funds may continue to flow your way. Unfortunately, such chicanery and the random effects of chance mean that the statistical significance in many published medical papers is often meaningless.

To find EBM-acceptable results, split the patients into lots of different groups, keep doing statistical tests, and you will be practically assured of significance. This process is called *subgroup analysis*. Obviously, with all these tests, there will be many negative or non-significant results. These are easily hidden, as selective reporting of results in EBM clinical trials is commonplace.[345,346] Study outcomes are often omitted, changed, or added.[347] Indeed, significant results from a clinical trial may simply reflect biased selection.

Typically, only the researcher knows how many statistical tests were done and this is not disclosed in the publication. However, this dodge is well known and it is possible that questions could be asked. To avoid such questions, another dodge can ensure a trial is successful, while using only a single statistical test.

The trick is to combine test results into a single *composite endpoint*. Instead of individually testing, say, a reduction in blood pressure, an improvement in sleep, and a reduction in pain, researchers combine them into a single parameter. This could be done by applying an equation to the results before they are tested. The outcome measure might be a logical combination, such as *a reduction in blood pressure* OR *more sleep* OR *less pain*. If a patient has any one or more of the three measures, this combination will get a positive result. Combining measures makes it easy to show that a drug has a beneficial effect. There is no restriction on the ways they can be combined: any algorithm is apparently acceptable. This means that with a little ingenuity, almost any drug trial could be presented as a glowing success.

The main advantages of using a composite endpoint are that statistical precision and efficiency will be increased.[348] The trial can be smaller and cost less, thus new treatments will get to market earlier. There are some awkward restrictions, however; for example, researchers might be required to decide on the way they are going to combine the measures *before they conduct the experiment*. Despite this, given earlier data, it is relatively straightforward to find a method that will help make any differences more significant. Also, having a composite end-point does not mean that the researchers cannot also test each of the parameters individually; they just need to explain why the significant factors are individually important.[349]

The idea that you can combine your results in an arbitrary algorithm, which will make it easier to get a significant result, is worrying. Indeed, if EBM trials were more rational, it would be a major concern—but this is just one more deficit. Dr James Prenton, Consultant Physician and Gastroenterologist at Scunthorpe General Hospital, England, has made the case against composite endpoints rather clearly:

> Composite end-points are a recipe for confusion and a source of misleading information. If the outcomes which seriously affect the lives of patients occur so infrequently that they are not sufficient to yield a statistically significant

difference, then this says a great deal about current medical research and, in particular, about large-scale randomized trials.[350]

Most clinical trials are wrong

At this point, we will let the reader into a not very well kept secret: the insiders know that EBM is a failure. Most published studies in EBM are wrong.

John Ioannides, Director of the Stanford Prevention Research Center and an international expert on medical study design, has provided a simple demonstration that the results of most clinical trials are false.[344] In EBM, it is more likely for a research claim to be false than true. Rather than being controversial, this challenge seems to be accepted. Once again, Bayesian statistics have been offered as a correction for the problem.[351] However, there are further issues. Initial reports of a drug's effects are often inflated.[352] This means the drug is reported to be more effective than later studies suggest (a form of regression to the mean). One in seven highly cited studies was contradicted by later investigations.[353]

Where there is a risk of bias, the chance of a misleading clinical trial is also high. In EBM trials, bias is the rule: it is predictable and there are numerous sources. Bias occurs when there is obvious manipulation, such as designing an experiment to have the power to show a required result. Then again, an experiment can be constructed to lose an important effect, such as a study of nutrition that uses inappropriate synthetic vitamins at inadequate doses.[354] Alternatively, the person doing the analysis knows which patients had the placebo and which had the treatment, allowing another possible source of bias.

Benjamin Djulbegovic and Iztok Hozo have tried to solve this problem within EBM.[355] Their approach is a form of cost-benefit analysis. They aim to determine something called the *acceptable regret*. Retrospectively, we find out if a medical decision was right or wrong. When it is wrong, it produces regret. If we had known earlier that the treatment had a terrible side effect, we might not have used it. Acceptable regret occurs when people would find the damage from a mistaken decision tolerable.[356]

In avoiding regret and justifying EBM, Djulbegovic and Hozo asked: "When should potentially false research findings become acceptable to society?"[355] Since any research finding is potentially false, the question is a little odd. Even odder is the idea of acceptability to society. Here we may take the word society to mean government, commercial medicine, or a large population. In the case of a patient, the primary question is what treatment is likely to be most effective for that particular person. It is the individual patient, their relatives and loved ones who will suffer the regret.

The realization that most clinical trial results are misleading will come as little surprise to doctors. The media is full of contradictory health claims, which are gradually bringing modern medical science into disrepute. As a result, some people are starting to view EBM as a joke. Hugh Davies compiled a list on Facebook of the "things that give you cancer".[357] These were risk factors that had been published by *The Daily Mail*, a national newspaper in the UK. Typically, such articles report recent "breakthroughs" in EBM, described for a popular audience. The A-to-Z of factors started with "age" and ran through "candlelit dinners", "gardens", and "water", concluding at "x-rays". There were twenty-eight factors beginning with the letter *C*—definitely a letter to be avoided! Couples might be hard-pressed to avoid these risks as, for example, "sex", "children", and "childlessness" were all causes of cancer. Even reading the article might cause you cancer, as using Facebook was on the list!

A second list was created on Facebook, which was even more amusing.[358] Many of the entries in this list had two links. The first to the *Daily Mail* article saying that the factor causes cancer and the second to a report in the same paper claiming it prevents it. So, for example, having a pet dog would both cause cancer ("a 29-fold increase"[359]) and lower the risk of lymphoma by a third.[360] Technically, both these statements could be accurate, but to the typical reader they are simply confusing.

EBM is bringing science into disrepute. Its methods are so questionable that it can be held up to public ridicule, while corporate medicine regards it with a level of zeal normally reserved for religions. Despite the EBM gold standard claims for randomised clinical trials, they are often wrong,[344] and the results often fail to be replicated,[361,362] clear signs of cargo-cult science.

Bad genes or bad science?

Medical researchers often ask us to believe that advances in genetics will soon overcome human disease.[363] The media carries frequent articles about scientists finding the gene for a particular disease, along with claims that this will lead to a cure. However, while the hype follows the medical literature, almost all of these claims are overblown, and many are simply wrong. There is no gene for cancer, for example.

Dr James Le Fanu, family doctor and well-known UK journalist, has suggested that the lack of progress in medicine over the last half century is a direct result of the use of "evidence-based" social and genetic medicine.[249] Despite the EBM hype, medical progress in preventing and treating illness has slowed in recent years.

In medical genetics, most publications are misleading. According to one report, five out of seven of the largest studies linking genes to cancer, over the period 1995 to 2003, did not perform better than chance; in other words, the genes supposedly linked to the disease could have been chosen randomly.[364] One paper reviewing this data described the remaining two studies, saying that they "barely beat horoscopes."[365] This comment might be amusing, except when we realise that the millions of dollars expended could have been used for real cancer research.

There are multiple possible associations between genes and diseases. Humans have about 25,000 individual genes. When a researcher searches for a link between a gene and a disease, sheer chance will produce many apparently significant associations. When a study linking a gene with an illness is repeated, the association may disappear.[366]

Such studies overestimate the genetic connection. Mostly, errors are caused by a failure to understand that results arose simply by chance or by selective misreporting in the literature.[367] While some of the disease-gene claims may be true,[343] replication of studies is essential for validation. Even if scientists confirm the claimed associations, discovering that a gene is associated with a disease is some way from finding an effective treatment.

Placebo control—weak and unethical

We are now in a position to take a critical look at the issue of placebo control. The technique is not foolproof; people in drug trials may guess whether they have received a drug or a dummy pill and, if their guesses are accurate, become unblinded. Drugs often have clear side effects, which inform the subject that they are not receiving the placebo.

Subjective results, such as perception of pain, are vulnerable to the placebo effect. Even the effects of opiate analgesics are influenced by a patient's expectation.[368] A drug's painkilling effect might be doubled if the patient has confidence in it, or it might be abolished completely if the patient has serious doubts. Such results are associated with physiological changes in the brain's response.

Many doctors believe strongly in the power of placebo effects, although this modern medical myth is not strongly supported by experimental results.[369,370] In fact, the lack of efficacy should have been obvious to all. However much a patient believes it, there is little evidence that a placebo or sugar pill will cause a definitive response. An example of a definitive response might be death—and we prefer to avoid an association between placebo and voodoo. Generally, the placebo effect is limited to conditions that have a psychological component. This conclusion is a direct consequence of the definition of a placebo as an *inert substance that has no pharmacological effect*.

Despite this, placebo control has been accorded almost mythical importance in medical experimentation. We recently had cause to explain that selection of studies for a meta-analysis based on having placebo controls was inappropriate. Goran Bjelakovic and others made a highly publicized claim, that antioxidant vitamins increase the risk of death.[371] A Bayesian scientist might explain that this conclusion is unlikely to be correct, as there is pre-existing data on the safety and benefits of antioxidants. However, we will ignore the context of the claim and concentrate on the researchers' choice of lack of placebo as a selection factor to reject studies.

The Bjelakovic study was a Cochrane "gold standard" review of the effect of vitamins on death from heart disease. We pointed out in a series of critical objections that a placebo could not cause or prevent death, and thus its use as a condition for selecting the studies was inappropriate.[372,373] The response of the authors was strange and attributed the placebo process with an increased range of magical properties:

> Placebo is not given to cause or prevent death. Placebo is given to blind participants, investigators, and assessors to avoid reporting bias, collateral intrusion bias, and outcome assessment bias.

Placebo controls do blind participants and experimenters so they do not know who is getting the treatment—but this is a moot point, if such knowledge will have no effect on the experimental outcome! Furthermore, contrary to suggestions by Bjelakovic and colleagues, placebo controls do not enable investigators to avoid bias in their reporting. Neither do they prevent intrusion of bias accompanying the treatment. The placebo also does not prevent biased analysis, or misreading and misrepresentation of the results. Studies of the placebo effect have shown that it does not have magical properties; we must therefore attribute the authors' response to wishful thinking.

The report's authors also suggested we re-read the papers on the placebo effect, which we did. The Cochrane Review of the placebo effect concludes the following:

> Placebo interventions are often claimed to improve patient-reported and observer-reported outcomes, but this belief is not based on evidence from randomized trials that compare placebo with no treatment.

and

> There was no evidence that placebo interventions in general have clinically important effects. A possible moderate effect on subjective continuous outcomes, especially pain, could not be clearly distinguished from bias.[374]

It would seem difficult to misread these statements. Life or death is a definitive outcome, to which the placebo effect does not apply. We are left to speculate as to why the Cochrane review authors insisted on placebo controls in a study of mortality, since the exclusion introduced bias into their results.

Eventually, such errors will be corrected in the independent medical literature. In this case, two German scientists, Joachim Gerss and Wolfgang Köpcke, described the suggestion of harm in the Cochrane review title as "questionable" and "inconsistent."[375] They stated that the result "can be explained by a higher proportion of male patients that were included in these trials compared to other trials" and that "none of these results can be regarded to supply evidence in a statistical sense." In the polite terms of scientific discourse, this amounts to a total rejection.

As well as being inappropriate, placebo-controlled trials can be unethical, as they rely on keeping patients in the dark as to whether or not they are receiving a genuine treatment. The Helsinki Declaration is the World Medical Association's international standard of medical ethics.[376,377] Rule 32 of the 2008 declaration is explicit:

> The benefits, risks, burdens and effectiveness of a new intervention must be tested against those of the best current proven intervention, except in the following circumstances:
> - The use of placebo, or no treatment, is acceptable in studies where no current proven intervention exists; or
> - Where for compelling and scientifically sound methodological reasons the use of placebo is necessary to determine the efficacy or safety of an intervention and the patients who receive placebo or no treatment will not be subject to any risk of serious or irreversible harm. Extreme care must be taken to avoid abuse of this option.

This means that the majority of EBM placebo-controlled drug trials are unethical. Clinical trials should compare new treatments with the most effective methods available. The use of placebos should be reserved for studies where there are no effective or current treatments. Unfortunately, drug companies using EBM methods often compare their new drug with a sham treatment. Even then, they frequently struggle to show that their new treatments outperform the placebo, despite their mechanisms for favouring the drug.

A rational patient would surely expect that a new drug would outperform an existing drug; ideally, it should be better than the best, as suggested by the Helsinki Declaration. It should give greater clinical benefit, have fewer side-effects, or, at least, cost less. However, the drug's side effects will not be established until it has been on the market for some time. So, a patient taking the latest drug is risking unknown side-effects, while paying for the opportunity to be a Guinea pig.

According to EBM, a new drug merely needs to be better than no treatment at all. This means the new drug may be less effective than existing treatments, although typically it will be more expensive. This brings us back to economics and Gresham's law. In economics, this is usually stated as "bad money drives out good money."[378] Corporate medicine has an equivalent mechanism, suggesting an analogous heuristic "bad new drugs drive out good old drugs." Introducing and marketing a new drug involves competing with existing treatments. Newer drugs are "proven", modern, and more profitable. They replace old treatments, but may be less effective. Ironically, use of placebo-controlled trials may mean medicine becomes less beneficial to patients.

Sadly, we are forced to conclude that the reason new drugs are tested against placebo is that they are not competitive with existing treatments. As suggested by the Helsinki Declaration, this is where medical ethics should come to the defence of patients and outlaw placebo-controlled drug trials.

Regulatory capture

In 2006, the US Food and Drug Administration (FDA) planned to eliminate any reference to the Helsinki Declaration.[379] The FDA objected that conforming to the suggested ethics would affect drug trials and make it difficult for pharmaceutical companies to introduce new products! Clearly, this objection would only apply to those products that were inferior to current treatments: improved drugs would still be approved. We might wonder why the FDA apparently wants to encourage the introduction of substandard treatments.

The answer could lie in a phenomenon known as *regulatory capture*, which happens when regulatory agencies become dominated by the industries they were intended to control. George Stigler, a Nobel Prize winning economist, described regulatory capture. Stigler explained how government agencies, formed to look after the interests of the general public, often end up supporting commercial interests.[380] This phenomenon is not restricted to medicine but is a troubling aspect of human society in general.

Deep capture describes how large corporate interests have a disproportionate ability to control and manipulate our exterior and interior situations.[381] Corporate medicine has taken regulatory capture to absurd limits. Large companies have unduly influenced the whole of medicine, from international bodies such as the World Health Organization, through government institutions like the FDA, down to the level of the individual doctor writing a prescription.

The FDA is the agency that regulates food and pharmaceuticals in the United States, supposedly for the benefit of the people and their wellbeing. Despite this, the FDA is often perceived as a defender of the pharmaceutical industry.[382] On closer inspection, we find that the FDA is funded by the industry it regulates; in 2002, it received about $300,000 in fees for each new drug approved.[383] The current application fee for a new drug is $1,542,000 if it includes

241

clinical data.[384] There is a clear conflict of interest: the more drugs the FDA approves, the more money it gets (and the better paid and more secure are its employees). Patients can suffer serious drug side effects as a result.[385]

Wasting resources

The resources spent on just one large EBM clinical trial could give a major boost to scientific medicine. The costs of clinical trials vary but are increasing.[386] A recent estimate was from $22,000 for a phase one exploratory trial to $48,000 for a phase three treatment trial.[387,388] However, these figures are *per subject,* not the whole experiment! A phase three trial of 1,000 patients could cost about $50 million. Let us assume a modest EBM clinical trial, costing nine million dollars and extending over three years. The outcomes are some vague and unreliable results on, say, the action of a single form of statin drug in coronary heart disease.

The money for this single EBM clinical trial would be enough to fund 100 PhD research students for three years at $90,000 each. One biochemistry student might be set to study the physiology of atherosclerosis and associated heart attack. A mathematics student could relate stress in the arteries to the distribution of atherosclerotic plaques. A computer science student might generate a database of patients with heart disease and matched controls from patient records. He might then use data mining techniques to check existing hypotheses about heart attack causation. A biophysicist might consider the role of antioxidants in plaque formation.

Our hypothetical research students produce 100 direct scientific studies, each addressing a particular question. Each student would aim for a minor breakthrough in understanding. Perhaps 300 research papers could be generated, with the potential for novel ideas or beneficial results. At the end of the period, the country potentially has 100 new PhDs in a range of disciplines, to provide a boost to research, development, and the future economy.

Theology and science

Clinical trials are not new: there is even a report in the Bible.[389] In the Old Testament, Daniel performs a trial with the aim of showing that a King was wrong to insist that only a meat and wine diet would make people strong. Using two groups, Daniel compared a vegetarian diet with the King's preferred fare.[390] Daniel's people were given vegetarian meals for 10 days, and compared to controls from the King's family, who ate meat and wine. The visitors apparently thrived on the vegetarian diet, appearing "fairer and fatter in flesh than all the children which did eat the portion of the King's meat." Although the experimental group was self-selected and controls were not chosen at random, the results refuted the King's hypothesis.

Despite this promising biblical start, clinical trials remain unsatisfactory. EBM's clinical trials are an imperfect medical test of limited value. Supporters of EBM might claim that their clinical trials are not perfect but that even a tarnished gold standard can, with effort, be polished to a shine. Unfortunately, EBM's clinical trials do not provide sufficient information content to address a patient's needs. Improved methods are possible: earlier, we described a simple Bayesian trial that a family doctor could perform. This direct approach avoids most of the issues plaguing EBM.

Main Points

- EBM's placebo-controlled drug trials are unethical.
- Multiple risk factors and outcomes ensure useless results.
- Multiple tests ensure significance.
- An EBM significant result often means almost nothing.
- Most EBM trial results are wrong.

A fool must now and then be right, by chance.

William Cowper

Meta-analysis as Pseudoscience

> Any system that achieves appropriate selection (to a degree better than chance) does so as a consequence of information received.
>
> W. Ross Ashby

Meta-analysis has been hailed as the ultimate gold standard of EBM. As we look more closely at meta-analysis, the real role of *best evidence* becomes apparent. *Best* really means *selected* information. EBM claims to select high quality studies based on perceived value. Unfortunately, high quality data can simply mean information that is both useful for corporate medicine and consistent with the needs of EBM. Strangely, it excludes solid data, while unpublished results may be included on a whim. In the following chapter, we demonstrate that, if its best evidence is meta-analysis,[49] EBM is an exercise in absurdity.

Not everyone agrees with us on this. Indeed, one UK broadcaster and medical doctor, Ben Goldacre, selected meta-analysis as his *Moment of Genius*, for the BBC radio programme of the same name. The programme asks contributors to describe what they consider the greatest turning points in the history of science. According to Goldacre, systematic review "saved more lives than you could possibly imagine." Goldacre could have chosen any of the great discoveries from medicine or science, but he chose systematic reviews.

Goldacre claims that systematic review, i.e. meta-analysis, removes the chance of people trawling the literature in search of papers to support their ideas and then ignoring any that go the other way. For example, by selecting positive studies and ignoring negative results, a reviewer could make even a poor treatment look good. By contrast, with a meta-analysis, apparently, you measure methodically *without looking at the results*. Goldacre seems to believe that meta-analysis is a great triumph of scientific rigor. Normally, we would ignore such a lapse in judgment by someone who is not a scientist. However, as a leading sceptic, Goldacre has made a reputation by criticizing others for far less trusting beliefs, such as the benefits of nutrition. Here we will explain how meta-analysis fails; read the details and decide for yourself.

The need for reviews

Sometimes, clinical trials give conflicting results. Suppose twelve trials have been conducted; perhaps eight have given positive results, two were negative, and the final two were inconclusive. One way round this is to combine the results into a meta-analysis or systematic review—a single statistical study incorporating all twelve trials. The claimed advantage is that the number of subjects is larger, which increases the power of the result. When a number of large-scale clinical trials are available, the effective sample size in a meta-analysis can be vast.

Typically, randomized placebo-controlled trials are selected for the analysis, although additional evidence is often included. The criteria for inclusion may be specified in advance but is often ignored. Superficially, meta-analysis allows an ultimate decision to be made using the available medical data. The critical failure relates to data selection. To quote the Oxford-based Bandolier group, systematic reviews: "select studies or reports for inclusion."[391] As a result, we did not find even one statistically valid meta-analysis in two of the world's leading medical publications.

The sock drawer

The core problem with meta-analysis is illustrated by the problem of selecting socks from a drawer. Suppose we have 100 socks in a drawer—fifty white and fifty black socks, all mixed together. When Bob wakes, it is not yet light, so he has to select a pair of socks and put them on, without seeing them. Since the socks are the same brand, made of the same material, and only differ in their colour, Bob cannot tell them apart. In this case, Bob has an even chance of selecting a pair of matching socks or an odd pair.

Bob calls to Alice, who is outside the door, and asks will she bet a dollar that he has odd socks on. If she guesses correctly, Bob will give her 2 dollars. Alice can happily bet with Bob on the chance of him selecting a pair of matching socks: since Bob has no information with which to select the socks, the game will be fair. The choice will be random—it is the same as betting on a coin toss. Alice can reasonably expect to come out ahead, since she will drop one dollar if she is wrong but will gain two dollars if she guesses correctly.

Thinking ahead, Alice plans to use the money on her next vacation and has a good estimate of how much she will have won. This is a good bet for Alice, because Bob is offering her odds of two to one, when the chance of a mismatched pair is fifty-fifty. Thanks to Bob's generous odds, Alice can expect to gain a dollar every two days.

Now, let us change the conditions slightly. Suppose Bob's black socks are made of wool and his white socks of nylon. Bob can now choose the socks he wears by touch. This extra information means that Bob will be able to tell the socks apart. Should Alice continue to bet with Bob, if he can feel a difference in the material? The bet is far less advantageous, as Bob's selection is no longer random: he now controls the colour selection. Suppose that Bob tells Alice that he is ignoring the feel of the socks. He explains that he is selecting the socks at random and assures her that he can be trusted—he is known for his honesty! Would you advise Alice take this bet?

If you think Alice should take the second bet, we suggest you might also like to contribute to her holiday funds and help cover her losses. Fortunately, Alice is less naïve and realizes the difficulty. Randomization is challenging. When people try to write down a random list, say of heads and tails, they produce a non-random sequence. It does not matter whether we believe Bob is honest and will not deliberately rip Alice off. The idea that he would be able to ignore the information on the different feel of the socks is implausible. Selection is powerful. Bob could easily sort the whole sock draw into matching pairs with complete accuracy, using touch alone. Alice could lose every bet and would be unwise to rely on Bob's generosity for her holiday funds.

This example is analogous to the choice of studies in meta-analysis. Researchers select studies and, contrary to the rather innocent beliefs of Ben Goldacre and others, the results are known in advance. The results of the selections are supposed to be unbiased. We are asked to trust the researchers' judgment and believe they are somehow impartial. Alice declined to play the rigged game, as she did not want to lose a few dollars. However, EBM demands that your health or even your life be wagered on the results of a prejudiced selection.

Actual Data

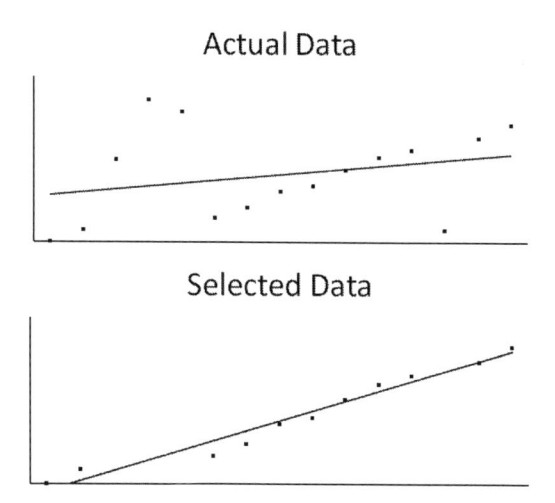

Selected Data

One of the first lessons for science students is do not select the best evidence – all data must be considered. The lines indicate how using just the "best" data gives a better, though misleading, fit.

GIGO (Garbage-In Garbage-Out)

> Given a large mass of data, we can by judicious selection construct perfectly plausible unassailable theories—all of which, some of which, or none of which may be right.
>
> Paul Arnold Srere

The current practice in meta-analysis is biased. Two of the most prestigious EBM publications allow authors to select the data and thus to generate reviews that may simply reflect their prejudice. Note that these two publications are not alone as, for example, Bandolier and the US Institute of Medicine's standards for systematic reviews also promote the errors we outline here.[392]

Journal of the American Medical Association

Let us start with the Journal of the American Medical Association (JAMA). This journal came to our attention when it refused to publish a letter describing errors we had found in one of its meta-analysis reviews. The rejection was strange, as the errors were obvious and fundamental. JAMA did not provide an alternative explanation for the errors and we were not told that we were incorrect. Our letter was not sent for review, the editor simply took the decision to reject. This is common practice with journals, as they get many more submissions than they can publish. However, our objection was important: we were claiming that the journal had published a paper that was completely wrong, misleading, and which could threaten people's health.

JAMA is acknowledged as a world-leading medical publication. Sadly, this does not mean the papers it publishes are all of excellent quality. We noted that at least one of its reviews was ridiculous. As we looked through a few more of the published reviews, we became more suspicious. We began to wonder whether *all* the published meta-analyses were flawed.

This possibility—that each and every JAMA review was flawed—became a topic of discussion among our academic friends interested in the topic. We discussed the issue with Dr Len Noriega, a specialist in artificial intelligence and decision science at Staffordshire University, England. Big Lenny, as he is affectionately known on campus, suggested we should have a quick look at the available data. To help us with this, we enlisted Andrew Hickey, a software engineer and (at that time) computer science student at Oxford University, who was also interested. Andrew offered to search through back issues of JAMA, to see just how many reviews had statistical problems. With suggestions for likely errors, he examined 38 papers that contained the term meta-analysis in the title or abstract, published in the years 2005-2006.

The results were shocking: not one review was statistically sound. The reviewers were free to select the studies that would give them the results they wanted. Like our example of Bob selecting socks by touch, the authors were choosing which studies they included. Suppose a researcher wanted to show a drug was more effective than vitamin E in preventing heart disease. If a study showed that vitamin E successfully prevented heart disease, it could be left out of the analysis and ignored. A story could always be provided to explain the exclusion. People, including scientists, have a predisposition for such *narrative fallacy*, which is the ability to fit a story or pattern to a series of facts, to explain events after they have occurred.[33]

The reviewers could hardly avoid being biased, as they had information about the results of the studies they were choosing. We ignored eight of the published studies, as they were not actually meta-analyses. One review of observational studies had poor blinding in study selection, but had included all reasonable studies.[393] A second study of refugees had some blind data extraction, but studies were openly selected.[394] The other 28 reviewers selected their clinical trials with no blinding. In total, 30 out of 30 meta-analyses were subjective, with potentially biased selection.

The authors of the reviews and the people selecting the data had access to the names of the original study authors, the full text of the studies, and the study results. Of the meta-analyses, six did not select independently, and four did not make the selection method clear. The selection involved "independent" researchers in the remaining 19 studies. However, it was not clear in what way they were considered independent. People who know the data cannot provide an independent selection. Just as Alice could not bet on Bob forgetting that he knew the colour of his socks, we cannot expect researchers to overlook results when selecting studies.

Selection bias dominated the meta-analyses. Astonishingly, in the JAMA reviews, *almost all the available data were excluded*. Out of 39,894 studies, only 962 (2.4%) were included, while the remaining 38,932 studies were ignored. This small number of included studies was particularly dangerous, as it makes it easier to exclude any unwanted results. How any rational person could expect such tiny samples of selected data to be representative, let alone "best", is beyond us.

As if this were not enough, there were further problems, which caused even more extreme bias. The reviewers handpicked particular study authors and contacted them, to provide additional information. In half (15/30) of the reviews, there was communication with study authors. In only three cases was it declared that authors or representatives from all the studies were contacted. In other words, the reviewers were free to obtain non-peer reviewed data for chosen studies of particular interest.

As we looked deeper, we noted that 14 reviews used additional unpublished or non-reviewed data. The reviewers apparently found it appropriate to ask selected scientists for extra information. Six included unspecified data from study authors they had chosen to contact. This was particularly peculiar logic. The meta-analyses were supposed to exclude studies that were not peer-reviewed or contained some apparent experimental defect. However, the reviewers covertly introduced suspect information through the back door! This is particularly disquieting, since such data could not be checked. Consider the implications carefully: we are being asked to believe private data, perhaps from drug companies, on commercially sensitive issues.

Narrative fallacy makes it easy for people to explain an event after it has occurred. History, for example, provides a plausible explanation for complex chaotic events, such as those leading up to the First World War. A story can be generated to explain any unusual set of circumstances. Similarly, if you are conducting a meta-analysis and want to exclude a certain group of studies from your review, it is always possible, if you know the details. If we asked Bob, on a particular day, why he had selected two black socks at "random", he might say he had not chosen as many black pairs as white pairs and he needed to balance up the numbers. The response is irrational, but is superficially plausible for someone consciously trying to produce a random sequence of socks.

In line with the suggestion of narrative fallacy, inconsistent reasons were given for excluding studies. Only 14 of the 30 meta-analyses in JAMA restricted their data to papers from peer-reviewed journals. Five reviews provided incomplete criteria on inclusion and exclusion. Only three reported that they used pre-prepared selection criteria before gathering the data, which should have been an essential requirement. This would not have helped much, however, because the reviewers were familiar with the data. Nevertheless, they could at least have gone through the motions of deciding why studies would be excluded.

Even pre-prepared data selection is not reassuring. If the authors knew the literature then, consciously or unconsciously, they could choose the selection criteria to achieve a desired result. Thus, they could have biased the criteria. Conversely, if they were not familiar with the literature, it might be argued that they should not be attempting the review. Even worse, authors of 25 of the meta-analyses could have chosen their criteria after the selection was made. The narrative fallacy applies once more: first exclude the study, then look for a reason why the study was no good, finally make that reason a criterion for exclusion. Our researcher may be honest but the self-justifying explanation becomes the story he remembers. Finally, in 19 of the reviews, the outcome measures were not identical from one study to another: the review was comparing apples with oranges."[395]

JAMA Meta-analyses Examined (2005-2006)	
Total number	38
Actual meta-analyses	30
Number of studies considered	39,894
Number of studies selected	962 (2.4%)
Independent selection	19 (63%)
Inappropriate selection	30 (100%)
Authors contacted	15 (50%)
Used only peer-reviewed studies	14 (47%)
Additional unpublished data used	6 (20%)
Selection criteria incompletely specified	5 (17%)
Outcome measures invalid	19 (63%)
Post hoc criteria possible	25 (83%)

All the meta-analyses published in the Journal of the American Medical Association, in the period 2005 to 2006, that we examined, were flawed.

Our investigation began because JAMA did not publish our objection to just one of its published reviews. Perhaps the editors realized that our criticisms could apply to all their published meta-analyses. The reviews appear to be lists of highly selected data, chosen to validate a particular medical viewpoint. This subjective interpretation is presented by JAMA as "proof".

Cochrane

We suspected that the practice of meta-analysis was bunkum, but thought that perhaps JAMA was an unusual case. Perhaps its high-ranking reputation was unjustified. Other EBM journals might be more objective. To test our suspicions, we decided to examine the Cochrane Foundation reviews. JAMA is a leading journal, but Cochrane Reviews are considered (by some) to be the touchstone of medical evidence. It turned out that the Cochrane meta-analyses are equally questionable.

The Cochrane Foundation reviews fail to meet minimum requirements. They select their data, facilitating bias and censorship of scientific results. Like those in JAMA, the studies included in their reviews cover only a small fraction of the total available information.

Cochrane validates data selection by suggesting that at least two people should do it. Two, preferably independent, people are expected to assess the eligibility of studies.[396] The two people must use methods that are transparent, minimize bias, and human error. By this stage, the reader may begin to wonder about the scientific naivety of such claims. They do not specify what makes two people independent enough to minimize bias and human error. Having two people, or even a whole committee, make the selection does not make it less subject to bias. Ironically, Cochrane goes to great lengths to point out the potential for errors that arise from non-blinding in the original clinical trials. Despite this, they ignore the selection bias in their own reviews. When we requested an explanation for these errors, the Cochrane Foundation declined a response.

In 2007, we examined 100 reviews in the Cochrane archives, chosen by searching on the term "meta-analysis". Five of the reviews were protocols or experimental designs, which simply provided a description of how an experiment was to be done. Of the remaining 95 reviews, only three had any blinding in selecting the clinical trials.

The first of these three had some blinding of the results; however, the selectors examined the abstracts to determine eligibility.[397] This means the people doing the selection had a summary of the trials, the results, and the conclusions. Since the abstract summarises the paper, this approach would not prevent bias. The second of the three was partially blinded to the names of authors, institutions, and funding sources. However, the selectors knew the study results.[398] In the last study, a third party removed the title, authors, and results, but the review's authors would presumably be competent in the field and familiar with the literature, so the blinding was almost inevitably ineffective.[399] Thus, selection bias could not be avoided, even in these three exceptional reviews, which had at least acknowledged the problem and tried to minimize the error. The vast majority did not even attempt to adhere to Cochrane's inadequate guidelines.

Most of the reviews were completely deficient. The remaining 92 of the 95 reviews had no blind study selection. In 90 reviews, both the names of the study authors, and their conclusions were available during study selection. The full study text was used in 91 reviews. Incredibly, additional non-peer reviewed and unpublished material was included in 65 of the reviews. So, they had selected evidence on the basis of published study quality and then included extra data from preferred authors, or perhaps those which provided the required answer.

Non-peer reviewed clinical trials were included in 67 of the reviews. Furthermore, six reviews included unpublished results from unnamed "experts". This is in breach of the basic philosophy of EBM, in addition to being improper. Only seven reviews made it explicit that the selection criteria were chosen before examining the data. Unconsciously or otherwise, 88 of 95 reviewers may have decided how to select the data after they knew the results.

All of the 95 reviews had inadequate study selection. Only about half of the reviews (47) stated the numbers of studies considered. In these, a mere 1.1% of total clinical trials were selected. The potential for bias is therefore obvious and large, or even inevitable. Finally, only 71 of the reviews measured the same outcomes. Once again, they were comparing apples with oranges: one trial might report a change in blood pressure, while another mentioned increased cholesterol.

Cochrane Meta-analyses	
Total number of studies	100
Actual meta-analyses	95
Partial blinding in selection	3 (3%)
Proportion of studies included	1.1%
No blinding in selection	92 (97%)
Authors names used in selection	90 (95%)
Full text used for selection	91 (96%)
Used additional unpublished results	65 (68%)
Used non peer reviewed trials	67 (70%)
Opinion/data from "experts" used	6 (6%)
Specific non post hoc criteria	7 (7%)
Clearly defined outcome measures	71 (75%)

Table summarizing problems with the first 100 systematic reviews (meta-analyses) published by the Cochrane Foundation in 2007.

Let us return to the bets between Alice and Bob. When Bob said he would ignore the fact that he could tell the colour of his socks because they were made of different materials, Alice did not believe Bob. She sensibly declined the bet: Alice was not naïve. If she had accepted the bet, Bob might have considered her a mug. Do you really want to bet your life on the choice of the Cochrane selectors, just because they tell you they are not biased? What about the lives of your family or close friends?

A drunkard's search

We have already discussed the general problems of data selection in EBM. Here we recall the old joke about a drunkard, who drops his car keys while unlocking his car one night. He walks 100 yards to the nearest streetlight and starts searching. A police-officer approaches.

Police-officer:	"What you doing?"
Drunkard:	"Looking for my keys."
Police-officer:	"Where did you drop them?"
Drunkard:	"Over there, down the road by the car."
Police-officer:	"So, why are you looking here?"
Drunkard (smugly):	"Because I can see better over here."

The drunkard's search is a cautionary tale for social[400] and behavioural[401] scientists. Searching in the "best" place is a flawed strategy.

Systematically wrong

> I have great suspicion that they don't know, that this stuff is [wrong], and that they're intimidating people.
>
> Richard Feynman (on applying mathematics to social science)

We have limited our criticism to the gross errors in the use of meta-analysis in preeminent journals. In so doing, we have ignored numerous other issues we noticed. Many other doctors and decision scientists view meta-analysis as nonsense. This is one example.

Tatyana Shamliyan and colleagues from the University of Minnesota, School of Public Health have looked at the quality of these so-called systematic reviews.[402] Shamliyan examined 145 meta-analyses. The results were:

- Fewer than half met each quality criterion.
- Only 49% reported study flow.
- 27% assessed grey literature (non-formal publications).
- Only 2% hid the sponsorship of individual studies.
- None hid the disclosure of conflict of interest by study authors.
- Only 37% planned formal quality evaluation of included studies.
- Quality was not linked with the journal, topic, or conflict of interest.

Dr Shamliyan was kind in her assessment: "Collaborative efforts from investigators and journal editors are needed to improve the quality of systematic reviews." We make a stronger assertion: current meta-analysis is unscientific, biased, and irrational.

Sceptics?

At the beginning of this chapter, we mentioned that Ben Goldacre chose systematic review as an outstanding development in rigorous science. He claimed that meta-analysis studies were selected without looking at the data, and so on. We suggest that Goldacre becomes a little more sceptical and does not take the claims of EBM at face value. We do not know of any evidence that suggests that systematic reviews have saved more lives than we can imagine, as he believes. Indeed, we are not at all sure how such a statement could be justified. We invite all sceptics to look closely at what is actually the case in EBM.

In our experience, proselytising sceptics are not very sceptical. They often attack soft targets, such as homeopathy, which fall outside the mainstream scientific paradigm. The establishment does not criticize people for attacking these easy targets. Occasionally, sceptics will attempt to appear more credible by, for example, suggesting that large drug companies cannot be trusted to perform unbiased trials; this is rather obvious and unlikely to lose them any brownie points.

A true sceptic would demand adherence to the scientific method. He would base his ideas on his own intellect. A real scientist would not care what others thought, particularly the experts. With EBM, rational sceptics might turn their noses up at large studies, and laugh at authorities who tried to promote something as flawed as meta-analysis. Our results indicate that meta-analysis is unreliable. We do not ask anyone to believe these findings: it is not necessary. While we state the case strongly, we think readers should make up their own minds.

A person attempting to replicate our results may find a little divergence, because they make different choices when searching through the reviews. However, the deficiencies in these gold standard reviews are so gross that we feel confident that a reader who takes the trouble to look over a few meta-analyses will be convinced. The Cochrane library is published online, so anyone can examine the published reviews to see how they were actually done.

Just inspect a couple and check them for yourself. Trust but verify: that's what good science is all about!

No scientific credibility

Independent scientists have examined the process of meta-analysis and are disturbed by its lack of reliability and integrity. EBM cannot claim to be rational and take meta-analysis seriously. Professor Charlton puts the position clearly, saying "meta-analysis is a logically incoherent technique of zero scientific credibility."[277] Charlton argues that the innocent enthusiasm of EBM supporters is distressing to those who understand statistics. These supporters have armour plated the confusion and developed an orthodoxy that is beloved of managers and politicians.

Even within EBM, the supporters of meta-analysis disagree over its objectivity and utility.[403] Meta-analysis is an embarrassment to EBM, despite being extolled as its most reliable evidence. The combination of meta-analysis with large-scale trials is contaminating the medical literature with a cargo-cult.

Losing the plot

The theory behind meta-analysis is limited. It typically uses simple linear statistics and is technically deficient. There are many more powerful methods available for reviewing data. As described earlier, Deep Blue, an IBM computer beat the World Chess Champion Gary Kasparov in 1996. Few who have played that game against a good computer chess program would doubt its ability. IBM went on to develop Watson, a computer system named after Thomas Watson, the company's first president. Watson (the computer) had software developed to play the TV quiz show game *Jeopardy!* Its artificial intelligence was able to interpret the limited grammar of the questions in English using natural language software. Watson competed in a two game match broadcast in February 2011. The computer beat Brad Rutter and Ken Jennings, two of the game's champion record holders. IBM is working with the University of Maryland to see how Watson might help in medical diagnosis and treatment.

Robert Weber, IBM's senior vice president for legal and regulatory affairs, has pointed out the potential for Watson-related computers to help with legal searches. He claims "we're pretty sure it would do quite well in a multistate bar exam!"[404] Indeed, similar software is already in use in legal cases.[405] In January 2011, data mining software helped analyse 1.5 million documents for less than $100,000. This may be compared with a $2.2 million search by a small army of lawyers and paralegals through six million documents. It is possible to automate processes, instead of spending months searching through millions of documents. The results can be available almost immediately instead of weeks later.

In the above paragraphs, we are merely making a comparison with meta-analysis, not promoting the use of computers and data mining. Meta-analysis is linear and is essentially limited to questions such as: on average, is a drug more effective than placebo when given to a very large group of people? For selected studies, it provides some limited statistics to help with the comparison.

Meta-analysis is supposed to replace human search and review. Scientists and doctors often assess the literature. However, human reviews are considered inferior by EBM, as they are (like meta-analysis) the subjective viewpoint of the reviewers. However, human reviewers have two great advantages. Occasionally, individuals develop new ideas and interpretations of the data. A classic case is Charles Darwin's reinterpretation of biology in terms of evolution. Meta-analysis crudely aggregates results. Humans can provide creativity, synthesis, and new theories. Groups of independent human reviewers have an emergent property—the wisdom of crowds.[406]

In 1906, Frances Galton, one of the founders of modern statistics, attended a country fair in the South West of England.[407] He noticed a competition to guess the weight of meat a fat ox would yield after slaughter. He asked for and received the slips of paper from about 800 participants after the competition was over. He found that the middle estimate was 1,207 pounds and the actual weight was 1,198 pounds. Amazingly, the crowd's average estimate was within 1% (9 pounds) of the correct weight. Galton realised this was not an accident. He used the result to illustrate how voting can provide a robust form of estimation.

Crowds have emergent behaviour. A school of fish or a flock of birds can engage in complex organised behaviour. The fish swoop around like a cloud, changing direction almost instantaneously. Each fish moves in a complex dance, avoiding collisions. A shark approaches the fish, which divide and swerve around the predator in a confusing swarm, only to recombine into the original amorphous school. This swarm behaviour arises from simple rules, such as "keep a short distance away from the nearby fish and move in the same direction as them."

Scientists have investigated the behaviour of groups of animals that show emergent intelligence.[408] A single ant displays limited behaviour but a colony can search out the best paths to nearby food sources and build bridges across streams with their bodies. Once again, this swarm intelligence emerges from simple rules. Software programs that copy the behaviour of ants and related swarms (ant algorithms) are used in practical problem solving.[409]

Similarly, groups of independent individuals can provide accurate and robust solutions. Doctors and scientists searching and reviewing the literature as individuals can have an overall positive effect that is more intelligent than a single individual. Some reviewers will be what Frances Galton described as "cranks" and will produce divergent outlier results. But these outliers are an essential part of the process that leads to a robust solution. Galton also explained over a century ago that the effect of outlier cranks was easily avoided.

Meta-analysis is not some outstanding method of decision making but a limited, linear, and rather simpleminded technique. Considering meta-analysis as an ultimate gold standard implicitly overrides human insight and the emergent group behaviour known as science.

Obfuscating the real solutions

In EBM, meta-analysis is the top of the evidence hierarchy. We can find no scientific justification for this elevated position. A more objective view is that meta-analysis is a mechanism for hiding bias and promoting the prejudice of reviewers. Meta-analysis provides poor quality data that lacks originality.

The gold-standard claims for meta-analysis seem to be based on the idea that they are the ultimate large-scale study. Despite the claims, meta-analysis is described by some critics as modern alchemy: an attempt to get something for nothing from clinical trials.[410] From our analysis, the situation is more dismal than even these disapprovals suggest.

Meta-analysis is simply a way for researchers to select the results they want, in order to confirm their prejudgments. It hides prejudice and gives it gold standard status. A meta-analysis is cheap and easy to perform. It does not require technical resources and a laboratory, just a computer, the internet, and perhaps a library. The required level of skill is low. Unfortunately, while meta-analysis is popular, its results are hogwash. Meta-analysis is fool's gold.

Main Points

- Meta-analysis is subjective and biased.
- Meta-analysis includes private non-peer reviewed data.
- Meta-analyses are misleading, even those in preeminent journals.
- Gold-standard EBM reviews are statistical nonsense.
- Statistics cannot replace human intellect in reviewing data.
- Acceptance of EBM review findings is irrational.
- Sceptics prefer supporting the *status quo* to scepticism.

> I have yet to see any problem, however complicated, which, when you looked at it the right way, did not become still more complicated.
>
> Poul Anderson

Predictable Irrationality

I can calculate the movement of the stars, but not the madness of men.
Isaac Newton (after losing a fortune in the South Sea bubble)

One way in which EBM benefits corporate medicine is by limiting unwanted information; it ignores exploratory data and evades unwelcome questions. Avoiding the question is an effective way of implementing censorship. In decision science, the false dilemma, or false dichotomy, is when only two alternatives are considered and other options are ignored.

The logical either-or fallacy is in widespread use in medicine. This is when someone provides two options and gives the impression that they are the only viable choices. Patients might be given two "best practice" treatment options, say radiation or chemotherapy, but are not informed of others. In a socialist health service, a cancer drug that might be more effective but expensive might not be mentioned. Conversely, private medicine might exclude low cost and low profit options. The ethics or politics of such situations are not the concern here, we are merely indicating that the information provided may be selective.

So-called "proven" treatments may be only marginally more effective than a placebo, or may be based on flawed studies. The proven drug may be less effective, have more side effects, or be more costly than the alternatives. Conversely, an unproven treatment may be effective and safe. If "unproven" has any meaning, it is merely a statement that EBM's large-scale trials have not been performed. There are many reasons for a treatment being unproven; most commonly, it is lack of resources or lack of potential profits.

Suppressing ideas

The effects of corporate medicine on a person's health are often hidden. A form of pervasive medical censorship harms us all.

People are provided with selected information, supported by institutional authority. We will describe the treatment of diabetes with diet, by way of illustration.

Diet was a standard treatment for diabetes centuries before Banting, Best, and Collip demonstrated that lack of insulin from the pancreas was the cause.[411] The introduction of insulin was a major breakthrough in the treatment of early onset diabetes. Insulin turned diabetes from an acute illness to a chronic disease. Diabetes remains a threat to life but treated diabetics live longer healthier lives than if they were untreated.

With increasing affluence, Type 2 diabetes has become more prevalent. Unlike the early onset form, people with Type 2 or late onset diabetes still have insulin in their blood. As the name suggests, late onset diabetes occurs as people became insulin deficient or resistant with age. However, late onset is becoming an inappropriate description, as increasingly Type 2 diabetes affects younger age groups. The primary cause of Type 2 diabetes appears to be changes in the modern diet.

While we were editing this chapter, the media announced a remarkable breakthrough and potential cure for Type 2 diabetes. It made the front page of national newspapers.[412,413] These reports concerned research undertaken by Professor Roy Taylor and colleagues of Newcastle University into the effect of low calorie diets on diabetes.[414] Eleven Type 2 diabetics had recovered their health after eight weeks on a low calorie diet. Previously, medicine had assumed that the illness was a life sentence of chronic disease. In fact, it has long been established that a change in diet can both reverse late onset diabetes and greatly help insulin dependent patients.

The university claimed that the "team has discovered that Type 2 diabetes can be reversed by an extreme low calorie diet alone."[415] This is not quite correct. We note, for example, that a 2007 documentary, *Simply Raw: Reversing Diabetes in 30 Days*, covered the reversal of diabetes by a less radical change in diet. Reversal of late onset diabetes by diet is a recognised treatment that has been adopted by many. In 2008, Dr Gabriel Cousens published a popular book on the topic, *There Is a Cure for Diabetes: The Tree of Life 21-Day+ Program*.[416] Thus, the Newcastle findings were hardly news. Our interpretation is that the team had essentially replicated the video in the form of a controlled trial. We have no specific criticism of the researchers—replication is important—but they should have been aware of the background data, including the video and earlier reports.

However, taking the EBM viewpoint, a documentary, books, and multiple clinical and case reports published over decades are "no evidence". Thus, because the Newcastle researchers came from a university and published in a peer-reviewed journal, they had made a "discovery" that could potentially lead to a breakthrough in treatment. As far as we can tell, the Newcastle researchers had not provided substantive new information. However, they were given the credit for the discovery of a well-known phenomenon. One criticism we do have of their research is that they misunderstood the nature of the effective diet. Calorie restriction is not the key issue, rather a change in food quality and quantity.

The problem for rational diabetic patients is that following the establishment approach would have left them chronically ill for years. Alternatively, they could have simply changed their diet and recovered quickly. Even Type 1 diabetics, with the most severe form of the illness, will greatly benefit. Unfortunately, the EBM medical advice was that such changes were unproven therapies. Patients electing to change their diet might be tolerated but were hardly encouraged.

We have known people with diabetes who we informed about how simple dietary changes could restore them to full health. They responded that they were getting excellent treatment from their doctors and dieticians at the local hospital. Not to put too fine a point on it, we watched them remain chronically sick, gradually lose their feet to infection and surgery, and finally die of complications. Although we provided the information, faith in the establishment and corporate medicine is powerful. Everyone has the right to make such decisions about their own health, but perhaps the medical establishment has an obligation to provide unbiased information.

Treatment of polio

Many unproven remedies have substantial supporting evidence. Often there are multiple case reports, trials that lack placebo controls, or others that are considered too small in EBM's world of mega-studies. The following example concerns the observations of a family doctor during a polio outbreak. Unfortunately, his observations were not structured as a clinical trial. In discussing this topic, we ask that the reader put preconceptions to one side and simply follow the story.

With some minor changes, the report might have been a rigorous indication for a potential treatment. Earlier, in our small Bayesian trial, we found that a small number of patients being treated by Dr Carlos, a hypothetical family doctor, could be analysed to provide a speedy estimate of the chance that a treatment will work. In the case we discuss here, the observations are a description of a single doctor's unusual experience.

Dr Frederick Klenner was a family physician in Reidsville, North Carolina, during the polio epidemics that achieved their maximum intensity around 1950. He developed a method of treating a range of diseases, using massive doses of vitamin C. About that time, vitamin C was thought to be protective against poliovirus and other infections. However, Klenner determined by clinical experiment that treatment of polio required doses orders of magnitude greater. With these colossal doses, he reported that patients recovered from polio in only three to five days. None of the treated patients suffered paralysis or showed continuing neurological symptoms.

In 1949, Klenner reported at a medical conference that massive doses of vitamin C could cure polio. At the time, poliomyelitis was epidemic and was a dominant medical concern, as it was killing and paralyzing children. The doctor would surely have expected his report to be welcomed. Instead, Klenner found that he was ignored. We should caution here that many EBM supporters equate high-dose vitamin C with pseudoscience. Despite this, we think the response should be rational and the data should determine such conclusions.

There are several reasonable responses to Klenner's claim. If people did not believe it, then they might challenge the veracity of his statement. Discussion at scientific conferences can be direct, frank, and aggressive. They could have suggested that perhaps the doctor had overlooked something and had come to the wrong conclusion. Alternatively, other doctors could have tested the claim, with their own small studies. There was no effective treatment for polio at the time, so testing the approach would have been ethical. We might at least expect the audience to have discussed the results. Surprisingly, the audience's response was to disregard the presentation and data. Perhaps they thought the idea was completely unbelievable and the presenter unreliable. After all, how could a simple vitamin produce such an effect? Whatever the reason, the absence of a response is thought provoking.

Klenner had been working with massive doses of vitamin C over a period of seven years. He realized that vitamin C was remarkably safe, and gave doses 1,000 times larger than normal. With these huge intakes, Klenner explained, he could cure patients and return them to complete health, without paralysis. He clarified that he had saved even critical patients, those with bulbar infection. Dr Klenner's claims did not seem to make any medical sense.

Typically, polio is a mild, flu-like infection. However, in a small proportion of those infected, the disease attacks the spinal cord, resulting in levels of damage that vary from muscle weakness to complete and permanent paralysis. Of the children who had paralysis, some would have direct infection of the brain, called bulbar polio. The bulbar region consists of several structures at the base of the brain. With bulbar polio, the head, neck, and breathing are affected. The child may be unable to talk, swallow, or breathe without assistance. Notably, nurses often had to suck out nasal and throat secretions, to prevent choking and death.[417]

At the annual meeting of the American Medical Association, Klenner described how he had saved patients with bulbar polio. We can quote him directly:

> ...if vitamin C in these massive doses—6,000 to 20,000 mg in a twenty-four hour period—is given to these patients with poliomyelitis, none will be paralyzed and there will be no further maiming or epidemics of poliomyelitis.[418]

Klenner was claiming he could eliminate the polio problem. He presented data showing that he could cure polio within three days. Since that time, there has been a controversy over the use of vitamin C in infectious disease. Nowadays, EBM simply rejects Klenner's results, based on the methods he used. However, his detractors did not test his claims in clinical trials, so we find such rejection to be potentially groundless.

Klenner's clinical observations

If challenged, Klenner might have welcomed the opportunity to justify his bold statement to the American Medical Association, as he was about to publish a paper on treating polio with vitamin C.[419] In the paper, he reported treating 60 cases of the disease. He described the clinical symptoms, including fever, a temperature of 101° to 104.6° F, headache, and pain at the back of the neck, in the lower back, between the shoulders, and in one or more extremity. Additional features were conjunctivitis, scarlet throat, nausea, vomiting, and constipation. These are classic symptoms of polio.

Two patients regurgitated fluid through their noses, which Klenner took to be a sign of the more dangerous bulbar infection. He reported that such patients may require postural drainage, oxygen, and, in some cases, a tracheostomy, in the first 36 hours, to allow the vitamin C time to deal with the infection. A doctor who did not realize this might risk the patient's recovery.

While these symptoms are indicative of polio, they may also apply to other diseases, such as influenza or meningitis. Rationally, we need to consider the chance that Klenner's patients actually had polio, as claimed. In 15 of the patients, Klenner confirmed his diagnosis of polio by means of lumbar puncture. He reported a cell count in the cerebrospinal fluid (CSF) from 33 to 125. The normal white cell count in CSF is between 0 and 5, so this sample of patients probably had an infection in the brain or spinal cord.

The cerebrospinal fluid is a clear watery fluid that bathes the brain and spinal cord. The brain floats in CSF, which cushions and protects it from mechanical injury. Collection of the patient's spinal fluid by lumbar puncture is a standard clinical test. A normal spinal tap should produce clear fluid. A straw or yellow–colour suggests the presence of excess protein, which can indicate cancer or inflammation. Blood–tinged or yellow to brown CSF suggests bleeding. A cloudy CSF is characteristic of infections. Analysis and culture of the cerebrospinal fluid is a definitive method of diagnosing infections of the brain and spinal cord.[420] Eight of Klenner's patients had been in contact with confirmed polio cases, and two of this group had spinal taps.

Dr Klenner seems to have had a good working knowledge of Bayesian statistics, since he states that, "A patient presenting all or almost all of the above signs and symptoms during an epidemic of poliomyelitis must be considered infected with this virus." We question the use of the word "must" but agree that his diagnosis was reasonable. There is a realistic probability that children with these symptoms were infected with polio, given that they were observed during a polio epidemic.

Unfortunately, Dr Klenner did not perform spinal taps on all his patients. He had several concerns, including the possibility that the procedure might promote infection. Klenner was conducting his own clinical research into vitamin C and infectious disease. Performing lumbar punctures would make it necessary to report each case he diagnosed to the health authorities. If he did this, they would no longer be his patients, as they would be transferred to a polio-receiving centre, in a nearby town. Dr Klenner believed he had a duty to keep treating them himself, as he thought his treatment could cure the patients and his results were consistent with this hypothesis.

Diagnostic criteria

Unsurprisingly, the criteria for diagnosis of polio have changed with time. Blood antibody tests for poliovirus are a potential aid to diagnosis.[427] Modern laboratories can recover poliovirus from stool samples or a throat swab. When poliovirus is isolated from a patient, it can be tested to find out if it is a wild form or was derived from polio vaccine.[421] A clinical diagnosis of paralytic poliomyelitis may be indicated by limp paralysis in one or more limbs. Tendon reflexes in the affected limbs can be reduced or absent. It is also necessary to rule out other possible causes and make sure that touch and mental functioning is normal.

A case is also considered to be substantiated if the individual has a neurologic deficit within 60 days of the initial symptoms, or has died. Officially, if there is no information available about the follow-up status, the case might also be considered confirmed.[422] Before the arrival of modern laboratory support, a clinical diagnosis was accepted.

Treatment

Klenner gave his polio patients massive doses of vitamin C in divided doses. Ideally, Klenner would have given all the children he treated intravenous vitamin C, as a sodium ascorbate infusion, so that greater amounts could be absorbed. However, intravenous treatment was impractical for some patients. Klenner seems to have been limited to giving injections, rather than continuous infusions.

In this approach, Klenner was remarkably astute. About 50 years later, we determined the half-life of high dose vitamin C in plasma to be about half an hour, using data published by the US National Institutes of Health. Until we clarified the issue, the half-life of vitamin C was thought to be somewhere between one and six weeks.[354] Surprisingly, Klenner's clinical approach was in agreement with current ideas of the dynamic-flow of high dose vitamin C in the body.[423]

The initial dose was 1,000 to 2,000 mg, increasing with age. Young children, up to four years old, were injected intramuscularly. Klenner did not have access to laboratory facilities to measure blood levels of the vitamin. He measured the patient's temperature at two hourly intervals. If the temperature did not drop two hours after the injection, he gave a second 1,000 or 2,000 mg injection. If the temperature went down, he would allow up to two more hours before the second dose. The injections were continued in this way for 24 hours. Patients treated at their homes received intravenous injections of 2,000 mg every six hours. These injections would have increased the blood levels only briefly. To help maintain blood plasma levels, an additional 1,000 to 2,000 mg was given orally, every two hours. Klenner knew that when vitamin C is taken by mouth, blood levels peak between two to four hours later.

After one day of treatment, the patients' temperatures were consistently lower. Klenner then switched to giving 1,000 to 2,000 mg injections, every six hours, for the next two days. When spinal taps were done, Klenner reported that the spinal fluid typically became normal after the second day of treatment. Within 72 hours, all patients had recovered. However, three patients relapsed, so the treatment was extended for another 48 hours or more, with doses of 1,000 to 2,000 mg every eight to 12 hours.

Risks of infection

The majority of people infected with poliovirus have no symptoms, or a mild fever, with gastrointestinal upset.[424] Only one person in ten to twenty infected people develop symptoms.[425] In those with symptoms, some (4-8%) are fortunate and recover without involvement of the brain or spinal cord.[426] The risk of becoming paralysed is reported to be one or two per hundred.[427,428] The risk of paralysis increases with age, varying from perhaps one in two thousand children to one in seventy five adults.[424] However, these rates of paralysis depend on the type of poliovirus. Type 1 poliovirus produces high rates of paralysis while Type 2 poliovirus is more benign and produces lower rates.[429] At the time of Klenner's study, Type 1 poliovirus caused about 85% of paralytic polio.[430]

Patients that survive an attack with symptoms of paralytic polio usually recover some motor function. However, permanent paralysis of one or two extremities is common and may be severe. Improvement of motor function usually starts shortly after the acute illness. In rare cases, increased paralysis can occur as late as three or four weeks after contracting the illness.[431] Most recovery occurs within about six months, with further improvement possible over the next year or two.[432]

Getting a reasonable prediction of the risk of death for those infected with polio is not straightforward. In the west, few people contract the illness these days. The death rate for patients with paralytic polio is reported to be 5-10%.[433] Typically, patients die because the muscles used for breathing stop functioning. The risk of death varies with age; perhaps 2–5% of children and 15–30% of infected adults with paralytic polio fail to survive.[426] These death rates are low compared with early epidemiological reports and may reflect the increase in vaccine-derived poliovirus, as opposed to the wild virus. They also may reveal the technological changes in treatment of those affected in the half century since Klenner's time. The relative mortality before immunization was higher than that following its introduction.[434] The death rate for polio in Virginia in 1950 is reported to be 5-10% of those infected.[435] The mortality varied with location and this may reflect differences in local hospitals and medical care.

Spinal polio, where the virus infects the spinal cord, is the most common form of paralysis-inducing disease. The higher the disease strikes in the spine, the more critical the paralysis. Bulbar polio can result in encephalitis and often leads to death, unless respiratory support is provided.[436] If such support was given, the death rate for bulbar polio in Klenner's time was reduced to 25% in children and to about 75% in adults.[437] When full medical ventilators are used, the death rate is further lowered to about 15%.[438] This description provides some background data to help assess Klenner's claims.

Analysing Klenner

Klenner's observations and claims were sufficiently unusual to be a matter for discussion over the following decades. Intuitively, if 60 patients have polio and all return to health in a few days, we potentially have a powerful treatment that could have saved many lives. Unfortunately, Klenner was unable to compare the likelihood of his patients' recovery with those of standard treatments. Had he tossed a coin to select and place half the patients in the hospital, he could have had a direct Bayesian comparison of the outcomes. This was not done, partly because Dr Klenner was convinced the outcome for his patients would be more favourable with his home-based treatment.

For fun, we will break the rules and apply probability to Klenner's results. In doing this, we are aware that it is not technically valid. The probabilities are uncertain. Klenner's experiment was done decades ago and the experiment cannot be replicated. In Klenner's day, the social conditions and nutrition were quite different, the viral strain has changed, and so on.

Current US Centers for Disease Control (CDC) figures for polio are given in the table below. However, Klenner's report was from before the introduction of vaccination and modern life support. The death rates from polio have changed with time. We have a rough estimate of 5-10% for the death rate in the Virginia epidemic in 1950.[435] However, there are indications that some of Klenner's patients had the more severe form of bulbar polio. We may reasonably allocate an expectation of death of 50% (0.5) in these patients, so we might expect that one of his two bulbar polio patients would have died. So the expected number of deaths in Klenner's sixty patients is between 4 ($\approx 0.05*58+1$) and 7 ($\approx 0.10*58+1$).

We can compute a probability that none of Klenner's patients would have died, had they not received the treatment. This probability is between about 1 in 60 (i.e. p<0.016) and 1 in 1,600 (i.e. P<0.0006). However, while these values are conventionally significant, they hide an important point.

Estimated Risk in 10,000 People With Polio		
Outcome		Rate
No Symptoms		9000-9500
Minor Illness		400-800
Brain Inflammation (Meningitis)		100-200
Paralysis		10-50
Spinal Forms	Spinal Infection	8-40
	Bulbo-Spinal	2-10
	Bulbar	0-1
Deaths (Paralytic polio)		0-15
Deaths (Bulbar polio)		0-1

Not only did none of Klenner's patients die, they were also free from paralysis and recovered quickly. We can ask what is the likelihood of Klenner's 60 patients all having polio symptoms but recovering quickly and completely. Some patients were reported to begin the treatment with severe disease, including bulbar polio, so our question is conservative. From the CDC data, we expect 3-4 out of every 10 patients with symptoms will have severe illness. Using these figures, we can estimate the probability of Klenner's group recovering so quickly by chance alone to be between about 1 in 2,000,000,000 and 1 in 20,000,000,000,000. (Though impressive, these figures are for illustrative purposes and should not be taken too seriously.)

Klenner's results are unusual but could have occurred by chance. Rare events sometimes happen. However, on its own, Klenner's report is interesting and has been the source of repeated speculation. The results are controversial because some doctors point out the potential for misreporting and error on Klenner's part, whilst others are impressed by the apparent improbability of his results.

Rejecting Klenner

The medical establishment rejected Klenner's result. Many polio experts were confident that vitamin C would not work against polio. Dr Albert Sabin, a leading researcher, claimed that vitamin C was not effective. Sabin had worked with Rhesus monkeys and low doses of vitamin C. He carried out these tests in response to results obtained by Dr Claus Jungeblut, who claimed that vitamin C had antiviral activity, specifically against polio. With hindsight, it now appears that Sabin did not replicate Jungblut's experiments properly but used lower doses of vitamin C.[354]

When Klenner presented his data, the physicians had a prior belief that vitamin C was ineffective against polio. In the light of this, it was possible to rationalize Klenner's results. The results may have appeared exceptional, but Klenner was making an exceptional claim. People generally interpret evidence to support their existing beliefs;[439] humans seem to operate in this way.

Klenner's results are frustrating. We have a hint that something important may have happened but the observations were not controlled. Alternatively, Klenner could have been mistaken and his report attributable to wishful thinking. If only Dr Klenner had planned his work according to Bayesian principles.

Replications

In the 1950s, other doctors tried Klenner's approach. If the dose was below Klenner's recommendations, the experiments failed. However, those who used massive doses reported similar results.

In 1952, Dr H. Bauer from Switzerland reported benefits with 10,000 to 20,000 mg of vitamin C per day. Similarly, in 1955, Dr Edward Greer, using 50,000 to 80,000 mg per day, recorded five serious cases of polio that responded. Before he died in 2009, Dr Abram Hoffer told us that an unpublished controlled trial of 70 young patients in the United Kingdom in the late 1950s replicated Klenner's observations. Patients given vitamin C recovered fully, but a number of the controls suffered permanent harm. We lack confirmation; this study was not published, as polio vaccination appeared to make the results obsolete. Many other doctors reportedly told Klenner that they had confirmed his results. Some of these doctors claimed to have cured themselves or their children.[440]

Up until his death in 1984, Klenner made similar astounding observations and claims for the action of vitamin C, in a wide range of viral infections, such as influenza, measles, and pneumonia. He claimed that vitamin C in massive doses was the antibiotic of choice in all viral illness and would be a major help in all infections.

The obvious question is whether Klenner was a crackpot or a genuine pioneer. During the sixty years since Klenner's early reports, many other clinicians have repeated and apparently confirmed his observations on massive doses of vitamin C. Notable examples are Dr Abram Hoffer, Dr Robert Cathcart, Dr Hugh Riordan, Professor Ian Brighthope, Dr Archie Kalokerinos, and Dr Tom Levy. Since the incidence of polio is now low, many of these replications concern the effect of massive doses of vitamin C in other infections, such as AIDS, influenza and herpes. The reports however are consistent, describing an unparalleled clinical effect, *provided the doses are adequately large and frequent.*

The response of the medical establishment has been to ignore these results. In the past 60 years, not one randomized clinical trial has been performed on the vitamin C doses that Klenner and others claim to be effective. Some readers may consider our last statement somewhat naïve. They would argue that the rational response of pharmaceutical companies, who fund most clinical trials, would be to ignore the reports of Klenner and others. They make their profits from selling expensive drugs, and little gain is likely from a simple, unpatentable vitamin. A family doctor or consultant generally is not a trained scientist and may be wary indeed of taking on the pharmaceutical giants.

One of our friends, Dr Robert Cathcart, reported similar observations on the efficacy of massive doses of vitamin C on thousands of patients. Cathcart told us that when he reported his clinical observations in this area, his colleagues simply thought he was mistaken. They assumed he was honest but was suffering from wishful thinking. However, he was never able to persuade them to try the experiment themselves.

Klenner's observations on polio occurred years ago; perhaps he and the other physicians were deluded. However, a recent example suggests that Klenner was correct and implies that EBM's influence on modern medicine is less than rational. Here, we relate a story that questions most people's comfortable and reassuring prejudices.

Life or death—a choice

> Now of the difficulties bound up with the public in which we doctors work, I hesitate to speak in a mixed audience. Common sense in matters medical is rare, and is usually in inverse ratio to the degree of education.
>
> William Osler

In 2009, Allan Smith, a 56 year-old New Zealand farmer, developed a severe case of swine flu. His story was covered in a series of television reports.[441] Mr Smith was prescribed an antiviral drug, Tamiflu, with antibiotic support. However, he continued to deteriorate. He developed pneumonia, as his lungs filled with infected fluid. Mr Smith was placed on ECMO (extracorporeal membrane oxygenation), a technique where blood is pumped from the body, passed through a membrane that allows gas transfer, and the oxygenated blood is returned to the patient. ECMO is given to newborn infants and during intensive care, to keep them alive for a short period when their lungs do not function, even with a ventilator.

Mr Smith was on the ECMO machine for nearly three weeks, before the hospital told his family he could not survive. This was a hopeless case and they wanted permission to switch off his life support.

Switching off the ECMO would amount to a death sentence. The hospital medical group for the case reported "The group is in unanimous agreement that Mr Smith should be removed from ECMO and allowed to die. Continuation is only prolonging his inevitable death." Just to add to his problems, the hospital had discovered that Mr Smith had hairy cell leukaemia. "The type of leukaemia Mr Smith has is potentially treatable if that is all he had. However, with his lung failure, Mr Smith cannot survive." There was no hope.

The Smith family had heard about the claims for massive doses of vitamin C and asked the doctors to try it. Allan Smith was alive, but switching off the machine would almost certainly end his life. The doctors initially refused the family's request to give vitamin C, as they thought it would not work. They told the family there was *no proof* that it would do any good.

Intravenous ascorbate (vitamin C) would be very low risk: certainly, it could not have done more harm than switching off the ECMO machine. However, the doctors were complying with the edicts of EBM. In these terms, "evidence-based" medicine is the use of "proven" treatments. The family's request might have seemed holistic, new age, or just plain silly.

The doctors were consistent in saying Mr Smith was effectively dead and the machine should be switched off. Their thinking was perhaps along the following lines: switching off a machine is an emotional event for loved ones and relatives. Of course, the family would not want the machine switched off—they were not qualified and might cling to any possible hope. There are always quack remedies but medicine should be "evidence-based". Furthermore, a good hospital should conform to best practice. And so on.

As the family explained, trying vitamin C would have given them the feeling that they had tried everything. They would not have to spend the rest of their lives regretting that they had not tried hard enough to save their father. The doctors would be helping the family come to terms with the decision to switch off the machine— even if the vitamin C did not work, as the doctors expected.

Despite the family's plea, Mr Smith's doctors were unwilling to go against EBM's belief system, according to which vitamin C is an *unproven* treatment. Smith's doctors might have been aware of the prejudice against the assumed pseudoscience of high dose vitamin C. If the vitamin C treatment proved effective and Mr Smith recovered, the doctors might have found it hard to explain their position. Why had they used an *unproven* treatment? Did they really believe it had worked? Is it ethical to promote quackery? We can sympathise with the physicians. From the doctors' point of view, their professional status and ethics required that they act according to the best evidence.

The Smith family were resourceful and insistent. With external medical support and their outright refusal to permit the removal of life support, the family at last persuaded the doctors to try intravenous vitamin C. It was agreed that if there was no improvement by the next Friday, life support should be terminated. By Wednesday, however, the patient was improving. At this point the hospital suggested, incorrectly, that the vitamin C was doing harm and causing problems with Mr Smith's kidneys and liver. We note in passing that liver damage is a side effect of Tamiflu, which they were happy to prescribe. The family contacted Dr Tom Levy, a world expert in the US, who provided clinical information.

Fortunately, New Zealand law was on the side of the family and the hospital was legally required to follow the family's wishes. Intravenous vitamin C at 25 grams per day began, late on 21st July. The following day, x-rays suggested that there were "air pockets" in the patient's lungs. This indicated recovery was advancing rapidly. Over the first three days, the dose was increased to 50 grams, twice a day. This 100-gram dose was continued for six days. Within the first three days of treatment, Mr Smith's lung function began returning. The recovery continued and ECMO was stopped on day five. Shortly afterward, Mr Smith began breathing without a ventilator.

Then, a new consultant physician decided to stop Mr Smith's vitamin C, and his condition worsened rapidly. Mrs Smith described the new physician's attitude towards vitamin C treatment:

> ...he was so adamant against it. He sat back in his chair. And rolled his eyes and crossed his arms and looked at the ceiling. And said, 'No, not putting him back on it. No. No.'

The family's battle had resumed. They managed to get permission for a single gram injection of vitamin C, to be given twice a day. This intake is ridiculously small and would most likely be ineffective. However, once again, this will have seemed a large dose to the hospital—one that was safe for the patient.

When Mr Smith was transferred to Waikato hospital, nearer to home, the family's problems restarted. The new hospital stopped the intravenous vitamin C. The family instructed a lawyer. The lawyer was dumbfounded by the antics of the hospitals. She argued that it was illegal and the family would go to the high court. Finally, the hospital agreed to give a low dose (two grams), instead of the 50 grams a day that was claimed to work.

With this low dose, Mr Smith slowly started to recover and was eventually able to consume additional vitamin C orally. The family gave him six grams of liposomal vitamin C a day and he began to recover quickly. Liposomes are tiny nanoparticles of fat, surrounding the vitamin C. Liposomal vitamin C is rapidly absorbed following oral administration. This form may be a more effective approach than intravenous administration in some instances, as liposomes can enter cells directly.

Last time we heard, Mr Smith was healthy and well, having returned to active life on his farm. He no longer has leukaemia.

Another unproven claim for massive doses of vitamin C is that they kill cancer cells.

An EBM explanation

Despite our willingness to see the point of view of the doctors, we still find their decisions irrational. Simple game-theory indicates that they should try the treatment. There are three main outcomes. If the treatment works, the patient's life is saved. If the treatment fails completely, the patient would have died anyway. The treatment is known to be low risk but if it caused harm it would be less damaging than switching off the machine: there is no treatment outcome with a lower payoff than switching off life support.

Mr Smith lived. The hospital observed the improvement and provided an explanation; they suggested that turning Mr Smith over in his bed had caused his recovery. This is equivalent to saying a miracle had occurred:

> Mr Smith is stable but still critical. He has improved over the past couple of days. Turning Mr Smith prone has probably made the biggest difference. His chest X-ray is better.

The hospital's prior expectation was that Mr Smith would "inevitably" die. They offered no hope and no treatment. Neither did they believe, before turning him in his bed, that this might save his life. Indeed, if simply turning the patient could cure him, there would have been no reason for turning off the ECMO machine. One of Mr Smith's sons expressed it well, when he responded to the doctors, saying "Why didn't you try that before even suggesting to turn the machine off?"

Doctors at these hospitals constrained by EBM would apparently rather believe in a miracle than update their belief system. As we have indicated, Littlewood's miracles not only happen, but should be expected. However, turning the patient remains an unlikely explanation. The simplest conclusion is that the intravenous vitamin C brought about the cure, as had been predicted by both the family and by experts.

The official response, given by the Auckland District Health Board Chief Medical Officer, Dr Margaret Wilsher, was that

> No evidence exists to confidently say that high-dosage vitamin C therapy is either safe or effective.[442]

This standard EBM response of "no evidence" is, of course, scientifically incorrect. In real science, evidence is not restricted to the results of selected clinical trials. There is a great deal of supporting data,[354] and a strong hypothesis. These data include Mr Smith's recovery.

In light of recent publicity, Dr Wilsher asked Auckland City Hospital's Clinical Practice Committee (CPC) to review the efficacy of high-dose vitamin C in the treatment of influenza and other critical illness. The CPC found *no evidence* that would allow it to say high-dose vitamin C treatment is either safe or effective. The safety aspect is clearly incorrect, as people have been taking large doses for decades without apparent harm. Furthermore, there is evidence—the CPC was simply ignoring it. In the words of Mai Chen, the family's lawyer, "intravenous vitamin C is a well-researched treatment." The hospital, however, resorted to the standard EBM claim:

> Only a suitably-constructed and approved clinical trial could establish the facts.

In short, this statement shows a complete lack of scientific understanding. Do they really believe that there is no other possible way to establish scientific facts? According to this restricted vision, only an EBM clinical trial, that has been officially approved and performed according to specified procedures, can provide relevant data. Sadly, this is what happens when EBM takes control of medicine.

Any data other than that sanctioned by EBM is described as "no evidence". To provide such evidence you need millions of dollars and several years to spend on a clinical trial. Indeed, we caution the reader that even if they have the time and money to conduct an EBM clinical trial, they had better not disagree with the status quo. The response to getting the "wrong" result is likely to be a claim that "it is only one trial" and is therefore an anomaly; a meta-analysis of multiple large-scale studies will be needed. A reasonable estimate of the time scale for such a venture might be 10 to 20 years, and a few hundred million dollars. The real purpose of EBM seems to be to prevent or delay unwanted research (POSIWID).

We first realised the extent of the irrationality arising from EBM when we wrote a book about vitamin C.[354] Whatever the reality of such therapies, the prevailing idea of science under EBM appeared to be nonsensical. In this example, Mr Smith's sons observed the sorry saga and noted the changes as the treatment was given or denied. They had their own interpretation. While admitting to not being medical experts, they noted that Mr Smith's recovery was directly proportional to the dose of vitamin C he was taking. When the intake was stopped or reduced, his progress diminished accordingly. The Smith family argue that you would have to be "a bit thick" not to realise what was going on. Once again, readers can make up their own minds.

Main Points

- Claims of "no evidence" usually indicate suppression.
- The term "unproven" is scientifically meaningless.
- Most surgery and much of modern medicine is "unproven".
- Demands for proof can delay medical progress by many years.
- EBM restricts doctors' options.
- When medicine gives up, you may as well try an unproven therapy.

> If I have not seen as far as others, it is because giants were standing on my shoulders.
>
> Hal Abelson

Simply Brilliant Heuristics

> If there is a problem you can't solve, then there is an easier problem you can't solve: find it.
>
> George Pólya

We need to get back to basics. Effective medicine depends on the expertise of individual doctors. However, institutional science has slowly been taking over. For the past half century, there has been an increase in the size of research teams. Now, large organised groups tackle medical questions. There is an assumption that the days of the lone scientist making major breakthroughs have past. According to this view, science has advanced so far that breakthroughs are difficult and progress is largely incremental.

This attitude is hardly new. It is reminiscent of the beginning of the 20th century. Lord Kelvin, one of the leading physicists of the time, is known for a lecture at the British Association for the Advancement of Science in 1900. He said

> There is nothing new to be discovered in physics now. All that remains is more and more precise measurement.

Two years later, Albert Michelson is reported to have said

> The most important fundamental laws and facts of physical science have all been discovered, and these are now so firmly established that the possibility of their ever being supplemented in consequence of new discoveries is exceedingly remote.[443]

This was shortly before Einstein and Poincaré's introduction of relativity, the beginnings of complexity theory, and the start of quantum mechanics, which revolutionized physics. Ironically, Michelson's experimental data were explained by the special theory of relativity. The problem with science is that breakthroughs are difficult and daunting. It can be more reassuring to believe everything of importance is already known, rather than admit the need for new ideas.

The rise of "big science" was influenced by the Manhattan project, which produced the atomic bomb. However, the critical physics needed for the bomb was known before the initiative, from the work of individual physicists and small teams. Building a nuclear weapon was largely engineering and technology. Putting astronauts into space was another engineering problem. The "rocket science" of the space program was new technology, though it was mainly based on the physics of Isaac Newton 250 years earlier.

Some projects in science need large-scale equipment. An example is the European Organisation for Nuclear Research, known as CERN, where the Large Hadron Collider is built into a 27 km long circular tunnel. As would be expected, over the years CERN has generated some important and fundamental results in particle physics. Currently, CERN is searching for the Higgs boson or god-particle. Notably, when British scientist Peter Higgs first described the theory of the particle, the editors of Physics Letters rejected the paper as apparently it was "of no obvious relevance to physics"![444] Higgs resubmitted the paper to Physical Review Letters with an added paragraph that introduced the particle. Other physicists developed the theory independently and published. So, the journal rejecting the paper could have cost Higgs credit for this major scientific achievement. The point is that the massive international scientific enterprise at CERN is currently occupied in searching for the particle first described by Higgs, a single physicist.

Individual researchers at CERN provide an excellent example of the importance of the lone scientist. Two breakthroughs of major importance, one in computer science and one in physics, were generated by specific people at CERN. The entire multibillion dollar funding of CERN could be justified by their results alone. However, the ideas developed from the initiative of individual genius. They are of a different quality that anything in EBM.

John Bell was one of the most impressive physicists we ever met. While on leave from CERN, Bell developed a key theory in quantum mechanics.[445] Bell's theory overturned an invalid mathematical proof by eminent mathematician, John von Neumann. Such was von Neumann's reputation that other physicists had simply accepted his results and overlooked the error. It took someone as iconoclastic as John Bell to check von Neumann's work carefully. Bell inspired a new generation of physicists to re-evaluate quantum mechanics.

One of the major developments in computer science also came from CERN. Tim Berners Lee and Robert Cailliau developed an incredibly simple idea while at CERN. Tim Berners-Lee was an independent computer contractor and he had a simple idea to link documents in a computer network with hypertext. Unsurprisingly at first, the idea gained little support from the organization. Initially, connecting documents across a network with something called hyperlinks might have seemed minor—an almost banal development. However, in a short time, this linking of documents in a computer network found widespread support and involvement. Tim Berners-Lee's idea became the World Wide Web and changed the world. Individual researchers and small groups are still providing the core developments in science, medicine, and engineering.

Becoming more rational

Rational decision making is challenging but most people can improve their ability. Patients look to doctors and other medical professionals to help them make rational decisions, often in life threatening situations. Perhaps all doctors—and patients for that matter—could begin by looking again at risk. We suggest reading *The Illusion of Certainty* by Erik Rifkin and Edward Bouwer.[446] The book originated when a PhD scientist needed to make a decision about the health of his 7-year old son and was concerned by the arbitrary nature of the medical decision. It provides a basic background to understanding risk in everyday life.

Sophistication in problem solving is often overrated. An approximate solution to the right problem is better than an optimal answer to the wrong question.[447] The second book we recommend is *Guesstimation: Solving the World's Problems on the Back of a Cocktail Napkin* by Laurence Weinstein and John Adam.[448] This book explains how to make rough Fermi estimates. A Fermi problem appears insoluble at first glance but can be solved rather simply. The name comes from Enrico Fermi, a Nobel Prize winning physicist who was adept at predicting the results of experiments using back of the envelope calculations. Fermi estimated the explosive power of the first atom bomb at Alamogordo by dropping pieces of torn paper and seeing where they landed.[449] A classic Fermi problem is "How many piano tuners are there in Chicago?"

Physicists often do Fermi calculations before an experiment to give themselves a rough estimate of the possible results. Suppose a biologist friend tells you the weight of a 20 year-old Indian elephant female is 7,700-9,900 lbs. and the male 11,000-14,000 lbs. It is possible to check that the result is within reasonable limits. You might not know the first thing about elephants, except that they are large and heavy mammals.

Suppose you are an adult male and weigh 180 pounds and think you have a volume similar to that of a single small elephant leg. Let's round the number up, to make the calculation easy, and say a small female elephant's leg weighs about 200 pounds. Since an elephant has four legs, a female will weigh at least 800 lbs., not counting the body or head. The head and neck is relatively large and probably has the volume of at least 2 legs (another 400 lbs.). The body is much larger than a leg: let's guess its volume is about 20 times bigger (8,000 lbs.). So the total weight of a female elephant is about is around 9,200 lbs. and a male slightly larger, say about 10%, so a male weighs about 10,000 lbs. Allowing for reasonable error (of about 30%) in the estimates, Indian elephants would weigh in the range say 6,500-13,000 lbs., which is similar to the biologists' figures.

We are not suggesting that estimating the weight of an elephant is particularly useful. However, the ability to approximate in this way will help in making medical decisions. The Fermi approach to estimation provides a way of checking that the reported results and importance of clinical trials are reasonable. Doctors and patients doing such estimates would quickly place EBM in context.

In considering an EBM trial, we suggest you estimate the size of the effect for an individual patient. Perhaps you might use the 80-20 rule. In this case, you might estimate whether a result is important using limits such as:

> At least 80% of the patients should achieve a minimum 20% benefit.

OR

> At least 20% of the patients should achieve at least 80% benefit.

Use of these or similar estimates would quickly tell if the treatment meets a rational patient's expectations. A rational patient would expect to have a good chance of a manifest benefit from taking the drug, rather than to pay and risk side effects just to contribute to a statistical average.

Doctors, not statistics

Most doctors do not enjoy statistics. More particularly, medical education is lacking in decision science and Bayesian statistics. The most intelligent and able doctors are typically unable to make a full rational analysis of the constant stream of new scientific data. Furthermore, even infinitely intelligent doctors would have insufficient time to read all the papers and attend all the conferences in their fields.

We have described earlier how leading mathematicians can have difficulty analysing a simple game. A practicing physician is not normally expected to understand fully the results of a meta-analysis. However, doctors could be trained to make rational decisions and to place conventional statistics where it belongs, with a minor role as descriptive support. Earlier, we described a simple Bayesian clinical trial, to inspire doctors to undertake real research. Bayes takes a little getting used to but it is worth the effort to counterbalance the complicated statistics used in EBM.

The first approach to analysing data can be graphical. Graphics can illustrate the size of a claimed effect and its importance. EBM avoids the visual inspection of descriptive statistics, as it would place minor results into a more practical context. Earlier, we suggested a decision tree as a simple but powerful approach to medical decision making. If doctors understood and employed these methods, medicine would be transformed. In this section, we are returning to the use of heuristics, rules for solving problems.

A heuristic many scientists use is that *the measured difference in an experiment should be obvious*. The classic cautionary tale of obscure and vague data is the N-Rays of French physicist René-Prosper Blondlot (1849-1930). Blondlot described how all objects gave off a barely visible radiation that could hardly be seen on phosphorescent detectors. One hundred and twenty other scientists confirmed the rays in about 300 research papers.[450] The N-rays did not actually exist but were of psychological origin; the scientists were fooling themselves.[451] Since that time, scientists have generally been careful that the studied effect should be obvious, large, and not at the limits of observation. This implies that the EBM results that require thousands or even tens of thousands of subjects to establish are questionable.

Doctors want results that make for practical decision-making. An archetypal doctor examining a patient will measure the pulse and use a thermometer to take the temperature. These are direct objective measurements. In taking these measurements, the doctor is using some simple rules to check the individual for signs of illness. Basic observations are made with an extensive understanding of physiology and pathology. There is a body of scientific knowledge with which to interpret the information.

Throughout its long history, medicine has used heuristics. Most physicians probably think of them as simple rule of thumb guides to practice, but they have been with us since at least Hippocrates.[452] Hippocrates left a series of such aphorisms to guide physicians, including:

- When sleep puts an end to delirium, it is a good symptom.
- Persons who are fat are apt to die earlier than those who are slender.
- Autumn is a bad season for persons with consumption (TB).
- Desperate diseases require desperate remedies.

Hippocrates suggestion that obese people have a shorter life expectancy is similar to modern health advice. Ross Ashby similarly left a series of aphorisms, such as

> Don't appoint, as the President's driver, an Englishman who has spent thirty years learning to drive on the left.

More generally, proverbs provide us with a series of often apparently contradictory instructions on living. The proverb "You're never too old to learn" conflicts with "You can't teach an old dog new tricks." These proverbs are not necessarily contradictory, their effective use depends on the context. Proverbs become useful heuristics only when employed intelligently, according to the problem and its environment.

Evidence is not expertise

Let us return to that much praised answer to a criticism of EBM: "the practice of evidence based medicine means integrating individual clinical expertise with the best available external clinical evidence."[10] These are weasel words and an attempt to avoid objections to EBM's naïve empiricism. From the point of view of information science, the claim is peculiar. The doctor's expertise dominates and the amount of information EBM provides that is relevant to an individual patient is generally tiny. The statement about EBM is equivalent to describing a harvest mouse sitting on an African bull elephant as "a mouse with a trifling appendage".

Any individual doctor is free to read and evaluate the selective evidence of EBM in its limited context. It may help with a particular case but, more likely, using it as a guide will lead to suboptimal treatment. We can characterize the benefits of EBM as a set of weak heuristics.

EBM generates rules of thumb that are typically long, complicated, and feeble. For example, the results of a clinical trial might suggest that "For a middle-aged affluent male of oriental extraction, living in the north west United States, with atherosclerosis, Type 2 diabetes and high LDL cholesterol, 10mg of the statin Obecalpine each day may be very slightly better on average, in terms of cardiac events but not life expectancy, than doing nothing—but we will not have established the side effects of this drug for the next decade."

Taken as a whole, EBM provides a collection of somewhat unrelated and complicated aphorisms of this form. They do not generalize well. They are not useful for prediction. The underlying premise is statistical and a statement belongs only to the population from which it was derived. Our hypothetical example does not apply to women, for example, nor other ethnic or age groups, nor people living in different locations. There is no central theme to EBM's results, other than they are statistical findings from a set of officially sanctioned trial and error studies.

Supporters of EBM apparently do not realize that their methods are out-dated. Statistics do not have the same problem solving capabilities as humans; doctors can outperform statistical averages. To show this we can use a graphic. The chart below uses a set of circles and triangles to plot two "risk factors" from a clinical trial.

Let us say the triangles represent sick people and the circles are healthy controls. The distributions have similar average values (means are zero) and they overlap. Overall the spread of values (standard deviations) will differ slightly with the triangles (sick people) being more concentrated around the centre.

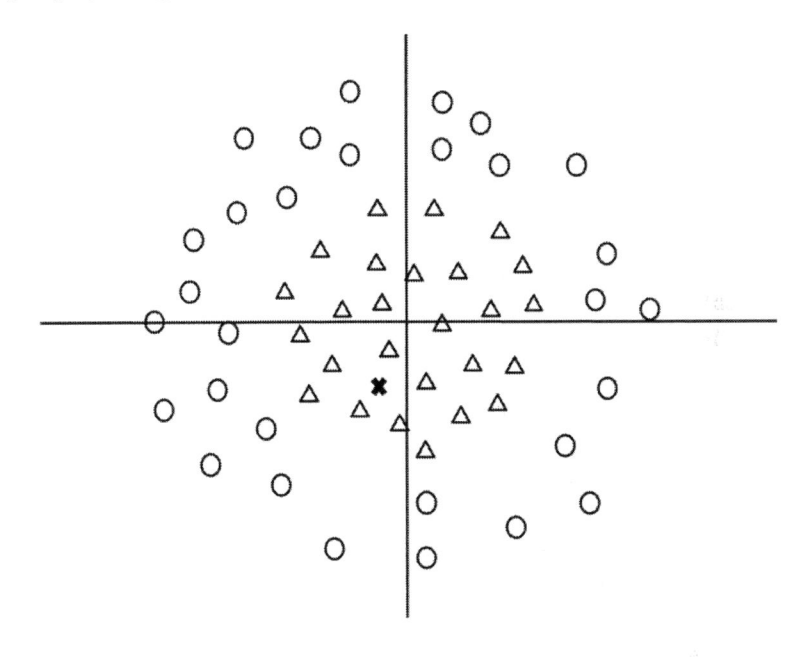

△ sick   O healthy   ✖ Bob Cross

Hypothetical illustration of two "risk factors" from a clinical trial

Many of the EBM's techniques simply measure the difference between the mean values, which in this case are identical. Occasionally the variation in values is considered, which might give some minor statistical indication that these two distributions differ in the way they are spread about. Using EBM's methods, we might say little more than the healthy people are more varied. Despite this limitation, most people can easily see that the triangles and disks make different patterns. The triangles are all contained in a disk near the centre while the circles form a surrounding ring (doughnut or annulus). Visually the two groups are distinct. There is no difficulty in grouping the different shapes and telling them apart.

Just looking at the data can be more powerful than the complicated but linear methods of EBM.

A doctor is concerned with diagnosing a single individual, who we have represented in the diagram as a cross. Let us call him Bob Cross, for fun. If asked whether Bob Cross belongs to the group of triangles (i.e. is sick) or the group of circles (i.e. is healthy), most people will conclude he is sick, as his cross lies within the group of triangles, at a distance from the circles. A non-linear method of classifying Bob Cross is to use the *nearest neighbour method*, which means we ask if the nearest other result is a triangle or a circle. A quick visual inspection of the diagram should immediately suggest this approach would give a definitive result in this case. In the same way, a doctor might remember having a patient with similar symptoms last year.

In diagnosing Bob Cross, we have just used nearest neighbour analysis, a form of pattern recognition. These non-linear methods are widespread in other disciplines. Roadside cameras for reading license plates, the bank's computer system for checking credit scores, fingerprint door locks, and security organizations' computer tracking of suspected terrorists all use pattern recognition. Surprisingly, formulate the question well, and even a simple nearest-neighbour approach can be highly accurate. These effective pattern recognition techniques are largely absent from EBM.

It is unclear in what sense the linear statistics of EBM add to individual clinical expertise, which requires pattern recognition. EBM merely provides a setting: it gives the doctor a little vague information on the average patient's response, though this is typically of limited use. The important aspect is the clinical expertise of the doctor.

We need now to consider that nature of this expertise. A standard definition is:

> By individual clinical expertise we mean the proficiency and judgment that individual clinicians acquire through clinical experience and clinical practice.[10]

We should add the knowledge gained during education and medical training. There should be some scientific knowledge, details of pathology, physiology, pharmacology, biochemistry, and so on. An established doctor will have years of professional training in addition to his degree. The totality of the doctor's expertise constitutes his requisite variety.

Supporters of EBM would have us believe that it is objective and more powerful than the "art" of diagnosis. There is ultimately an art to a doctor's diagnosis, but it is constrained by rational decision making. Doctors differ when making diagnoses. For example, doctors may disagree in classifying a case of diabetic retinopathy as mild or severe. In EBM, this variation is taken as a sign of subjectivity in their response;[453] the doctors are not assessing their patients objectively and reproducibly, or they would display a high level of consistency. Presumably, in a "scientific" EBM world, the doctors would be in close agreement, despite the patient's individual characteristics.

If this lack of variation in medical decision-making were to become standard, a patient would get the same treatment, whichever doctor they chose. As patients, we find this idea disturbing. Getting a second opinion is a minimum option for a patient's independent quality control. Moreover, as scientists, we do not see how what would in effect be a single physician, practicing a fixed form of authorized medicine, could accommodate biological variation.

Physicists and other scientists reading this may also feel uncomfortable. Some physicists do not believe in an expanding universe, others have a non-standard interpretation of quantum theory, and others think string theory is a form of pseudoscience. Real science involves differing opinions, not an imposed consensus. There is a reason for this variation. The population of scientists needs to have sufficient variety to make progress. The difference in belief and the associated disputes drive scientific advancement. In other words, variation in the doctor's response may be a healthy sign that medicine contains independent agents, rather than "sheeple".

Trisha Greenhalgh has described the use of "maxims" in tandem with the narrative of the patient's history.[453] To Greenhalgh, a maxim is a rule of thumb, for example: "Diarrhoea in previously well children is generally viral and self-limiting." She suggests that maxims provide a powerful approach to combining the results of science with the art of a doctor's decision-making. However, to Greenhalgh, EBM is the science that provides the "gold standard" of data. The art comes from clinical proficiency and judgment.[454,455,456] Greenhalgh suggests the dissonance between science and the doctor's art arises when an EBM approach is emphasized, rather than an integrated approach. Our interpretation differs, as we do not consider EBM to be scientific.

In the end, Greenhalgh describes the use of narrative: the patient's story. Of course, listening to a patient and getting their history is hardly new. It only becomes a novel approach when doctors have become imbued with the EBM philosophy. A patient's diagnosis relies on the reasoning of the individual doctor. Ultimately, the skilled doctor's expertise may seem like magic, or at least an art. However, there are underlying methods that provide this expertise. The doctor has learnt by induction. With time and experience, trainee doctors and health professionals can develop such skills.

Effective problem solvers learn to use an inductive approach, built upon heuristics and pattern recognition. Decision science describes this process. Alone it will not make a person a great diagnostician or theoretical physicist, but it may help ensure that doctors are at least competent.

Simple rules

A heuristic is more than a maxim, proverb, or rule of thumb. The word derives from the Greek for discover. Heuristics are guides to problem solving. They can be algorithms as well as sayings. A child might learn not to touch a hot stove with the heuristic *touching the stove—it is hot and hurts*. This may be shortened by parents to pointing to the stove (or other source of heat) and saying "No, hot!" rather loudly. At the other end of the scale, mathematicians and theoretical physicists often use heuristics in their search for novel solutions to complex problems.

How to solve it

In 1945, the mathematician George Pólya wrote a classic book called *How To Solve It*, which explained how to use heuristics in cracking difficult problems.[457] There is a two-volume follow up text on heuristics for mathematics and plausible reasoning.[458] The text begins with the phrase: "Experience modifies human beliefs", which readers may recognise as a description of Bayes. This form of inductive reasoning is at the heart of real science and rational thinking. Pólya has influenced mathematics and computer science for decades. His suggested heuristics for solving problems could also be useful in evaluating medical data:

- Begin by understanding the problem
    Specify what are you are asked to find
    Restate the problem in your own words
    Is there a picture or a diagram that might help understanding?
    Do you have enough information to find a solution?
    Check you understand all the words used to state the problem
    Do you need to ask a question to get the answer?
- Plan your approach
    Guess and check
    Make an ordered list
    Use direct reasoning: eliminate possibilities
    Use symmetry
    Consider special cases
    Look for patterns
    Solve a simpler problem or use a model
    Work backwards—check out a solution
- Carry out your plan
    This part is usually straightforward. An EBM-style cookbook approach would fit in here—but one that is tailored specifically to model the problem.
- Check the result and see if it could be better
    You may, for example, have found that antacids are effective—does this mean that ulcers are not an infection?

The heuristic approach has great potential for medical decision-making. In fact, heuristics provide a partial explanation for the art of medicine. Clinical intuition is based on heuristic reasoning[459] and pattern recognition. Rules of thumb can provide an adaptive toolbox for clinical decision-making.[460] Clinically, simple heuristics are more useful than EBM.

Interpreting evidence

Heuristics provide a tool kit for interpreting EBM studies. Here are some suggested guidelines for doctors who are considering scientific papers and results. These may be a useful start for a heuristic toolbox, aimed at finding the real meaning behind "evidence-based" trials.

- Firstly, think for yourself. Do not rely on the study authors' interpretation of the data. Such claims are often misleading.
- The paper's topic should be stated simply and clearly. If not, try to restate the problem. Just asking a straightforward question can often clarify the issues.
- In drawing conclusions from the data, ask what you can be sure is valid. If there is any other possible explanation, acknowledge it.
- If an effect is small, it is generally irrelevant, regardless of statistical significance levels. The benefit of a treatment should be substantial. Before you spend your time reading, look at the claimed results: the effect should be large. For example, an average reduction in cold symptoms from 7 days to 6 days is minor—don't waste effort on trivial improvements. Conversely, if an apparently terminal pneumonia victim might be restored to health in three days using penicillin, this is a large and obvious effect.
- If an effect cannot be demonstrated without statistics, it is probably too weak to be of use in treating an individual. A medical scientist may tell you that substantial effects are difficult to discover and that this criterion is unreasonable. We disagree. Clinical researchers who are not looking for effects large enough to be useful in treating individual patients are wasting resources.
- The reported results should apply to an individual patient. A heuristic might be that an average patient should have a fifty-fifty chance of receiving reasonable benefit. Alternatively, use the 80-20 rules above.
- Do not relax the criteria of requiring a substantial effect in a high proportion of patients for serious illness. Patients should not be short changed just because they have severe disease. Researchers or doctors may claim that for some diseases, such as terminal cancer, a small benefit in a few patients is a major advance. Don't take much notice. A small improvement in a small proportion of patients is a small benefit, no matter what the disease.

- If results are presented as percentages, risk ratios, odds ratios, or other relative values, mistrust them. Convert the figures to actual results. If ten patients are treated, how many will benefit?
- Check if the results apply only to a specific group, such as males over 75 years of age, who have recently had a heart attack. If so, make sure conclusions are not generalised beyond this group.
- Check whether results apply to a specific dosage, formulation, or treatment. If so, make sure conclusions are not generalised beyond these.
- Make sure you understand the meaning of all the words used in the paper. Often papers use specialized jargon to obscure the meaning. Typically, when restated, a complex or convoluted sentence hides a simple statement.
- Be suspicious of large studies: if a study is large, it probably has little relevance to an individual patient. Results from large-scale clinical trials are useful to drug companies and governments, not patients.
- Papers describing multiple risk factors or outcomes provide little information. Ask yourself how many statistical tests were used. See if you can estimate how many statistical tests could possibly have been performed and not reported. Remember that the authors may have tested each risk factor and outcome combination.
- If the paper tested subgroups, the results may not be valid. It is possible to segment a large data set into multiple subgroups, for example the number of females aged between 35 and 47 years with red hair. Each subgroup allows additional statistical tests and many such comparisons could have been made. How many possible subgroups might have been tested?
- An important criterion for evaluating a study is whether it is compatible with established science. A clinical trial should be evaluated in terms of current knowledge, including findings in the basic sciences, such as biochemistry, physiology, and pathology. Any result in statistical medicine that disagrees with basic science is highly questionable and probably wrong.
- No particular experimental procedure should be regarded as having a special validity in all cases. Randomized clinical trials are just one way of conducting an experiment. It is at least as easy to mess up a big randomized trial as any other experiment!

With time, you can get used to Bayes theory and find it easy—certainly easier than the over-complication of EBM's statistics. In case of doubt, convert all probabilities and results into fractions of a large population and build a decision tree. Start with the incidence of the disease in the population, and continue from there to examine the full implications of the research.

Socrates' cave

Imagine a brilliant doctor who is trying to be "evidence-based". Imagine that the doctor was trained well but is suffering from amnesia. She can remember little of her education and less of her subsequent career. However, more recent memories, such as her master's degree in medical statistics, are exceptionally clear. Following the MSc, she did a second master's degree in "evidence-based" medicine. Our doctor is in the odd position of being an expert in EBM and statistics, with apparently no clinical expertise or medical training.

The Greek philosopher Plato described how Socrates provided an allegory that applies to such situations. Plato's analogy of the cave describes a group of people who are chained in a cave, unable to see anything but shadows on the wall. They can view a projection of a small section of the world and occasionally they hear associated talking and noise. The people gradually get to think of the shadows as real things. It is all they know. They develop an understanding of the shadows and build up knowledge of how they behave. A person who most accurately predicts which shadow comes next and how it might behave is highly praised. Their culture depends entirely on the behaviour of the shadows.

Next, Socrates explains what happens when a prisoner is released to experience the real world. Initially, the prisoner believes the shadows on the wall to be more genuine than reality. Gradually, the prisoner realizes the difference between the external reality and its shadow. Reality has colour, is three dimensional, and is highly varied. The information content of the real world is so much greater than that of the shadows.

Having become adjusted to reality and learned its nature, the prisoner returns to the cave. The enlightened prisoner now has the problem of explaining how much richer is the actual experience of reality than the limited shadow world of the cave. The philosopher suggests that the enlightened prisoner might disparage the praise and honours awarded for predicting the behaviour of shadows. Socrates proposes that the returning prisoner would be a poor player of the game and the other prisoners might conclude that the outside world has corrupted him and reality has no value. Socrates explains they might even kill the enlightened prisoner who tries to pass on his apparently absurd knowledge.

Returning to our amnesic doctor—with her extensive knowledge of statistics and EBM, she knows about medical shadows. The shadows are the statistical averages from clinical trials and meta-analyses. The information content is reduced. Results are selective and data are filtered to yield vague generalizations. She knows what disease is associated with which set of symptoms. Like most people, she knows that a longitudinal study of boxers suggests they have a high incidence of brain damage.[461] She does not infer that being hit about the head repeatedly can damage the brain, because the result is equally correlated with boxers wearing those funny little silk shorts, gum protectors, and thick leather gloves.

A simple approach

A simple approach is often more powerful than the most advanced statistical techniques. An art expert does not need all the available information to tell whether a painting is genuine—a quick glance from across a dimly lit room may suffice. The image does not need to be the best possible, it just needs to contain the relevant information. He takes one look at the painting and within a moment reports that it is a fake. But ask the expert how he knows it's a fake and his answer will probably be unconvincing: "It doesn't look quite right" or "The colours are wrong" or some other statement that conveys little information. The expert typically doesn't know and cannot explain how he came to a decision.

The physicist Richard Feynman was noted for his ability to solve problems but the solutions appeared to come from nowhere. Feynman's genius was once described by the mathematician Marc Kac:

> There are two kinds of geniuses: the 'ordinary' and the 'magicians'. An ordinary genius is a fellow whom you and I would be just as good as, if we were only many times better. There is no mystery as to how his mind works. Once we understand what they've done, we feel certain that we, too, could have done it. It is different with the magicians. Even after we

understand what they have done, it is completely dark. Richard Feynman is a magician of the highest calibre.[462]

Experts like Feynman do not exercise their genius through calculation or long lists of rules, but by a form of pattern recognition. Feynman did not calculate the path of an electron in his head—he knew how electrons behaved. When you start to learn chess, you need to know the rules for how each piece can move. The rook can only move in straight vertical or horizontal lines and the bishop along the diagonals. As a player gains expertise, the rules change to those of strategy, such as take control of the centre of the board. Novice chess players do a lot of calculations: if I move my bishop to that square, his rook will take it, but my pawn will take his rook, and then his queen could take my pawn… and so on.

By contrast, some grandmasters remember every chess game they ever played, as well as those of all the world championship contenders for perhaps a century. They open with one of numerous standard openings, pulled from memory. Many moves into the game they appear to look at the pattern of pieces across the board, comparing it visually with thousands of previous games. It is move 12 in game 11 of the Alekhine vs Capablanca world championship match in 1927, only the white king's pawn is advanced one square, for example. Grandmasters occasionally play exhibition matches blindfolded, against multiple good players, perhaps twenty games at once. Going from board to board, they immediately recognize the pattern and select between the two obvious moves.

Overrated experts

It does not always pay to follow expert advice. Make sure the guidance is reasonable. Consider an experiment in which a simple rule, or heuristic, is used to predict the relative size of cities in the United States. Gerd Gigerenzer relates an experiment whereby he asked American and German students to predict which of two cities were larger. The American students were from Chicago University, with presumably a good knowledge of the geography of the United States. As might be expected, the German Students had more limited recognition of US cities. They knew some of the city names but little else. However, Gigerenzer reports that all the German students recognised that San Diego was larger than San Antonio, compared with only 62% of the American students. The German students recognized the name of San Diego but not San Antonio, so they chose that city, as it seemed likely that it was larger. The US students recognized both city names but presumably had too much background information to make an accurate choice.

A similar experiment was done to predict 32 FA cup football (soccer in American English) games in England. This study compared Turkish with British participants. The Turkish people knew little about the English football league, while the British participants were far more familiar. The Turkish participants, however, were almost as accurate as the British, predicting the outcome of matches correctly in 63% (20) of the 32 matches compared with 66% (21) correct British predictions. Once again, simple name recognition performed rather accurately. In predicting a result between, say, Manchester United and Port Vale, the Turkish participants knew the name of United and reasoned that it was more famous and therefore likely to be the better team.

Simple but sophisticated

Simple methods and rules can often outperform the most advanced statistical techniques. Let us consider another example. *Multiple regression* is one of the most powerful standard statistical techniques: it uses all the data and is an EBM "gold-standard" method, weighing and combining parameters in an optimal linear fashion. Large-scale trials are sometimes analysed using multiple regression techniques. So, how well does it compare in practice to simple heuristics?

Gigerenzer and colleagues performed a comparison between the two methods, over a set of 20 different environments, ranging from fish fertility to high-school dropout rates.[463] They found that that multiple regression worked well, with 68% prediction accuracy, using an average of 7.7 parameters (equivalent to risk-factors in EBM terminology). Surprisingly though a simple heuristic, Take-the-best, worked even better: it used only 2.2 parameters and returned a prediction accuracy of 73%.

Although it used less data and was faster, the Take-the-best heuristic was more accurate. Five percent extra may not sound like much, but each small increase in accuracy of prediction is progressively more difficult to achieve. You can get 50% accuracy for free by flipping a coin, but each increase above this is

297

progressively more demanding and harder to achieve. Importantly, Gigerenzer and his group simplified the Take-the-best heuristic into a stripped down rule suitably called Minimalist. Even Minimalist had a prediction accuracy of 65%. These results are typical for studies of decision rules—simple algorithms often make accurate predictions.

There is a caution in our tale of Take-the-best and multiple regression. The accuracy was also estimated on the data that was used for training the system. On the training data, multiple regression came out top, with a 77% accuracy (compared with 75% for Take-the-best, and 69% for Minimalist). Multiple regression seemed more accurate on old data than it was in real prediction. This is consistent with the general experience of decision scientists—in practise, complicated techniques are often over-determined and are not as accurate as they appear. The implication should be clear: EBM-style methods often indicate drugs in clinical trials are more effective than they are in the real world with patients.

Choice is individual

Rationality means having good sense and sound judgement; rational decisions are based on modelling the situation. A rational and affluent passenger who wanted to satisfice their need to travel from London to New York might choose any airline that would provide a comfortable, short, safe journey. For the less affluent, cost is more important than time or comfort, and a round-about route with a budget carrier is rational. In either case, passengers might not care about irrelevant "risk factors", such as whether the aircraft was painted red or the pilot was Scandinavian. In economics, rational people are those maximising the utility of their choices, which means getting the most benefit for themselves. Similarly, rational patients want treatments that work effectively, safely and quickly, for them personally. The typical patient wants to recover from their illness and live a long, healthy life.

Simplicity saves lives

Imagine a person is rushed into an emergency unit in a hospital with a suspected heart attack. There are two options. The doctor can measure 19 different parameters, such as blood pressure, as the patient arrives. These results can be combined using statistical software with the most powerful analytical techniques to help the physician reach a decision. Alternatively, the physician can ask three questions:

Question 1

Is the minimum systolic blood pressure over 24 hours above 91?

> The systolic pressure is the higher of the two pressures normally measured, i.e. in a blood pressure of 120/80; 120 is the systolic pressure and 80 is the diastolic pressure. If the answer to this question is no (i.e. the patient's blood pressure is low), he is considered to be at **high risk**. Otherwise, go to Question2.

Question 2

If the patient is 62 and a half years or less, the patient is **low risk**. Otherwise go to Question 3.

Question 3

If the heart rate is above 100 beats per minute (called sinus tachycardia) the adult is at **high risk**, otherwise the patient is at **low risk**.

These questions form a decision tree and were derived from a careful analysis of the data.[464] When compared with more complex approaches, these three simple questions performed as well—and often better—than more involved, expensive, and technically complex solutions. This solution involves only simple non-invasive measurements and provides an effective method of heart attack prediction.

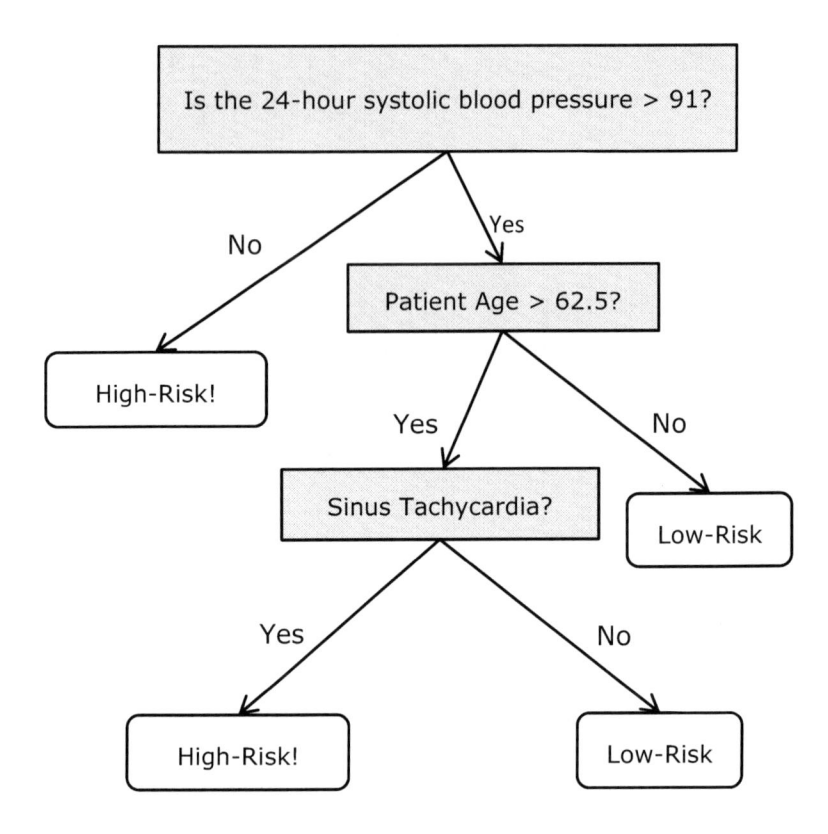

```
                    ┌─────────────────────────────────────────┐
                    │  Is the 24-hour systolic blood pressure > 91?  │
                    └─────────────────────────────────────────┘
                           /                    \
                        No                       Yes
                       /                            \
            ┌──────────────┐              ┌──────────────────┐
            │  High-Risk!  │              │  Patient Age > 62.5?  │
            └──────────────┘              └──────────────────┘
                                            /              \
                                         Yes                No
                                         /                    \
                              ┌──────────────────┐      ┌──────────────┐
                              │ Sinus Tachycardia? │     │   Low-Risk   │
                              └──────────────────┘      └──────────────┘
                                /           \
                             Yes             No
                             /                 \
                  ┌──────────────┐      ┌──────────────┐
                  │  High-Risk!  │      │   Low-Risk   │
                  └──────────────┘      └──────────────┘
```

Note that while these questions are simple, the process of determining which questions to ask and building the decision tree takes some effort. We provided a brief description of how to go about constructing a decision tree earlier. Once the tree has been developed, however, such simple rules are practical and effective, and easy enough to use in a busy emergency department.

Main Points

- EBM's statistics are arbitrary.
- Rational decision making is at least as rigorous as EBM.
- Simple techniques can be as effective as complicated decision methods.
- EBM's linear statistics are severely limited.
- Heuristics are remarkable effective.

> Once upon a time statisticians only explored. Then they learned to confirm exactly - to confirm a few things exactly, each under very specific circumstances. As they emphasized exact confirmation, their techniques inevitably became less flexible.
>
> The connection of the most used techniques with past insights was weakened. Anything to which a confirmatory procedure was not explicitly attached was decried as 'mere descriptive statistics', no matter how much we had learned from it.
>
> John Tukey

Worshiping a Cult

There is no nonsense so gross that society will not, at some time, make a doctrine of it and defend it with every weapon of communal stupidity.

Robertson Davies

The British Medical Journal recently published the results of a reader survey, carried out to determine "the greatest medical breakthrough since 1840." The top five results were sanitation (clean water and sewage disposal), followed by antibiotics, anaesthesia, vaccines, and discovery of the structure of DNA. Not one of these involved a large-scale, double-blind, randomised controlled trial. Even Dr John Snow, father of modern epidemiology (the nearest thing to EBM in this list), carried out a pragmatic experiment to test his theory that a water pump in Broad Street, London was spreading cholera. He removed the pump's handle, and found that the incidence of new cases of the illness dropped dramatically. Snow did not use modern statistics but plotted the cases on a map and used his judgement.

Science does not exist on experiment alone, hypothesis and theory are equally essential. Often, when talking to doctors about medical studies, we are faced with the challenge "But that's just *theory*!" Modern medicine does not appreciate theory. One reason for this may be that throughout much of its history, medicine has been crippled by deference to authority—a phenomenon sometimes called "eminence-based medicine".

Earlier, we described Claudius Galen, surgeon to the gladiators and physician to several Roman Emperors. Modern medicine sometimes describes Galen as generating incorrect theories. However, wrong theories should not pose a problem, unless they are imbued with overwhelming authority. William Harvey helped destroy Galen's perceived authority.

Harvey is credited with discovering the circulation of the blood. Before Harvey, people thought that blood was created in the liver and transported by the heart and blood vessels to the various parts of the body, where it was destroyed. Inspired by the physics of Galileo, Harvey took a scientific approach.[465] He tied off arteries and noticed that they expanded with blood on the side nearest the heart but collapsed on the far side, as blood drained from the vessel. When he tied off veins, however, he found they did the opposite. This suggested that blood was flowing away from the heart in the arteries and back to the heart in the veins. Furthermore, there were valves in the veins and these allowed blood to travel in one direction only—back towards the heart.

Harvey also used the Fermi approach: a simple back of the envelope calculation showed that the heart pumped more blood than it seemed possible for the body to create and destroy. In a short period, the heart would pump a greater volume of blood than the whole body. When Harvey followed the path of the blood vessels, he saw that they branched and became ever smaller, until he could trace them no farther. The simplest explanation was that the heart was pumping the blood around the body, in a cycle: from heart, to arteries, to smaller arteries, to somewhere unknown (capillaries), to small veins, then larger veins, and back to the heart.

The circulation of the blood is a theory and is perhaps the single most important finding in cardiovascular medicine. If you doubt this assertion, would you agree to be operated on by a surgeon who did not know how the blood circulates? Harvey's model is so widely accepted that doctors may take it for granted. However, theories such as the circulation of the blood are the result of the sort of investigation that is missing from current medicine. In EBM, Harvey's work might be dismissed as providing low-grade information. For a start, it depends on methods from the bottom of the EBM evidence hierarchy. Harvey made observations on animals; his work was bench science and calculation. He worked from first principles, to generate a model, from which he made generalizations. Harvey did not perform a large-scale trial with thousands of subjects.

Emergent solutions

The history of medicine shows that it was most successful when it embraced innovation and employed a true scientific approach. Solutions to health problems emerged naturally from the apparent chaos surrounding them. Managers and other bureaucrats may wish to remove such chaos by promoting formalised methods (such as EBM) but a degree of turmoil is essential to science—it reflects variety and unexpected findings. Science filters knowledge out of disorderly investigations. Progress comes from unexpected directions. Had Fleming managed his laboratory, used standard methods and kept the place spotlessly clean, his petri dishes might not have become contaminated with Penicillium. Even if they did, he might have sent them for sterilization, rather than appreciating the importance of the event.

Unlike EBM, science does not rely on reaching a consensus. Scientific pioneers tend to be independent and unconventional. Charles Darwin, despite making one of the major breakthroughs in the history of science, never received a knighthood. His theory of evolution was controversial and remains so, to this day. Although the theory arose from two scientists, Darwin and Wallace, each worked independently. Similarly, the race for the human genome depended on an imaginative way of copying DNA, worked out by Kary Mullis, who made the mapping of the human genome possible. The genome sequencing itself was repetitive calculation, based on incremental accumulation of data. We can think of no major breakthrough in the history of medicine that was made by a committee—autonomous and independent thinking is essential to science.

Before EBM, the authority for clinical decisions resided with each individual doctor. If doctors were uncertain about a diagnosis, they might get a second opinion. Doctors knew the patients' medical history, and had extensive relevant training and skill. In cybernetic terms, they had the variety necessary to achieve an effective decision. An individual doctor was not completely autonomous, clinics and hospitals had organizational structures and often enforced detailed internal policies. However, not too long ago, these policies emerged from discussion between medical professionals, influenced by patients. Professional and managerial policy was based on the experience and practice of individual health professionals. In management terms, the organizational policy was bottom-up, rather than top-down.

"Evidence-based" medicine condemns the experience and observations of medical professionals as anecdotal. EBM's supporters claim to be quantitative and scientific. However, statistics do not provide an effective approach to management. Management science is based on cybernetics[254] and the related fields of game theory, operational research, quantitative methods, and so on. With the

Tarnished Gold

introduction of social and statistical medicine, culminating in EBM, governments have extended their control over medicine and health.[466,467] Patients became clients, consumers of products and services. Now that it is established, EBM will be difficult to dislodge. EBM's claims and propaganda have gained a grip on the minds of politicians and managers.[468] Supporters of EBM have a record of ignoring criticism.

To reiterate: EBM is not based on scientific evidence,[5,469] nor is it scientifically defensible. It represents the introduction of authoritarianism into medical practice.[470] EBM is not supported by empirical data or cohesive theory. It is a mere proposal, which asserts that its selective statistical evidence is the "best". EBM is following its own political agenda.[306] Moreover, there is little evidence to support the teaching of EBM in universities.[471] "Evidence-based" medicine claims to be a paradigm shift in medicine, but it is simply a form of statistical social science.[472] Furthermore, doctors are sifting through papers according to EBM's self-referential "critical appraisal", which they mistakenly believe validates quality.

EBM fails to conform to the scientific method and merely provides some practical tests of limited use. It can determine whether on average a drug works in a population of people. It compares drugs with placebos, which is unethical but helps corporate medicine promote new, profitable but potentially less effective treatments. EBM's methods do not help to explain how a drug works or provide information about how it may be improved.

False reckoning

Proponents of EBM do not want people looking too closely at its philosophy. It claims to subject medical claims to scientific experiment. However, there is little or no data supporting the idea that EBM trials are more effective than the alternatives. In fact, taking a Bayesian approach is at least as good as any other method, including EBM. We have provided a simple Bayesian trial, to show how easy, inexpensive and effective clinical trials could be. The deceptively simple Bayesian trial overcomes most of the problems with "evidence-based" medicine. EBM's approach has serious limitations, which are exposed by such comparisons.

EBM's proponents have presented little or no direct scientific data to demonstrate that their hierarchy of evidence is valid. Lawyers, not scientists, specified the relative importance of the data in EBM. The idea that EBM is clinically useful has little direct supporting evidence. Declaring that EBM is scientific, when it is actually an overly-complicated cargo-cult methodology, may influence doctors by promoting fear and logical confusion.

A natural consequence of these problems is that EBM's contribution to medical research is likely to be minor. We suggest it might be re-labelled as simply *"official medical statistics"* or perhaps *"legal medicine"*. Its results may provide some indication of how many people are having heart attacks in a large population. EBM studies may have some value in suggesting the overall benefit of a treatment to an entire population. However, they are obstructive to an individual patient wishing to return to health.

A pathway to rational medicine

> The basic formula for decision-making is: Use what you know to narrow the field as far as possible: after that, do as you please.
>
> W. Ross Ashby

The practice of medicine could become rational and more scientific. Medicine could be based on data, without authoritarian control of the doctor restricting patient choice. We are not concerned with utopian dreams but with doctors being allowed to practice wisely and with freedom.

Once doctors and patients realise that almost any evidence will be wrong for some people, they can start making rational decisions once more. To achieve this requires that both doctors and patients demand that any "evidence-based" medicine is *demonstrably rational at the level of the individual patient*. Options must be presented objectively, in simple Bayesian terms, and the decision left to the doctor-patient partnership. As Ashby suggested, use the available data to assess and present the possible options; help the patient make a balanced but free choice.

When it's irrational to be rational

Most clinical decisions are made in the absence of full and complete information. A doctor has to make decisions under conditions of uncertainty. The uncertainty arises because not all the information that would ideally be required is available. Doctors have limited knowledge and a limited amount of time and energy to expend on each decision. A rational approach under these conditions is *bounded rationality*.

Bounded rationality is important when decision-making is based on limited information. Nobel Prize winning scientist Herbert Simon first proposed the bounded rationality approach. Simon made fundamental contributions to a range of disciplines, including economics, computer science, and psychology; he is one of the founding fathers of artificial intelligence. His main area, however, was decision-making. In economics, previous models had assumed a population of rational beings, who were infinitely intelligent and possessed all the information they might require to make a decision. This assumption is clearly inappropriate in the real world. As we have explained, people work with the knowledge they have to obtain a satisfactory result, they satisfice.

To take a simple example, the attempt to get all the information possible to choose between a chocolate or vanilla ice cream cone could require more energy and time than is available in a single life. Importantly, the ice cream would have melted by the time the decision was made. It is key not to expend more effort on making a decision than the solution is worth. Medical decisions are obviously important, but doctors have lots of patients, restricted time, and limited resources. Thus, most doctors end up using expertise and *ad hoc* rules of thumb. It is generally accepted that consistent use of heuristics might lead to more effective medical care.[473] What is not often realised is that the use of heuristics is good science.

Humans evolved simple fast-and-frugal, or quick-and-dirty if you prefer, decision making. These facilitated our survival and the construction of human society. For example, when faced with a big cat, our ancestors must have made a quick decision to run or fight. They did not stop to appreciate the beauty of the tiger's stripes and the elegance of its movement. Quite likely, the issue came down to whether the potential prey could outrun his companions, to avoid being the one eaten. There are confounding issues, such as how quickly our ancestors could run, but, critically, those who could make rapid, effective decisions were more likely to survive.

You exist and are able to read this because your ancestors could make decisions quickly, with a minimum of information.[474] The necessity for rapid decisions in life threatening situations has not gone away, and is not limited to medicine; heuristics are essential to survival. For example, driving a car depends on fast decision-making, using limited data. If you are a driver, you have avoided thousands of potential automobile accidents. Learners use heuristics such as, if in the US, drive on the right side of the road. In the UK, Japan and some other countries, the heuristic changes to drive on the left. With time, the driver's expertise increases and the heuristics become automatic.

It is possible for a car to be driven by a computer, using cybernetic methods, although programming the computer is difficult. It is not easy to get a complete set of instructions or to include all the necessary data. Heuristics help but are often incomplete. Human expertise, in driving, as in medicine, comes with practice. However, the statistical methods used in EBM were long since rejected as inadequate and inappropriate for such applications. For instance, driver statistics would not help a person to find their way safely from Boston to New York on a specified day. The journey requires specific decisions, based on particular information.

EBM's problems are greater still. Like a driver's choices, a doctor's decisions are often made under time constraints, in a life-threatening environment, and with incomplete information. To continue the analogy, EBM is like a back seat driver, barking conflicting instructions, which the doctor could well do without!

EBM as the new astrology

For centuries, medicine was influenced by astrology.[475] Even in Victorian England, astrology was considered important in medicine.[476] Victorian women were assumed to be less than honest about their sexual activity, so the way to assess this aspect of their health was by using an astrologer to determine their sexual past.

In times past, astrology was considered to be good science.[477] One of the reasons it lost its influence was that people began to see it as irrational. For example, there is no obvious mechanism connecting the movements of distant objects in space with a person's blood pressure. Thus, astrology does not meet the scientific paradigm. However, its effects are testable. In 2005, Schwendimann and colleagues investigated the relationship between patient falls and lunar cycles, and found no apparent connection.[478] The key element here is refutation—an astrological prediction can be tested and refuted.

Contrary to popular belief, therefore, astrology could almost be considered a scientific discipline. Astrological predictions or hypotheses may have a low probability of being correct. Nevertheless, in principle they can be tested experimentally and shown to be wrong, in accordance with the scientific method. So, we could theoretically convert astrology into a valid scientific discipline—though one that, like EBM, lacks a coherent scientific theory of how it might work.

In a recent large-scale, EBM-style study, Peter Austin demonstrated a positive relationship between some astrological signs and diseases.[479] The real aim of the study was to demonstrate problems with statistical methods in medicine. Austin's large-scale study included all 10,674,945 people, between the ages of 18 and 100 years, living in Ontario in the year 2000. Subjects were randomly assigned to equally sized groups and were sorted according to their star sign. Austin checked whether people from a particular star sign were more likely to have one of 223 common illnesses than those from another sign. The researchers found two significant connections between astrological sign and hospitalization. These subjects had a significantly higher probability ($p<0.05$) of finding themselves in hospital, compared with people born under all the remaining signs combined. People born under Leo were more likely to suffer gastrointestinal haemorrhage ($P=0.0447$), while Sagittarians had a greater incidence of fracture of the humerus ($P=0.0123$). As the authors were aware, these positive results were misleading: the experiment was conducted to illustrate a problem with EBM clinical trials, which it did, in an amusing manner.

Austin tested 24 statistical associations. After increasing the significance level to account for multiple tests, none of the identified associations remained. In other words, the link to astrological signs was simply a random result. The implication is to be similarly wary of EBM's large-scale statistical trials.

Fatal Errors

Analyse data just so far as to obtain simplicity and no further.

Henri Poincaré

Let us briefly review the problems with EBM. Any one of these problems will cause a snowball effect, degrading the medical literature with increasing rapidity. The initial effects of EBM were small. However, as EBM has become more popular, the number of invalid or simply irrelevant papers in the literature has grown.

The issues outlined are fundamental, they imply that EBM is not science and should not be taken seriously. The various problems with

EBM are independent and combine to destroy the discipline as a rational enterprise. Any one issue might be overcome but, taken as a whole, they demonstrate the failure of statistical medicine.

1. We can begin with the ecological fallacy. It is an error to use group statistics to predict the outcome in an individual. This is elementary statistics. EBM uses aggregate statistics and attempts to apply them to individual patients. It breaks a fundamental statistical rule. Pattern recognition methods should be used to address an individual patient.
2. Throughout its theory and implementation, EBM breaks the first law of cybernetics. Ashby's law of requisite variety applies to the information needed for diagnosing and treating a patient. The aggregate statistics and risk factors of EBM are inadequate to address the doctor-patient problem. If we are generous to EBM, it might provide a weak background context for clinical practice.
3. The large-scale randomized trials and meta-analyses of EBM are not appropriate for clinical medicine. These methods fail the good regulator theorem—they do not model the doctor-patient problem. A trial should model an individual doctor treating an individual patient. The appropriate trial would fulfil the Goldilocks requirement of being neither too small nor too large. We described a simple trial in which a family doctor treated single patients using Bayesian statistics.
4. Related to the Goldilocks requirement is EBM's use of over-determined methods. The large-scale methods of EBM model the background noise. Often, they are concerned with tiny effects in large populations. The result is over-determined, which give drugs an appearance of overall benefit, the falsehood of which is often revealed subsequently.
5. The trials in EBM are large and deficient. Even simple probability problems depend subtly on the precise way they are described. Large trials generally involve crude measurement and complex arbitrary statistics. They are sensitive to even minor variations in the way they are carried out. Patients leaving, early termination of the trial, or even what the participants know, can influence the outcome. EBM's methods do not accommodate or adequately control clinical trials. Bayesian methods are more appropriate, robust, and overcome EBM's arbitrary use of statistical criteria.

6. EBM is in clear breach of the curse of dimensionality. This breach is a curse placed on the health of patients. EBM is multifactorial. Multiple risk-factors are common when science lacks knowledge and uncertainty reigns. "Multifactorial" is an inappropriate claim, unless the researchers have determined the dimensionality of the problem.
7. EBM does not adhere to the scientific method. It is a poor induction system, unable to make breakthroughs or even reasonable progress. It does not approach Solomonoff Induction. EBM is simply an *ad hoc* set of inappropriate trials, often aimed at increasing authoritarian control and company profits, rather than improving health.
8. EBM has no underlying rational structure, it lacks coherence and theoretical underpinnings. EBM is debasing science and failing to progress medicine. There is a lack of effective replication and refutation, which are the key factors driving scientific progress.
9. EBM claims that meta-analysis is more rigorous than a standard literature review. Meta-analysis is a simple linear statistical method. Such statistics cannot compete with human ingenuity in performing a scientific review. The application of meta-analysis is selective. Only approved studies are included and other data are excluded. Low quality unpublished data is incorporated whenever it appears useful to the reviewer. Even in high quality journals, meta-analysis as practiced is replete with errors and bias. Meta-analysis is a biased and subjective interpretation of the data, hidden in statistical mumbo-jumbo.
10. EBM selects its data. A major feature of EBM consigns it to the wastebasket. It is not valid to select the "best" data, as the result is cargo cult science. Because of this selection, EBM has the appearance of science but is nonsense. It is not possible to know in advance which evidence is "best". Until the problem is cracked, any relevant information may hold the key to the solution.
11. EBM uses pre-computer and related statistical methods for separating groups. The apparently advanced statistics of EBM are out-of-date. It has singularly failed to apply appropriate Bayesian statistics, decision science, and prediction. Its insistence on concentrating on differences between large groups is an indication that the treatments and effects studied are insignificant to an individual patient.

12. The real clinical problem is prediction in an individual patient. The patient wants an accurate diagnosis and a treatment that is effective and will work for them. EBM avoids the critical problem of individual patient prediction. By avoiding this issue, EBM has little or no real-world relevance to practicing doctors or patients.
13. EBM falsely claims that large-scale trials are important for medical practice. The trials need to be large, because they study clinically unimportant effects. The number needed to treat is low. Significance is rigged using power calculations, subgroup analysis, multiple outcomes, and so on. The results from most of these trials are known to be wrong. But even if they were correct, they would have little value to anyone outside a government or large medical company.
14. EBM wastes research funds. Using scarce resources on large-scale trials slows progress. A single large-scale trial could be replaced by numerous PhD studies or 1970s-sized trials. The chance of finding effective treatments would increase proportionately. The loss of precision in determining slight treatment effects in large populations is irrelevant.
15. Placebo-controlled drug trials are unethical. New drugs should be tested against the most effective current therapies. The purpose of placebo-controlled trials is to introduce poor but profitable therapies. The slight benefits of such new drugs are likely to be overwhelmed by hidden side effects, awaiting discovery. This issue speaks for itself: EBM supports the development of treatments that may be slightly better than nothing.
16. EBM encourages totalitarian medicine. It is displacing the doctor-patient unit as the ultimate decision-making authority. Peer review is used as censorship. EBM is a self-referential closed system, where critical appraisal means checking whether a study conforms to its rules. So-called evidence-based medicine wrongly claims the authority of medical and scientific gold-standards.
17. There is no such thing as *scientific proof*. All treatments are scientifically unproven. EBM repackages and uses concepts from legal proof, in an attempt to impose a medical dictatorship. It pretends court judges are scientific authorities, in order to enforce health restrictions. There is no place in science for such abuse of social power. EBM enables corporate medicine to redefine science as a form of advertising. "Evidence-based" medicine implements restrictions on medicine for the benefit of professionals,

corporations, and governments. EBM reflects what Ivan Illich described as a conspiracy against the public, patients, and laity.[480]
18. EBM inhibits progress by restricting scientific and clinical innovation. Find a cure for cancer and, unless you have tens of millions of dollars or can promise massive profits for a pharmaceutical company, it will remain "unproven". The trials will not be performed and all other data will be described as "no evidence".

There are numerous additional objections to EBM but these will suffice. The rational conclusion is that EBM is a corrupt cargo-cult.

Laugh or Cry?

Democritus (about 460-370 BC), a Greek known as the laughing philosopher, is sometimes considered the father of modern science.[481] A strict determinist and materialist, he created an early version of the atomic theory and thought the earth was round.

However, the people of Abdera were concerned about his behaviour: Democritus was laughing incessantly, without apparent cause. They thought he might have gone mad. They sent for his friend, Hippocrates, to check whether he was sane.

Hippocrates found Democritus sitting under a tree, laughing. Hippocrates talked to Democritus for some time before returning to the townspeople and announcing that Democritus was not mad—he simply could not stop laughing at the irrationality of the world.

About the Authors

Dr Steve Hickey holds a PhD in Medical Biophysics from the University of Manchester, England; he is a Chartered Biologist and a Member of the Society of Biology. His PhD was on the development, aging, function and failure of the intervertebral disk. Following his PhD, he carried out research in the fields of medical imaging and biophysics. His later research included pattern recognition, artificial intelligence, computer science, and decision science. He has published hundreds of scientific articles in a variety of disciplines. Dr Hickey is the author of books on science, health, vitamins, and cancer. He is co-author, with Hilary Roberts, of Ascorbate: The Science of Vitamin C; Cancer: Nutrition and Survival; Ridiculous Dietary Allowance; and The Cancer Breakthrough.

Dr Hilary Roberts gained her PhD in the effects of early-life undernutrition from the Department of Child Health at the University of Manchester, England. She holds degrees in computer science, physiology and psychology. Following her PhD, she carried out research into the development of expert systems, at Manchester Business School, England. She is co-author, with Steve Hickey, of Ascorbate: The Science of Vitamin C; Cancer: Nutrition and Survival; Ridiculous Dietary Allowance; and The Cancer Breakthrough.

Glossary

Agency Problem. When an agent (e.g. lawyer, doctor, dentist, hospital) that is supposed to be acting in your interests works for its own benefit.

Ashby's Law. Ashby's law of requisite variety is the First Law of Cybernetics and states that only variety can destroy variety. This means that an effective solution to a problem contains at least the amount of information needed to describe it.

Bit. A unit of information with the value of zero or one.

Bayesian Statistics. A form of statistics in which new information is used to update existing beliefs. It is conceptually simpler than the frequentist statistics and arbitrary confidence limits used in EBM and equally, if not more, valid. Named after Thomas Bayes (1702–1761), a mathematician and priest. (See Frequentist Statistics.)

Bayes' Theorem. A single short equation that determines the whole of Bayesian statistics. Bayes' theorem is also called Bayes' Rule, Bayes' Equation, or Bayes' Law.

Black Swan. Metaphor for a rare, unpredictable, but sometimes inevitable major event.

Bottom Up. Starting from the component parts, when building or designing a system. (See Top Down.)

Cargo Cult. A sacred practice in tribal societies arising from contact with technologically advanced cultures. Cults use magic, religious rituals and practices in an attempt to obtain the benefits (the "cargo") of the advanced technology.

Cargo-Cult Science. Ritualistic imitation of science. It gives the appearance of science but lacks simple reproducible experiments and refutation. Typically, it relies on selective consideration of hypotheses, theories, experimental methods, and results.

Clinical Proof. In EBM, this means some legally acceptable supporting evidence is available, especially from a large-scale clinical trial.

Clinical Trial. A test involving human patients. A modest form of experiment. (See RCT)

Complexity. Describes high information content and disorder. A long random string is complex, because there are a large number of characters and the next character in the sequence cannot be predicted from the earlier characters.

Confidence Limit or confidence interval. Specifies an arbitrary limit to the variation of a parameter. Typically, it is a subjective value.

Critical Appraisal. In EBM, this means checking if a clinical trial or review conforms to EBM rules; thus it is a circular argument supporting EBM's methods.

Curse of Dimensionality. When adding risk factors decreases the accuracy and utility of your result. The solution has more than an optimal number of parameters or risk factors. (See also: Good Regulator, Over-fitting, Intrinsic Dimensionality, Over determined).

Cybernetics. The study of control and communication, particularly in machines and living systems. The mathematician Norbert Wiener (1894–1964) introduced the approach using results and concepts from a number of existing disciplines.

Data. An amount of information. Data is usually considered the plural of datum (a piece of information or bit).

Decision Science. Discipline concerned with the rationality and optimality of choices: making the "best" decision. Like its close relative, game theory, it is useful in mathematics, economics, philosophy, artificial intelligence, pattern recognition, and computing.

Deduction. An inference in which the conclusion has no further information than was contained in the initial data, i.e. a tautology. A calculation in pure mathematics is a deduction.

Dimensionality. The number of parameters, risk factors, or outputs. (See also Intrinsic Dimensionality).

First Law of Cybernetics. See Ashby's law.

Game Theory. The mathematics of competitive situations or games. In a game, the outcome of a player's choice depends critically on the actions of other players. Game theory is a central part of military theory, business analysis, and biology.

Goldilocks Requirement. Implies an effective solution is neither oversimplified nor overcomplicated. (Analogous to "Not too hot, not too cold, but just right!")

Group Think. When a person's ideas conform to the requirements of harmony in a decision-making group. A form of conformity.

Ecological Fallacy. The error of applying group statistics to a particular case. Applying the results from a standard clinical trial to a particular patient is inaccurate and ineffective.

Entropy. Lack of order or predictability. In information theory, entropy is a logarithmic measure of the information in a particular message.

Evidence. Information offered in support of a belief or hypothesis; legally acceptable data.

Evidence-based Medicine. 1. Form of medicine based on legal requirements; statistical medicine. 2. Defined by supporters as the conscientious, explicit, and judicious use of current best evidence in making decisions

Tarnished Gold

about the care of individual patients. See Evidence.

Fast and Frugal. A term applied to problem solving techniques that are efficient and easy to apply; an alternative name for "quick and dirty" methods.

Feedback. When an action by a system changes its environment and the induced change is fed back into to the system. There is a circular flow of information between the system and its environment. Positive feedback amplifies, whereas negative feedback dampens. Systems with feedback are the main subject of cybernetics.

Frequencies. Can be used as a more intuitive measure of probability. E.g. A 5% probability, (p-value = 0.05), can be stated as odds of 20 to 1 against. Always convert medical probabilities to frequencies.

Frequentist Statistics. These form the basis of EBM and interpret probability as the limit of its relative frequency in a large number of trials. Inductive inference based on this approach is generally arbitrary, as in the use of p-value confidence limits. (See Bayesian Statistics.)

Good Regulator. An effective controller, theory, or explanation. Every good regulator of a system must be a model of that system. This Goldilocks theorem is general and applies to all regulating and self-regulating systems. For example, a homeostatic system in biology must be a good regulator in order to maintain stability.

Heuristic. A rule of thumb for problem solving. (See Fast and Frugal.)

Induction. Also called inductive reasoning or inductive logic. Derives conclusions from examples and is used to make predictions. E.g., since all previous polar bears are white you might induce that the next polar bear you see will also be white. In everyday English, an educated guess is inductive reasoning. Science is an inductive process.

Information. An ordered sequence of symbols that form a message. (See variety.)

Information Content. Non-redundant information. The amount of information contained in a message, rather than the portion that is predictable.

Intrinsic Dimensionality. The smallest number of independent parameters needed to describe a system or data. (See Curse of Dimensionality.)

Kolmogorov Complexity. A measure of how complicated a statement is. (See Complexity.)

Mantra-trial. In EBM, a "well-designed, large-scale, double-blind, randomized, placebo-controlled, clinical trial". See RCT.

Meta-analysis. A statistical method for combining results from clinical trials in a systematic review. The methods involved are typically oversimplified linear techniques and the data is selected, introducing bias. (See Systematic Review and Selection.)

Multifactorial. Resulting from more than one factor, as in a disease with many contributory risk factors. A multifactorial approach often suggests underlying uncertainty. (See Intrinsic Dimensionality, Over-determined, Over-fitting).

Multivariate. When more than one variable (i.e. factor) is being considered.

Negative Feedback. When the output of a system opposes changes to the inputs. The signal is damped and the system tends to be stable. Negative feedback is important for adaptive systems. (Negative is not a pejorative term in this context.)

NNT. See Number Needed to Treat.

No Evidence. In EBM, this often means that there is no data of the EBM-approved kind. It does not imply that there is no scientific data. The claim is usually misleading, as it is not a general statement about the available information. (See Selective Evidence.)

No Scientific Evidence. Similar to "no evidence". In EBM, this means that there is no selected (EBM-approved) data. The statement is often wrong or irrational. Generally, some observational, experimental, or other replicable data is available, or a testable hypothesis has been suggested. (See Selective Evidence.)

Number Needed to Treat. The number of patients that need to be treated for one to receive benefit. An ideal drug would have an NNT of 1. A drug with an NNT of ten would mean that only one in ten patients would benefit. (What NNT would you find reasonable when paying for the drug, being treated, and risking side effects?)

Over-determined. Systems having more variables (risk factors) than degrees of freedom Many EBM trials are over-determined and thus unproductive. (See Intrinsic Dimensionality, Over-fitting).

Over-fitting. When a statistical model fits the background noise or random error, rather than the underlying pattern. Results in apparently excellent models that explain the known data, yet predict badly when applied in the real world. Over-fitting is common in over-determined systems.

Pattern Recognition. The identification and classification of patterns in data sets. In computing and the mathematical sciences, pattern recognition is the basis of machine intelligence. Pattern recognition is use to predict the class of an individual case, e.g., to identify a particular animal as a cat or to diagnose a patient's illness as conjunctivitis.

Placebo. A dummy or sham treatment, a "sugar pill". The placebo's ingredients in many studies are not stated. Placebo drug trials are typically unethical (see text).

Positive Feedback. The opposite of negative feedback. The output of a system enhances changes to the inputs. The signal is amplified and the system tends to be unstable. Despite the name, positive feedback can disturb a system; an explosion is an example of a system in positive feedback.

Power. A measure of the ability of a clinical trial to determine that a specific finding or result is significant. (See Significance.)

Probability. A measure of the ability to make accurate predictions. Probability is a measure of uncertainty or lack of knowledge. It varies between 0 (complete lack of predictive information) to 1 (complete predictive information).

Proof. A mathematical and legal concept that is excluded by the scientific method. There is no such thing as scientific proof. (See Scientific Proof, Clinical Proof.)

P-value. An arbitrary value for a probability. A p-value has no intrinsic rational justification but is used as a criterion of statistical significance. A p-value of <0.05 is conventional in medical research and means the odds that the result occurred purely by chance is less than twenty to one against.

Random. Unpredictable: a measure of uncertainty or ignorance. In tossing a perfect coin, the result is random. There is no useful information as heads or tails are equally likely. The expected accuracy of prediction for a sequence of tosses is thus 50%.

Randomized. Selected at random. In a randomized trial, the patients are assigned to groups randomly, e.g., by tossing a coin.

Randomized Controlled Trial. A mantra or EBM gold-standard trial: a well-designed, large-scale, placebo-controlled, randomized clinical trial.

RCT. See Randomized Controlled Trial.

Requisite Variety. The minimum amount of variety (or information) needed to fully describe or solve a problem.

Risk. The probability of an event multiplied by its impact or consequences. In specifying a risk, both the probability and the effect need to be stated, such as a 10% risk of death or a 90% risk of complete recovery.

Risk Factor. A parameter (e.g. cholesterol) statistically associated with an effect (e.g. heart disease). Risk factors derived from populations should not be applied to individuals. (See Ecological Fallacy.)

Scientific Method. An open-minded data based approach to learning, based on testing ideas (hypotheses) using reproducible experiments. Hypotheses are updated through experimental results and only impossible ideas are discarded.

Scientific Proof. An oxymoron, proof is not allowed by the Scientific Method.

Selection. A powerful method of specifying classes in data. Any selection other than random selection requires information and introduces bias.

Selective Evidence. Looking at only part of the available data and thus introducing bias. (See Selection.)

Significance. A statistical value meeting an arbitrary requirement (confidence limit). Note that statistically significant does not mean important, valid, or useful.

Simplicity. A simple statement has low information content. Simplicity is the opposite of complexity. This is a complicated idea. (See Complexity.)

Solomonoff Induction. The gold standard for inductive systems and a mathematical description of the scientific method.

Statistics. The collection and analysis of numerical data. Typically, it uses probability theory to estimate population parameters and make inferences on samples of data. (See Frequentist Statistics, Bayesian Statistics.)

System. A set of interacting, communicating or interdependent constituents that form an integrated whole. Thermodynamics, systems theory, cybernetics, dynamical systems, decision science, complex systems, and many other disciplines all use the concept. Systems are easy to recognise but difficult to define.

Systems Science. The interdisciplinary study of complex systems in nature, technology, and the social sciences.

Systematic Review. In EBM, a literature review that conforms to some standard methods. These reviews are typically selective and therefore subject to bias. (See Meta-analysis.)

Top Down. Building or designing from the overall system to its component parts. (See Bottom Up.)

Turing Machine. A theoretical computer, described by Alan Turing (1912–1954). A Turing machine controls symbols on a strip of tape, according to a table of rules. The concept defines modern computing. Modern digital computers are Turing machines.

Unproven. In EBM, this means a hypothesis does not meet institutional or legal requirements. NB: All science is unproven. (See Proof.)

Variety. The total number of distinct states of a system. The term can be used in an equivalent way to information. (See Information Content, Requisite Variety).

Wisdom of Crowds. A phenomenon whereby a collection of independent agents or people can outperform single experts in their accuracy of decisions.

Index

American Medical Association ... 6, 13, 84, 247, 251, 265

aphorisms 285, 286

Ashby's law

   Law of requisite variety.... *38, 39, 44, 46, 115, 130, 132, 134, 154, 232, 310, 315, 316*

astrology 308

Bandolier 89, 90, 162, 245, 247

Bayes 26, 27, 86, 108, 115, 135, 145, 146, 148, 284, 290, 294, 315

Bayesian statistics. 5, 26, 38, 84, 88, 99, 106, 108, 116, 117, 235, 266, 284, 310, 311, 315

Bayesian trial.... 106, 110, 117, 119, 147, 243, 264, 305

belief system 26, 27, 127, 137, 139, 143, 275, 277

black swan 33, 34, 37, 138, 143

bounded rationality 156, 307

causality 61, 64

censorship 170, 171, 201, 202, 252, 261, 312

Cochrane Foundation . 6, 169, 252, 254

confirmation bias *198*

Critical Appraisal *159, 223, 316*

Curse of dimensionality .. *225, 228, 230, 232, 311*

cybernetics 6, 8, 21, 22, 38, 77, 131, 132, 183, 304, 310, 317, 320

decision tree 99, 101, 102, 104, 105, 284, 294, 299, 300

Deep Blue 41, 257

determinism 68

drunkard's search 255

Ecological fallacy ... 24, 25, 26, 27, 28, 44, 46, 310

Ecological Fallacy 316, 319

emergent behaviour 68, 258

entropy 112, 113

Epicurus 138, 141, 146, 147

epidemiology 13, 16, 29, 54, 63, 67, 89, 152, 302

evidence hierarchy 58, 163, 180, 198, 259, 303

extraordinary claims 37

false negative 94, 97, 101

false positive 94, 97

Fermi problem 282

Flat Earth Society 49

fractals 92, 142

game theory 16, 21, 40, 45, 155, 304

Garbage-In Garbage-Out 247

gold standard ... 25, 53, 58, 84, 146, 149, 150, 151, 205, 207, 224, 236, 238, 243, 244, 256, 259, 260, 289, 320

Goldilocks ... 38, 130, 229, 310, 316

good regulator 43, 44, 134, 310, 317

hypothesis .. 47, 129, 138, 141, 143,

321

146, 151, 173, 199, 200, 201, 221, 243, 267, 278, 302, 318

information content 4, 42, 111, 112, 113, 114, 122, 243, 294, 295, 315

information theory 38, 68, 316

JAMA 248

legal system 16, 49, 50, 69, 181

Lindley's Paradox 84

Littlewood's miracles 33, 277

mammogram 26, 96, 97

medical screening 89, 90, 95

meta-analysis 4, 142, 162, 220, 238, 244, 245, 246, 247, 248, 250, 252, 255, 256, 257, 258, 259, 260, 278, 284, 311

Monty Hall . 73, 74, 75, 76, 77, 224

multifactorial 20, 61, 62, 63, 119, 225, 226, 311, 318

Multiple regression 297, 298

no evidence 17, 106, 169, 181, 239, 263, 278, 279, 313

Occam's razor .. 119, 120, 121, 126, 146, 225

parsimony 119, 225

pattern recognition .. 21, 28, 29, 30, 32, 43, 45, 109, 231, 288, 290, 291, 296, 316, 318

placebo control. 167, 175, 237, 238

Power Studies *219*

prediction 30, 89, 109, 117, 130, 137, 144, 148, 229, 231, 269, 286, 297, 298, 299, 308, 311, 312, 319

randomization 128, 166

recognition heuristic 83

refutation ... 51, 137, 142, 144, 150, 151, 204, 308, 311, 315

replication 139, 144, 145, 148, 161, 208, 213, 221, 237, 263, 311

Requisite Variety 38, 319, 320

rules of thumb .. 5, 20, 45, 286, 307

satisfice 156, 298, 307

sensitivity 24, 94, 158

social science . 13, 21, 67, 116, 255, 305

Socrates Cave 294

Solomonoff Induction 146, 148, 149, 150, 151, 311, 320

specificity 16, 94

Supreme Court 55, 56, 57

systematic review. 4, 152, 162, 215, 244, 245, 256, 317

Take-the-best 297, 298

Taleb distribution 34, 35, 36

trust but verify 19, 145, 208

Turing machine 149, 150, 320

Twenty Q 31

20Q 113, 230

unproven therapy 279

variety .19, 38, 39, 42, 44, 112, 113, 114, 115, 122, 130, 132, 134, 136, 154, 183, 193, 199, 231, 288, 289, 304, 310, 315, 317, 319

W Ross Ashby 61

Watson 119, 173, 201, 257

wisdom of crowds 155, 258

References

[1] Eddington A. (1958) Philosophy of Physical Science, University of Michigan Press.
[2] Charlton B.G. Miles A. (1998) The rise and fall of EBM, Q J Med, 91, 371–374.
[3] Guyatt G. (1991) Evidence-based Medicine, *ACP J Club,* 114(suppl 2), A16.
[4] Evidence-Based Medicine Working Group (1992) Evidence-based medicine: a new approach to teaching the practice of medicine, *JAMA,* 268(17), 2420-2425.
[5] Haynes R.B. (2002) What kind of evidence is it that Evidence-Based Medicine advocates want health care providers and consumers to pay attention to? BMC Health Services Research, 2, 3, doi: 10.1186/1472-6963-2-3.
[6] Hitt J. (2001) Evidence-Based Medicine, New York Times Magazine, Dec 9th.
[7] Montori V.M. Guyatt G.H. (2008) Progress in Evidence-Based Medicine, JAMA, 300(15), 1814-1816; Commentary and summary of Evidence-Based Medicine: A New Approach to Teaching the Practice of Medicine, Evidence-Based Medicine Working Group, JAMA, 1992, 268(17), 2420-2425.
[8] BMJ (2007) Medical milestones, 334, suppl_1, 6 January, website extra.
[9] Dearlove O. Sharples A. O'Brien K. Dunkley C. (1995) Many questions cannot be answered by evidence based medicine, Letters, BMJ, 311, 257-258.
[10] Sackett D.L. Rosenberg W.M.C. Gray J.A.M. Haynes R.B. Richardson W.S. (1996) Evidence based medicine: what it is and what it isn't, BMJ, 312(7023), 71-72.
[11] Spence D. (2010) Why evidence is bad for your health, BMJ, 341, c6368.
[12] Straus S.E. McAlister F.A. (2000) Evidence-based medicine: a commentary on common criticisms, CMAJ, 163(7), 837-841.
[13] Upshur R.E.G. VanDenKerkhof E.G. Goel V. (2000) Meaning and measurement: an inclusive model of evidence in health care, Journal of Evaluation in Clinical Practice, 7(2), 91–96.
[14] Bellman R. (1957) Dynamic Programming, Princeton University Press.
[15] Bellman R. Dreyfus S. (1962) Applied Dynamic Programming, Princeton University Press.
[16] Rust J. (1997) Using Randomization to Break the Curse of Dimensionality, Econometrica, 65(3), 487-516.
[17] Andrews D.W.K. Whang Y. (1990) Additive Interactive Regression Models: Circumvention of the Curse of Dimensionality, Cowles Foundation Paper 771, Econometric Theory, 6(4), 466-479.
[18] Fuller L.K. Shilling L.M. (1997) Dictionary of Quotations in Communications, Greenwood, Westport, Connecticut.
[19] Whitehead A.N. (2007) The Concept of Nature: The Tarner Lectures Delivered in Trinity College, BiblioBazaar, Charleston, SC.
[20] Robinson W.S. (1935) Ecological correlations and the behavior of individuals, Journal of the American Statistical Association, 30, 517-536.
[21] Greenhalgh T. (1997-2010) How To Read A Paper: The Basics Of Evidence Based Medicine, BMJ Books.
[22] Greenhalgh T. (1999) Narrative based medicine: Narrative based medicine in an evidence based world, BMJ, 318(7179), 323–325.
[23] Video (2011) 7 Billion: Are You Typical? National Geographic Magazine, youtube.com, March 2nd.
[24] Gladwell M. (2007) Blink: The Power of Thinking Without Thinking, Back Bay Books.
[25] Unspecified authors (1999) Encyclopedia Americana, vol 10, Grolier.
[26] Unspecified authors (1971) Webster's Third New International Dictionary, G&C Merriam.

[27] Unspecified authors (1989) Oxford English Dictionary, second edition, Vol1, Oxford University Press.
[28] McCrum R. Cran W. MacNeil R. (1992) The Story of English, Penguin.
[29] Zechmeister E.B. Chronis A.M. Cull W.L. D'Anna C.A. Healy N.A. (1995) Growth of a functionally important lexicon, Journal of Reading Behavior, 27(2), 201-212.
[30] Dilley D.C. Siegel M.A. Budnick S. (1991) Diagnosing and treating common oral pathologies, Pediatr Clin North Am, 38(5), 1227-1264.
[31] Littlewood J.E. (1953) A Mathematician's Miscellany, Methuen.
[32] Taleb N.N. (2000) Fooled by Randomness: The Hidden Role of Chance in the Markets and in Life, W. W. Norton & Company, London, UK.
[33] Taleb N.N. (2007) The Black Swan: The Impact of the Highly Improbable, Random House.
[34] Wolf M. (2008) Why today's hedge fund industry may not survive, Financial Times, 18 Mar.
[35] Kay J. (2003) A strategy for hedge funds and dangerous drivers, Financial Times, 16 January.
[36] Taleb N.N. (2007-2010) Technical Papers Associated with The Black Swan: The Impact of the Highly Improbable, NYU Poly.
[37] Hitchens C. (2009) God Is Not Great: How Religion Poisons Everything, Twelve books.
[38] Ashby W.R. (1956) An Introduction to Cybernetics, Chapman & Hall. This book is currently available as a free download from the Principia Cybernetica website.
[39] Beer S. (1979) The Heart of Enterprise, John Wiley, London and New York.
[40] Siegfried T. National Academy of Sciences (2006) A Beautiful Math: John Nash, Game Theory, and the Modern Quest for a Code of Nature, Henry Joseph Press, Washington.
[41] Schaeffer J. Björnsson Y. Burch N. Kishimoto A. Müller M. Lake R. Lu P. Sutphen S. (2005) Solving Checkers, International Joint Conference on Artificial Intelligence, 292-297.
[42] Schaeffer J. Burch N. Björnsson Y. Kishimoto A. Müller M. Lake R. Lu P. Sutphen S. (2007) Checkers is solved, Science, 317(5844), 1518-1522.
[43] Willams R. (1998) Biochemical Individuality: Basis for the Genetotrophic Concept, McGraw-Hill, New York.
[44] Conant R.C. Ashby W.R. (1970) Every good regulator of a system must be a model of that system, Int. J. Systems Sci, 1(2), 89-97.
[45] Scholten D.L. (2010) Every good key must be a model of the lock it opens, goodregulatorproject.org.
[46] Wein S. (2000) Cancer, unproven therapies, and magic, Oncology (Williston Park), 14(9), 1345-1350.
[47] Miller v. Minister of Pensions (1947) T.L.R. 474; 2 All E.R. 372; War Pensions Appeals, vVol. 1, 615.
[48] Simon, R.J. Mahan L. (1971) quantifying burdens of proof—a view from the bench, the jury, and the classroom. Law and Society Review, 5, 319–330.
[49] Miller W.M. Miller C.G. (2005) On evidence medical and legal, Journal of American Physicians and Surgeons, 10(3), 70-75.
[50] Laville S. Jones S. Weaver M. (2009) Prisoner has murder conviction quashed after 27 years, guardian.co.uk, Wednesday 18 March, accessed 29th Sept 2009.
[51] Frumkin D. Wasserstrom A. Davidson A. Grafit A. (2009) Authentication of forensic DNA samples, Forensic Science International: Genetics, 17 July, 10.1016/j.fsigen.2009.06.009.
[52] Popper K. (1963) Conjectures and Refutations, Routledge and Keagan Paul, London.
[53] Doll R. Hill A.B. (1950) Smoking and carcinoma of the lung; preliminary report, Br Med J., 2(4682), 739-748.
[54] Smith G.D. Egger M. (2005) The first reports on smoking and lung cancer – why are they consistently ignored? Bull World Health Organ, 83(10), Genebra, doi:10.1590/S0042-96862005001000020.

[55] Zhou H. Calaf G.M. Hei T.K. (2003) Malignant transformation of human bronchial epithelial cells with the tobacco-specific nitrosamine, 4-(methylnitrosamino)-1-(3-pyridyl)-1-butanone, Int J Cancer, 106(6), 821-826.

[56] Rubin H. (2002) Selective clonal expansion and microenvironmental permissiveness in tobacco carcinogenesis, Oncogene, 21(48), 7392-7411.

[57] D'Agostini F. Balansky R.M. Bennicelli C. Lubet R.A. Kelloff G.J. De Flora S. (2001) Pilot studies evaluating the lung tumor yield in cigarette smoke-exposed mice, Int J Oncol, 18(3), 607-615.

[58] Coggins C.R. (2002) A minireview of chronic animal inhalation studies with mainstream cigarette smoke, Inhal Toxicol, 14(10), 991-1002.

[59] Witschi H. Espiritu I. Ly M. Uyeminami D. (2005) The chemopreventive effects of orally administered dexamethasone in Strain A/J mice following cessation of smoke exposure, Inhal Toxicol, 17(2), 119-122.

[60] Curtin G.M. Higuchi M.A. Ayres P.H. Swauger J.E. Mosberg A.T. (2004) Lung tumorigenicity in A/J and rasH2 transgenic mice following mainstream tobacco smoke inhalation, Toxicol Sci, 81(1), 26-34. Epub 2004 May 24.

[61] Witschi H. (2003) Induction of lung cancer by passive smoking in an animal model system, Methods Mol Med, 74, 441-455.

[62] Lemjabbar H. Li D. Gallup M. Sidhu S. Drori E. Basbaum C. (2003) Tobacco smoke-induced lung cell proliferation mediated by tumor necrosis factor alpha-converting enzyme and amphiregulin, J Biol Chem, 278(28), 26202-26207.

[63] Davis D. (2007) The Secret History of the War on Cancer, Basic Books, New York.

[64] Oxman AD, Chalmers I, Liberati A. (2004) A field guide to experts, BMJ, 329(7480), 1460-1463.

[65] Tweedale G. (2007) Hero or villain?--Sir Richard Doll and occupational cancer, Int J Occup Environ Health, 13(2), 233-235.

[66] Beckett C. (2002) Illustrations from the Wellcome Library, An Epidemiologist at Work: The Personal Papers of Sir Richard Doll, Medical History, 2002, 46, 403-421.

[67] Singmaster D. (1985) The legal values of Pi, The Mathematical Intelligencer, 7(2), 1866-7414.

[68] Solomon S.M. Hackett E. J. (1996) Setting boundaries between science and law : Lessons from Daubert v. Merrell Dow Pharmaceuticals, Inc., Science, Technology, & Human Values, 21(2), 131-156.

[69] Supreme Court of the United States (1993) DAUBERT et ux., individually and as guardians and litem for DAUBERT, et al. v. MERRELL DOW PHARMACEUTICALS, INC. certiorari to the united states court of appeals for the ninth circuit, No. 92-102. Argued March 30, Decided June 28.

[70] Planning Committee (2003) Daubert: The most influential supreme court ruling you've never heard of, A Publication of the Project on Scientific Knowledge and Public Policy, coordinated by the Tellus Institute, Boston, MA.

[71] Hogben L. (1957) Statistical Theory, The Relationship of Probability, Credibility and Error, Allen and Unwin.

[72] Feldman E.J. (1980) Psychosomatic factors in duodenal ulcer disease, Brain Research Bulletin, 5, Supp 1, 39-42.

[73] Kalaghchi B. Mekasha G. Jack M. Smoot D.T. (2004) Ideology of Helicobacter pylori Prevalence in Peptic Ulcer Disease in an Inner-city Minority Population, Journal of Clinical Gastroenterology, 38(3), 248-251.

[74] Nobel Foundation (2003) Robert Koch and tuberculosis, Koch's famous lecture, Dec 9, nobelprize.org, accessed, 20th Nov 2009.

[75] Berger P.L. Luckmann T. (1966) The social construction of reality, Contemporary sociological theory, by Calhoun C.J. Gerteis J. Moody J., (2007) Wiley-Blackwell.

[76] Brown P. (1995) Naming and Framing: The social construction of diagnosis and illness, Journal Of Health And Social Behavior, Vol. 35, Extra Issue: Forty Years of Medical Sociology: The State of the Art and Directions for the Future, 34-52.

[77] Lipton R. Ødegaard T. (2005) Causal thinking and causal language in epidemiology: it's in the details, Epidemiol Perspect Innov, 29(2), 8.

[78] de Mesquita B.B. (2009) The Predictioneer's Game: Using the Logic of Brazen Self-Interest to See and Shape the Future, Random House, New York.

[79] Tam C.C. (2006) Causal thinking and causal language in epidemiology: a cause by any other name is still a cause: response to Lipton and Ødegaard, Epidemiol Perspect Innov, 3, 7, doi: 10.1186/1742-5573-3-7.

[80] Parascandola M. Weed D.L. (2001) Causation in epidemiology, J Epidemiol Community Health, 55, 905–912.

[81] Charlton B.G. (1996) Attribution of causation in epidemiology: chain or mosaic? J Clin Epidemiol, 49(1), 105-107.

[82] Krieger N. (1994) Epidemiology and the web of causation : has anyone seen the spider? Social Science & Medicine, 39(7), 887-903.

[83] Susser M. (1991) What is a cause and how do we know one? A grammar for pragmatic epidemiology, Am J Epidemiol, 133(7), 635-648.

[84] Olsen J. (2003) What characterises a useful concept of causation in epidemiology? J Epidemiol Community Health, 57, 86-88.

[85] Cialdin R.B. (1998) Influence: The Psychology of Persuasion, Collins.

[86] Baron R. S. Vandello J.A. Brunsman B. (1996) The forgotten variable in conformity research: Impact of task importance on social influence, Journal of Personality and Social Psychology, 71(5), 915-927.

[87] Bond R. Smith P.B. (1996) Culture and conformity: A meta-analysis of studies using Asch's (1952b, 1956) line judgment task, Psychological Bulletin, 119(1), 111-137.

[88] Vazsonyi A. (2002) Which door has the cadillac: adventures of a real-life mathematician, iUniverse.com.

[89] Rosenhouse J. (2009) The Monty Hall Problem: The Remarkable Story of Math's Most Contentious Brain Teaser, Oxford University Press, USA.

[90] Tierny J. (2008) Findings, and behind door no. 1, a fatal flaw, Science, New York Times, April 8.

[91] Brehm J.W. (1956) Postdecision changes in the desirability of alternatives, Journal of Abnormal Psychology, 52 (3), 384 -389.

[92] Chen, M. K. (2008). Rationalization and cognitive dissonance: Do choices affect or reflect preferences? Cowles Foundation Discussion Paper No. 1669, New Haven, CT: Yale University, Cowles Foundation for Research in Economics.

[93] Chen M.. Risen J.L. (2009) Is choice a reliable predictor of choice? A comment on Sagarin and Skowronski, Journal of Experimental Social Psychology, 45(2), 425-427.

[94] Sagarin B.J. Skowronski J.J. In pursuit of the proper null: Reply to Chen and Risen (2009), Journal of Experimental Social Psychology, 45(2), 428-430.

[95] Berry D. (2006) Bayesian clinical trials, Nature Reviews, Drug Discovery, **5**(1), **27-36**.

[96] Gigerenzer G. Todd P.M. & ABC Research Group (1999) Simple Heuristics that Make Us Smart, Oxford University Press, New York.

[97] Lindley D.V. (1957) A statistical paradox, Biometrika, 44(1-2), 187-192.

[98] Fontanarosa P.B. Lundberg G.D. (1998) Alternative Medicine Meets Science, 280, 1618-1619.

[99] Perneger T.V. Agoritsas T. (2011) Doctors and Patients' Susceptibility to Framing Bias: A Randomized Trial, J Gen Intern Med, Jul 27. [Epub ahead of print].

[100] Lopez R.E. Holle R.L. (1995) Demographics of lightning casualties, Semin Neurol, 15, 286-295.
[101] Ridker P.M. Danielson E. Fonseca F.A.H. Genest J. Gotto A.M. Kastelein J.J.P. Koenig W. Libby P. Lorenzatti A.J. MacFadyen J.G. Nordestgaard B.G. Shepherd J. Willerson J.T. Glynn R.J. for the JUPITER Study Group (2008) Rosuvastatin to prevent vascular events in men and women with elevated C-reactive protein, NEJM, 359(21), 2195-2207.
[102] Thabane L. (2003) A closer look at the number needed to treat (NNT): a Bayesian approach, Biostatistics, 4(3), 365-370.
[103] Manuel D.G. Kwong K. Tanuseputro P. Lim J. Mustard C.A. Anderson G.M. Ardal S. Alter D.A. Laupacis A. (2006) Effectiveness and efficiency of different guidelines on statin treatment for preventing deaths from coronary heart disease: modelling study, BMJ, doi:10.1136/bmj.38849.487546.DE.
[104] Bandolier (2007) Statins, medicine.ox.ac.uk/band47/b47-2.html, accessed 30th March 2010.
[105] Anon (2010) Developing evidence-based screening policies for the UK National Screening Committee, sph.nhs.uk, accessed 7th Feb, 2011.
[106] Reynolds J.D. Dobson V. Quinn G.E. Fielder A.R. Palmer E.A. Saunders R.A. Hardy R.J. Phelps D.L. Baker J.D. Trese M.T. Schaffer D. Tung B. the CRYO-ROP and LIGHT-ROP Cooperative Group (2002) Evidence-based screening criteria for retinopathy of prematurity, natural history data from the CRYO-ROP and LIGHT-ROP studies, Arch Ophthalmol, 120, 1470-1476.
[107] Mitchell L. (2009) Evidence-based screening tools helpful in assessing child development, J Okla State Med Assoc, 102(2):61.
[108] Bandolier (1994 - 2007) Evidence-Based Journalism, bandolier.ac.uk, accessed 8th Feb 2011.
[109] Bandolier (1994 - 2007) Screening Whitelist, bandolier.ac.uk, accessed 8th Feb 2011.
[110] Wright C.J. Mueller C.B. (1995) Screening mammography and public health policy: the need for perspective, Lancet, 346, 29-32.
[111] Correspondence to Wright Mueller (1995) Lancet, 346, 436-439.
[112] Horton K.M. (2005) Whole-body CT screening, Online Supplement to Applied Radiology, appliedradiology.com, August.
[113] Brenner D.J. Hall E.J. (2007) Computed tomography-an increasing source of radiation exposure, N Engl J Med, 357, 2277-2284.
[114] Slovis T.L. Berdon W.E. (2002) Panel discussion, Pediatr Radiol, 32, 242-244.
[115] Stanley R.J. (2001) Inherent dangers in radiologic screening, AJR Am J Roentgenol, 177(5), 989-992.
[116] Mandelbrot B.B. (1982) The Fractal Geometry of Nature, W.H.Freeman.
[117] Gullino P.M. (1977) Natural history of breast cancer: progression from hyperplasia to neoplasia as predicted by angiogenesis, Cancer, 39(6), 2697-2703.
[118] Brawley O.W. (1997) Prostate carcinoma incidence and patient mortality: the effects of screening and early detection, Cancer, 80(9), 1857-1863.
[119] Gøtzsche P.C. Olsen O. (2000) Is screening for breast cancer with mammography justifiable? The Lancet, 355, 129-134.
[120] Chapman J.A. Miller N.A. Lickley H.L. Qian J. Christens-Barry W.A. Fu Y. Yuan Y. Axelrod D.E. (2007) Ductal carcinoma in situ of the breast (dcis) with heterogeneity of nuclear grade: prognostic effects of quantitative nuclear assessment, BMC Cancer 7, 174.
[121] Page D.L. Dupont W.D. Rogers L.W. Jensen R.A. Schuyler P.A. (1995) Continued local recurrence of carcinoma 15-25 years after a diagnosis of low grade ductal carcinoma in situ of the breast treated only by biopsy, Cancer, 76, 1197-1200.
[122] Patnaik J.L. Byers T. Diguiseppi C. Dabelea D. Denberg T.D. (2011) Cardiovascular disease competes with breast cancer as the leading cause of death for older females diagnosed with breast cancer: a retrospective cohort study, Breast Cancer Res, 13(3), R64, Epub ahead of print.

[123] Eddy D.M. (1982) Probabilistic reasoning in clinical medicine, in Kahneman D. Slovic P. Tversky A., Judgment under Uncertainty: Heuristics and Biases, Cambridge University Press.
[124] Gigerenzer G. (2002) Reckoning With Risk, Penguin.
[125] Nyström L. Andersson I. Bjurstam N. Frisell J. Nordenskjöld B. Rutqvist L.E. (2002) Long-term effects of mammography screening: updated overview of the Swedish randomised trials, Lancet, 359(9310), 909-919. Erratum Lancet, 360(9334),724; comments: J Fam Pract, 2002, 51(6):513; Lancet, 360(9329), 337-338, author reply 339-40; Lancet, 360(9329), 337, author reply 339-340; Lancet, 360(9329), 338-339, author reply 339-340; Lancet, 360(9329), 339, author reply 339-340; Lancet, 360(9329), 339, author reply 339-340; Lancet, 359(9310), 904-905; Lancet, 362(9379), 246-247.
[126] Roberts M.M. (1989) Breast screening: time for a rethink? BMJ, 299(6708), 1153-1155.
[127] Jöns K. (2004) E2. A joint European strategy against breast cancer: challenges and perspectives European Journal of Cancer Supplements, 2(3), 6-7.
[128] Unspecified authors (2002) 7th Handbook on Cancer Prevention, IARC, Lyons.
[129] Advisory Committee on Breast Cancer Screening (2006) Screening for Breast Cancer in England: Past and Future, NHSBSP Publication no 61.
[130] Blanks R.G. Moss S.M. McGahan C.E. Quinn M.J. Babb P.J. (2000) Effect of NHS Breast Cancer Screening Programme on Mortality from Breast Cancer in England and Wales, 1990-8: Comparison of Observed with Predicted Mortality, BMJ, 321, 665-669.
[131] Huff D. (1991) How to Lie with Statistics, Penguin.
[132] Sutherland S. (2007) Irrationality, Pinter & Martin.
[133] Weinstein L. Adams J.A. (2008) Guestimation, Princeton University Press.
[134] Bland M. (2009) The tyranny of power: is there a better way to calculate sample size? BMJ, 339, 1133-1135.
[135] Shannon C.E. Weaver W. (1949) The Mathematical Theory of Communication, University of Illinois Press.
[136] Strathern P. (2005) A Brief History of medicine, Robinson, London.
[137] Darwin C. The Origin of Species, Gramercy, New York.
[138] Watson J.D. Crick F.H. (1953) Molecular structure of nucleic acids; a structure for deoxyribose nucleic acid, Nature, 171 (4356), 737-738.
[139] Franklin R. Gosling R.G. (1953) Molecular configuration in sodium thymonucleate, Nature, 171 (4356), 740-741.
[140] Aquinas T. Pegis A.C. (1997) Basic Writings of Saint Thomas Aquinas: God and the Order of Creation, Hackett Publishing.
[141] Russell B. (1967) History of Western Philosophy, Simon & Schuster.
[142] Wiles A. (1995) Modular elliptic curves and Fermat's Last Theorem, Annals of Mathematics, 141(3), 443–551.
[143] Popper K.R. (1992) The Logic of Scientific Discovery, 2nd edition, Routledge.
[144] Solomonoff R. (1960) A Preliminary Report on a General Theory of Inductive Inference, Report V-131, Zator Co., Cambridge, Ma.
[145] Kolmogorov A.N. (1965) Three approaches to the quantitative definition of information, Problems of Information and Transmission, 1(1), 1-7.
[146] Li M. Vitanyi P. (1997) An Introduction to Kolmogorov Complexity and Its Applications, Springer.
[147] Isaac R. (1998) The Pleasures of Probability, Springer, New York.
[148] Cochrane A. (1984) Sickness in Salonica: my first, worst, and most successful clinical trial, BMJ, 289, 22-29.
[149] Hawkin D.M. (2004) The Problem of overfitting, J. Chem. Inf. Comput. Sci., 44, 1-12.
[150] Nisbet R. Elder J. Miner G. (2009) Handbook of Statistical Analysis and Data Mining Applications, Academic Press.

[151] Alpaydin E. (2010) Introduction to Machine Learning (Adaptive Computation and Machine Learning), MIT Press.
[152] Japkowicz N. Shah M. (2011) Evaluating Learning Algorithms: A Classification Perspective, Cambridge University Press.
[153] Checkland P. (1999) Systems Thinking, Systems Practice: Includes a 30 Year Retrospective, John Wiley & Sons.
[154] Weiner N. (1948) Cybernetics: Or the Control and Communication in the Animal and the Machine, MIT Press.
[155] Canny M.J. (1985) Ashby's law and the pursuit of plant hormones: a critique of accepted dogmas, using the concept of variety, Australian Journal of Plant Physiology, 12(1), 1-7.
[156] Seth, A.K. (2002) Distinguishing adaptive from non-adaptive evolution using Ashby'slaw of requisite variety, Proceedings of the 2002 Congress on Evolutionary Computation, CEC '02,, vol 2, 1163-1168.
[157] Beer S. (1984) The viable system model: its provenance, development, methodology and pathology, The Journal of the Operational Research Society, 35(1), 7-25.
[158] CNN (1995) Driver in bus-train crash says light did not turn green, CNN News, Oct 27.
[159] National Transportation Safety Board (1996) Highway/Railroad Accident Report: Collision Of Northeast Illinois Regional Commuter Railroad Corporation (METRA) Train And Transportation Joint Agreement School District 47/155 School Bus At Railroad/Highway Grade Crossing In Fox River Grove, Illinois, On October 25, 1995, Record ID 9764.
[160] Ohio Pupil Transportation Safety Committee (2006) Safety News and Views, 2(3), p 7.
[161] Search conducted on 1th Nov 2010 at 19:09.
[162] Fukunaga K. (1992) Introduction to Statistical Pattern Recognition (Computer Science and Scientific Computing), Academic Press.
[163] Murty M.N. Devi V.S. (2011) Pattern Recognition: An Algorithmic Approach, Springer.
[164] Legg S. (1997) Solomonoff induction (Technical Report CDMTCS-030). Centre of Discrete Mathematics and Theoretical Computer Science, University of Auckland.
[165] Legg S. (2008) Machine Super Intelligence, Doctoral Dissertation submitted to the Faculty of Informatics of the University of Lugano.
[166] Hutter M. Legg S. Vitanyi P.M.B. (2007) Algorithmic probability, Scholarpedia, 2(8):2572.
[167] Conan Doyle A. (2008) The sign of the four, Complete Sherlock Holmes, Wordsworth Editions, Ware, UK.
[168] Moyal A. (2002) Platypus, Allen & Unwin, St Leonards, Australia.
[169] Fields W.B. (2005) Hickam's Dictum versus Occam's Razor: A Case for Occam, Award Winner: Research, Innovations and Clinical Vignettes Competition at the Society for Hospital Medicine's Annual Meeting in Chicago.
[170] Hilliard A.A. Weinberger S.E. Tierney L.M. Midthun D.E. Saint S. (2004) Clinical problem-solving. Occam's razor versus Saint's Triad, N Engl J Med, 350(6), 599-603.
[171] Russell B. (1976) The Problems of Philosophy, Oxford University Press, New York.
[172] Cox R.T. (2001) Algebra of Probable Inference, The Johns Hopkins University Press.
[173] Bickel P.J. Docksum K.A. (2000) Mathematical Statistics: Basic Ideas and Selected Topics, Vol I, 2nd Edition, Prentice Hall.
[174] Kirchherr W. Li M. Vitanyi P. (1997) The miraculous universal distribution, The Mathematical Intelligencer, 19(4), 1866-7414.
[175] Turing A.M. (1937) On computable numbers with an application to the Entscheidungs problem, Proc Lond Math Soc, Series 2, 42, 230-265.
[176] Good I.J. (2000) Turing's anticipation of empirical Bayes in connection with the cryptanalysis of the naval enigma, Journal of Statistical Computation and Simulation, 66(2), 101-111.

[177] Kuhn T.S. (1996) The Structure of Scientific Revolutions, University Of Chicago Press.
[178] Harari E. (2001) Whose evidence? Lessons from the philosophy of science and the epistemology of medicine, Australian and New Zealand Journal of Psychiatry, 35(6), 724-730.
[179] Cochrane A.L. (1999) Effectiveness and Efficiency: Random Reflections on Health Services, Royal Society of Medicine Press, London, UK.
[180] Hill G.B. (2000) Archie Cochrane and his legacy: an internal challenge to physicians' autonomy? Journal of Clinical Epidemiology, 53(12), 1189-1192.
[181] Cochrane Collaboration (2009) Archie Cochrane: the name behind the Cochrane Collaboration, Cochrane.org, accessed 12 October.
[182] Sackett D.L. Haynes R.B. Tugwell P. (1985) Clinical Epidemiology: A Basic Science for Clinical Medicine, Little, Brown and Company.
[183] Anon (1995) Evidence-based medicine, in its place, Lancet, 346, 785.
[184] Straus S.E. Richardson W.S. Glaziou P. Haynes R.B. (2000) Evidence Based Medicine: How to Practice and Teach EBM, 2nd edition, Churchill Livingstone, Oxford, UK.
[185] Healy B. (2006) Who says what's best? US News & World Report. September 3.
[186] Holmes D. Murray S.J. Perron A. Rail G. (2006) Deconstructing the evidence-based discourse in health sciences: truth, power and fascism, Int J Evid Based Healthc, 4, 180–186.
[187] Marchetti P. Centor R.M. Donnell R.W. Poses R.M. (2007) Does "Evidence-Based Medicine" Diminish the Physician's Role? The Problem Is in the Application, Medscape Med Students, 9(1), Section 1, medscape.com accessed 11 Oct 2009.
[188] Kuehn B.M. (2011) IOM sets out "gold standard" practices for creating guidelines, systematic reviews JAMA, 305(18), 1846-1848.
[189] Hayek F. (1945) The use of knowledge in society, American Economic Review, XXXV, 4, 519-530.
[190] McArdle M. (2011) Pharma Spending Less on Finding New Drugs, The Atlantic, Jun 28.
[191] Gigerenzer G. Selten R. (2002). Bounded Rationality: The Adaptive Toolbox, MIT Press.
[192] Goozner M. (2004) The $800 Million Pill: The Truth behind the Cost of New Drugs, University of California Press.
[193] Soros G. (2010) The Soros Lectures: At the Central European University, Public Affairs.
[194] Johnson E. (2011) Cancer Society spends more on fundraising than research, CBC News, Jul 6.
[195] Beer S. (2004) What is cybernetics? Kybernetes: The International Journal of Systems & Cybernetics, 33(3-4), 853-863.
[196] EBM Glossary (2008), Bandolier.com, accessed Dec 30.
[197] Horwitz R.I. (1996) The dark side of evidence-based medicine, Cleve Clin J Med, 63(6), 320-323.
[198] Straus S.E. McAlister F.A. (2000) Evidence-based medicine: a commentary on common criticisms, CMAJ, 163(7), 837-841.
[199] Shakespeare W. (~1600) Hamlet, Act 3, scene 2.
[200] Timmermans S. Mauck A. (2005) The promises and pitfalls of evidence-based medicine, Health Aff (Millwood), 24(1), 18-28.
[201] Wootton D. (2007) Bad Medicine: Doctors Doing Harm Since Hippocrates, Oxford University Press.
[202] Hill A. Spittlehouse C. What is critical appraisal? Bandolier Extra, What is Series, 3(2), 1-8.
[203] Loewy E.H. (2007) Ethics and Evidence-Based Medicine: Is There a Conflict? MedGenMed, 9(3), 30.
[204] Anon (1987) 100 years ago, British Medical Journal, 294(6570), 474.
[205] Racette S. Vo T.T. Sauvageau A. (2007) Suicidal decapitation using a tractor loader: a case report and review of the literature, J Forensic Sci, 52(1), 192-194.

[206] Smith G.C.S. Pell J.P. (2003) Hazardous journey, Parachute use to prevent death and major trauma related to gravitational challenge: systematic review of randomised controlled trials, BMJ, 327, 1459-1461.
[207] Feynman R.P. (1966) What is science? fifteenth annual meeting of the National Science Teachers Association, New York City, printed in The Physics Teacher, 7(6), 1968, 313-320.
[208] NHMRC (1999) A guide to the development, evaluation and implementation of clinical practice guidelines, Australian Government National health and Medical Research Council publication.
[209] Belsey J. Snell T. (2001) What is evidence-based medicine? Bandolier Extended Essay, 1(2), 1-6.
[210] Phillips B. Ball C. Sackett D. Badenoch D. Straus S. Haynes B. Dawes M. (2001) Levels of Evidence, Oxford Centre for Evidence Based Medicine, May, CP30.
[211] Concato J. Shah N. Horwitz R.I. (2000) Randomized, controlled trials, observational studies, and the hierarchy of research designs, N Engl J Med, 342, 1887–1892.
[212] Benson K. Hartz A.J. (2000) A comparison of observational studies and randomized, controlled trials, N Engl J Med, 342, 1878–1386.
[213] Koch E. Otarola A. Kirschbaum A. (2005) A landmark for Popperian epidemiology: refutation of the randomised Aldactone evaluation study, Journal of Epidemiology and Community Health, 59, 1000-1006.
[214] Anon (2003) The importance of size, Trials and systematic reviews, Bandolier Extra, January, 1-10.
[215] Press W.H. Teukolsky S.A. Vetterling W.T. Flannery B.P. (2007) Numerical Recipes 3rd Edition: The Art of Scientific Computing, Cambridge University Press.
[216] Knuth D.E. (1997) Art of Computer Programming, Volume 2: Seminumerical Algorithms, Addison-Wesley Professional.
[217] Hróbjartsson A. Gøtzsche P.C. (2001) Is the placebo powerless? An analysis of clinical trials comparing placebo with no treatment, N Engl J Med, 344(21), 1594-1602.
218 Maizels M. Blumenfeld A. Burchette R. (2004) A combination of riboflavin, magnesium, and feverfew for migraine prophylaxis: a randomized trial, Headache, 44(9), 885-890.
[219] Zempleni J. Galloway J.R. McCormick D.B. (1996) Pharmacokinetics of orally and intravenously administered riboflavin in healthy humans, Am J Clin Nutr, 63(1), 54-66.
[220] Blaylock R.L. (1996) Excitotoxins: The Taste That Kills, Health Press, Santa Fe, NM.
[221] Horton R. (2000) Genetically modified food: consternation, confusion, and crack-up, Med J Aust, 172(4), 148-149.
[222] Smith R. (2006) The Trouble with Medical Journals, Royal Society of Medicine Press.
[223] Jennings C. (2006) Quality and value: The true purpose of peer review, Nature, doi:10.1038/nature05032.
[224] Jefferson T. Rudin M. Brodney Folse S. Davidoff F. (2007) Editorial peer review for improving the quality of reports of biomedical studies. Cochrane Database of Systematic Reviews, Issue 2. Art. No.: MR000016.
[225] Ziman J.M. (1994) Prometheus Bound: Science in a Dynamic 'Steady State', Cambridge University Press.
[226] Josephson B.D. (2005) Vital resource should be open to all physicists, Nature, 433, 800, doi:10.1038/433800a; Published online 23 February.
[227] Smith R. (2006) Peer review: a flawed process at the heart of science and journals, J R Soc Med, 99(4), 178–182.
[228] Rennie D. (2003) Misconduct and journal peer review, in: Godlee F, Jefferson T, eds. Peer Review In Health Sciences, BMJ Books, London.
[229] Riedel S. (2005) Edward Jenner and the history of smallpox and vaccination, Proc (Bayl Univ Med Cent), 18(1), 21–25.

[230] Siegelman S.S. (1998) The genesis of modern science: contributions of scientific societies and scientific journals, Radiology, 208, 9-16.
[231] Ipsen D.C. (1985) Isaac Newton: reluctant genius, Hillside, Enslow, NJ.
[232] Milnor J. (2000) The Poincaré Conjecture, claymath.org, accessed 1st Sept 2010.
[233] Lobastova N. Hirst M. (2006) World's top maths genius jobless and living with mother, Daily Telegraph, 20th Aug.
[234] Maron B.A. (2007) Sudden death from collapsing sand holes, N Engl J Med, 356, 2655-2656.
[235] Vandenbroucke J.P. (2001) In Defense of Case Reports and Case Series, Ann Intern Med, 134, 330-334.
[236] Begaud B. Moride Y. Tubert-Bitter P. Chaslerie A. Haramburu F. (1994) False-positives in spontaneous reporting: should we worry about them? Br J Clin Pharmacol, 38(5), 401-404.
[237] McBride W.G. (1962) Thalidomide and congenital abnormalities, Lancet, 2, 1358.
[238] Editorial (1999) Exotic diseases close to home, Lancet, 354, 1221.
[239] Venning G.R. (1982) Validity of anecdotal reports of suspected adverse drug reactions: the problem of false alarms, Br Med J, 284, 249-252.
[240] Tubert P. Bégaud B. Péré J.C. Haramburu F. Lellouch J. (1992) Power and weakness of spontaneous reporting: a probabilistic approach, J Clin Epidemiol, 45(3), 283-286.
[241] Ioannidis J.P.A. (2008) Why most discovered true associations are inflated, Epidemiology, 19(5), 640–648.
[242] Fugh-Berman A. McDonald C.P. Bell A.M. Bethards E.C. Scialli A.R. (2011) Promotional tone in reviews of menopausal hormone therapy after the women's health initiative: an analysis of published articles, PLoS Med, 8(3): e1000425.
[243] Ross J.S. Hill K.P. Egilman D.S. Krumholz H.M. (2008) Guest authorship and ghostwriting in publications related to rofecoxib: a case study of industry documents from rofecoxib litigation, JAMA, 299(15), 1800-1812.
[244] Gøtzsche P.C. Kassirer J.P. Woolley K.L. Wager E. Jacobs A. Gertel A. Hamilton C. (2009) What should be done to tackle ghostwriting in the medical literature? PLoS Med, 6(2): e1000023.
[245] Feynman R.P. (1974) Cargo cult science, some remarks on science, pseudoscience, and learning how not to fool yourself, Caltech commencement address, Engineering and Science, 37(7), 10-14.
[246] Charlton B.G. (2000) The new management of scientific knowledge: a change in direction with profound implications. In: NICE, CHI and the NHS reforms: enabling excellence or imposing control? Ed. A. Miles, J.R. Hampton, B. Hurwitz, Aesculapius Medical Press, London, pp 13-32.
[247] Meggitt M. (1967) Uses of literacy in new guinea and melanesia, In: Bijdragen tot de Taal-, Land- en Volkenkunde, 123(1), Leiden, 71-82
[248] Leighton R. Feynman R.P. (1992) Surely You're Joking Mr Feynman: Adventures of a Curious Character, Vintage.
[249] Le Fanu J. (2002) The Rise and Fall of Modern Medicine, Basic Books, Jackson, TN.
[250] Nobel Committee (2011) The Nobel Prize in Physics 1923, Nobelprize.org, nobelprize.org/nobel_prizes/physics/laureates/1923, 21 Feb 2011.
[251] Feynman R.P. (2001) What Do You Care What Other People Think?: Further Adventures of a Curious Character, W. W. Norton.
[252] Feynman R.P. (1986) Appendix F — Personal observations on the reliability of the Shuttle, Report of the Presidential Commission on the Space Shuttle Challenger Accident, In compliance with Executive Order 12546 of February 3.
[253] Mendelsohn R. (1990) Confessions of a Medical Heretic, McGraw-Hill Contemporary.
[254] Beer S. (1981) Brain of the Firm, John Wiley, London and New York.

[255] Weingarten G. (2007) Pearls before breakfast, Can one of the nation's great musicians cut through the fog of a D.C. rush hour? Let's find out, Washington Post, April 8.

[256] Hovland C.I. Weiss W. (1951/2) The influence of source credibility on communication effectiveness, The Public Opinion Quarterly, 15(4), 635-650.

[257] Peters D.P. Ceci S.J. (1982) Peer-review practices of psychological journals: The fate of published articles, submitted again, Behavioral and Brain Sciences, 5(2), 187-255.

[258] Goldstein D.G. Gigerenzer G. (2002) Models of Ecological Rationality: The Recognition Heuristic, Psychological Review, 109(1), 75–90.

[259] Rodriguez-Paz J.M. Kennedy M. Salas E. Wu A.W. Sexton J.B. Hunt E.A. Pronovost P.J. (2009) Beyond "see one, do one, teach one": toward a different training paradigm, Qual Saf Health Care, 18, 63-68.

[260] Blass T. (1989) The man who shocked the world, Psychology Today Magazine, 35:(2), Mar/Apr.

[261] Milgram S. (1963) Behavioral study of obedience, J Abnorm Psychol, 67, 371-378.

[262] Blass T. (1999) The Milgram paradigm after 35 years: Some things we now know about obedience to authority, Journal of Applied Social Psychology, 29(5), 955-978.

[263] Twenge J.M. (2009) Change over time in obedience: the jury's still out, but it might be decreasing, Am Psychol, 64(1), 28-31.

[264] Burger J.M. (2009) Replicating Milgram: Would people still obey today? Am Psychol, 64(1), 1-11.

[265] Lockley S.W. Landrigan C.P. Barger L.K. Czeisler C.A. Harvard Work Hours Health and Safety Group (2006) When policy meets physiology: the challenge of reducing resident work hours, Clin Orthop Relat Res, 449, 116-127.

[266] Quine L. (2002) Workplace bullying in junior doctors: questionnaire survey, BMJ, 324, 878–879.

[267] Davis D. (2007) The Secret History of the War on Cancer", Basic Books, New York.

[268] Roberts S.J. (1983) Oppressed group behaviour: implications for nursing, Advances in Nursing Science, 5(4), 21-30.

[269] Wyklicky H. Skopec M. (1983) Ignaz Philipp Semmelweis, the prophet of bacteriology, Infect Control, 4(5), 367-370.

[270] Lankford M.G. Zembower T.R. Trick W.E. Hacek D.M. Noskin G.A. Peterson L.R. (2003) Influence of role models and hospital design on hand hygiene of health care workers, Emerging Infectious Diseases, 9(2), 217-223.

[271] Janis I.L. (1982) Groupthink, Houghton Mifflin.

[272] Harvey J.B. (1988) The Abilene Paradox: the management of agreement, Organizational Dynamics, Summer, 17–43.

[273] Rikkers L.F. (2002) The bandwagon effect, Journal of Gastrointestinal Surgery, 6(6), 787-794.

[274] NICE (2009) NICE and the NHS, nice.org.uk, accessed 11 Oct 2009.

[275] Fletcher P. (2000) Do NICE and CHI have no interest in safety? Opinion of the book NICE, CHI and the NHS reforms. Enabling excellence or imposing control? Adverse Drug React Toxicol Rev, 19(3), 167-176.

[276] Miles A. Hampton J.R. Hurwitz B. (2000) NICE, CHI and the NHS reforms: enabling excellence or imposing control? Aesculapius Medical Press, London.

[277] Charlton B.G. (2000) The new management of scientific knowledge: a change in direction with profound implications. In: NICE, CHI and the NHS reforms: enabling excellence or imposing control? Ed. A. Miles, J.R. Hampton, B. Hurwitz, Aesculapius Medical Press.

[278] Charlton BG. (1993a). Management of science, Lancet 342, 99-100.

[279] Jha A. (2010) Government proposes to scrap need for scientific advice on drugs policy, The Guardian, 6 December.

[280] Hickey S. Roberts H. Ridiculous Dietary Allowance, Lulu Press, Morrisville, NC.
[281] Lazarou J. Pomeranz B.H. Corey P.N. (1998) Incidence of adverse drug reactions in hospitalized patients: a meta-analysis of prospective studies, JAMA, 279(15), 1200-1205.
[282] Kohn L.T. Corrigan J.M. Donaldson M.S. (2000) To Err Is Human, Building a Safer Health System, Committee on Quality of Health Care in America, Institute of Medicine, National Academy Press.
[283] Brennan T.A. Gawande A. Thomas E. Studdert D. (2005) Accidental Deaths, Saved Lives, and Improved Quality, 353(13), 1405-1409.
[284] McCannon C.J. Schall M.W. Calkins D.R. Nazem A.G. (2006) Saving 100 000 lives in US hospitals, BMJ, 332, 1328-1330.
[285] Berwick D.M. Calkins D.R. McCannon J. Hackbarth A.D. (2006) The 100 000 lives campaign, setting a goal and a deadline for improving health care quality, JAMA, 295, 324-327.
[286] Hackbarth A.D. McCannon C.J. Berwick D.M. (2006) Interpreting the "lives saved" result of IHI's 100,000 Lives Campaign, Joint Commission Benchmark, 8(5), 1-11.
[287] Tanne J.H. (2006) US campaign to save 100 000 lives exceeds its target, BMJ, 332(7556), 1468.
[288] Trossman S. (2006) Campaign meets and exceeds goal of saving 100,000 lives, Am Nurse, 38(4), 1- 10.
[289] Sandrick K. (2007) Quality exponential: the journey from 100,000 to 5 million lives, Trustee, 60(10), 18(1), 14-16.
[290] McCannon C.J. Hackbarth A.D. Griffin F.A. (2007) Miles to go: an introduction to the 5 Million Lives Campaign, Jt Comm J Qual Patient Saf, 33(8), 477-484.
[291] Wachter R.M. Pronovost P.J. (2006) The 100,000 Campaign: A scientific and policy review, Jt Comm J Qual Patient Saf, 32(11), 621-627.
[292] Ross T.K. (2009) A second look at 100 000 lives campaign, Qual Manag Health Care, 18(2), 120-125.
[293] Nickerson R.S. (1998) Confirmation bias: a ubiquitous phenomenon in many guises, Review of General Psychology, 2(2), 175-220.
[294] Easterbrook P.J. Berlin J.A. Gopalan R. Matthews D.R. (1991) Publication bias in clinical research, Lancet, 337(8746), 867-72.
[295] Hopewell S. Loudon K. Clarke M.J. Oxman A.D. Dickersin K. (2009) Publication bias in clinical trials due to statistical significance or direction of trial results, Cochrane Database Syst Rev, Jan 21, 1, MR000006.
[296] Lovelock J. (2000) Gaia: A New Look at Life on Earth, Oxford University Press.
[297] Watson A.J. Lovelock J.E. (1983) Biological homeostasis of the global environment: the parable of Daisyworld, Tellus B, 35(4), 284-289.
[298] Saunders P.T. Koeslag J.H. Wessels J.A. (2000) Integral rein control in physiology II: a general model, J Theor Biol, 206(2), 211-220.
[299] Saunders P.T.J. Koeslag H. Wessels A. (1998), Integral rein control in physiology, J. Theor. Biol., 194, 163–173.
[300] Dickersin K. Straus S.E. Bero L.A. (2007) Evidence based medicine: increasing, not dictating, choice, BMJ, 334. Suppl 1, s10.
[301] Thomas L. (1978) Biomedical Science and Human Health, The Yale Journal Of Biology And Medicine, 51, 133-142.
[302] Feinstein AR. (1995). Meta-analysis: statistical alchemy for the 21st century, Journal of Clinical Epidemiology 48, 71-79.
[303] Charlton B.G. (1996) Megatrials are based on a methodological mistake. British Journal of General Practice 46, 429-431.
[304] Charlton B.G. (1996). The uses and abuses of meta-analysis, Family Practice, 13, 397-401.

[305] Charlton B.G. (1997) Restoring the balance: evidence-based medicine put in its place. Journal of Evaluation in Clinical Practice 3, 87-98.
[306] Goodman NW. (1999) Who will challenge evidence-based medicine? Journal of the Royal College of Physicians of London. 33, 249-251.
[307] Noah T. (2011) The Make-Believe Billion, How drug companies exaggerate research costs to justify absurd profits, slate.com, Posted Thursday, March 3.
[308] DiMasi J.A. Hansen R.W. Grabowski H.G. (2003) The price of innovation: new estimates of drug development costs, Journal of Health Economics, 22, 151–185.
[309] Love J. (2003) Evidence Regarding Research and Development Investments in Innovative and Non-Innovative Medicines, Consumer Project on Technology, September 22, 2003
[310] Lighta D.W. Warburton R. (2011) Demythologizing the high costs of pharmaceutical research, BioSocieties, 6, 34–50, doi:10.1057/biosoc.2010.40.
[311] Bland M. (2009) The tyranny of power: is there a better way to calculate sample size? BMJ, 339, 1133-1135.
[312] Gest H. (2004) The Discovery of Microorganisms by Robert Hooke and Antoni van Leeuwenhoek, Fellows of the Royal Society, Notes and Records of the Royal Society of London, 58(2), 187-201.
[313] Rahimtoola S.H. (1985) Some unexpected lessons from large multicenter randomized clinical trials, 72(3), 449-451.
[314] Horrobin D.F. (2003) Are large clinical trials in rapidly lethal diseases usually unethical? Lancet, 361, 695–697.
[315] Sever P.S. Dahlöf B. Poulter N.R. Wedel H. Beevers G. Caulfield M. Collins R. Kjeldsen S.E. Kristinsson A. McInnes G.T. Mehlsen J. Nieminen M. O'Brien E. Ostergren J. (2003) Prevention of coronary and stroke events with atorvastatin in hypertensive patients who have average or lower-than-average cholesterol concentrations, in the Anglo-Scandinavian Cardiac Outcomes Trial--Lipid Lowering Arm (ASCOT-LLA): a multicentre randomised controlled trial, Lancet, 361(9364), 1149-1158.
[316] Carey J. (2008) Do Cholesterol lowering drugs do any good? Business Week, Cover story, January 17.
[317] Taylor F. Ward K. Moore T.H.M. Burke M. Davey Smith G. Casas J.P. Ebrahim S. (2011) Statins for the primary prevention of cardiovascular disease, Cochrane Database of Systematic Reviews, Issue 1. Art. No.: CD004816. DOI: 10.1002/14651858.CD004816.pub4.
[318] Geison G.L. (1995) The Private Science of Louis Pasteur, Princeton University press, NJ.
[319] Debré P. Forster L. (2000) Louis Pasteur, The Johns Hopkins University Press.
[320] Judson H.F. (2004) The Great Betrayal: Fraud in Science, Houghton Mifflin Harcourt.
[321] Schulz K.F. Grimes D.A. (2005) Sample size calculations in randomised trials: mandatory and Mystical, Lancet, 365, 1348–1353.
[322] Halpern S.D. Karlawish J.H.T. Berlin J.A. (2002) The Continuing Unethical Conduct of Underpowered Clinical Trials, JAMA, 288, 358-362.
[323] Altman D.G. (1980) Statistics and ethics in medical research III, How large a sample? BMJ, 281, 1336-1338.
[324] Angell M. (2005) The Truth About the Drug Companies: How They Deceive Us and What to Do About It, Random House, New York.
[325] Krumholz S.D. Egilman D.S. Ross J.S. (2011) Study of Neurontin: Titrate to Effect, Profile of Safety (STEPS) Trial, A Narrative Account of a Gabapentin Seeding Trial, Arch Intern Med, 171(12), 1100-1107.
[326] Micklethwait J. Wooldridge A. The Company: A Short History of a Revolutionary Idea, Modern Library, New York.
[327] DSS (2010) Decision Support Systems Online Calculator, Two samples using average values, dssresearch.com/toolkit/sscalc/size_a2.asp, accessed 7th Sept.

[328] Feynman R.P. (1999) The Meaning of It All, Penguin Books.
[329] Gigerenzer G. (2204) Mindless statistics, Journal of Socio-economics, 33, 587-606.
[330] Glantz S. (1994) A Selection of OSHA Comments on Lung Cancer, Responses of tobacco industry witnesses to questions on whether active smoking causes lung cancer or other diseases, tobacco.org/Documents/osha/oshaglantz.html, accessed 10 Nov 2009.
[331] Thomas A. Lavrentzou E. Karouzos C. Kontis C. (1996) Factors which influence the oral condition of chronic schizophrenia patients, Spec Care Dentist, 16(2), 84-86.
[332] Jow G.M. Yang T.T. Chen C.L. (2006) Leptin and cholesterol levels are low in major depressive disorder, but high in schizophrenia, J Affect Disord, 90(1), 21-27.
[333] Daumit G.L. Dalcin A.T. Jerome G.J. Young D.R. Charleston J. Crum R.M. Anthony C. Hayes J.H. McCarron P.B. Khaykin E. Appel L.J. (2010) A behavioral weight-loss intervention for persons with serious mental illness in psychiatric rehabilitation centers, Int J Obes (Lond). 2010 Nov 2. [Epub ahead of print]
[334] de Leon J. Dadvand M. Canuso C. White A.O. Stanilla J.K. Simpson G.M. (1995) Schizophrenia and smoking: an epidemiological survey in a state hospital, Am J Psychiatry, 152(3), 453-455.
[335] Bouaziz N. Ayedi I. Sidhom O. Kallel A. Rafrafi R. Jomaa R. Melki W. Feki M. Kaabechi N. El Hechmi Z. (2010) Plasma homocysteine in schizophrenia: determinants and clinical correlations in Tunisian patients free from antipsychotics, Psychiatry Res, 30, 179(1), 24-29.
[336] Friedman J.I. Wallenstein S. Moshier E. Parrella M. White L. Bowler S. Gottlieb S. Harvey P.D. McGinn T.G. Flanagan L. Davis K.L. (2010) The effects of hypertension and body mass index on cognition in schizophrenia, Am J Psychiatry, 167(10), 1232-1239.
[337] Sowden G.L. Huffman J.C. (2009) The impact of mental illness on cardiac outcomes: a review for the cardiologist, Int J Cardiol, 132(1), 30-37.
[338] Indyk P. Motvani R. (1998) Approximate Nearest Neighbors: Toward Removing the Curse of Dimensionality, in ACM Symposium on Theory of Computing, STOC, April.
[339] Berchtold S. Böhm C. Kriegel H. (1998) The pyramid-technique: towards breaking the curse of dimensionality, Proc. Int. Conf. on Management of Data, ACM SIGMOD, Seattle, Washington.
[340] Theodoridis S. Koutroumbas K. (2008) Pattern Recognition, Academic Press.
[341] Fukunaga K. (1992) Introduction to Statistical Pattern Recognition (Computer Science and Scientific Computing), Academic Press.
[342] Chan A. Altman D.G. (2005) Identifying outcome reporting bias in randomised trials on PubMed: review of publications and survey of authors, BMJ, 330(7494), 753, doi: 10.1136/bmj.38356.424606.8F.
[343] Ioannidis J.P. (2003) Genetic associations: false or true? Trends Mol Med, 9(4), 135-138.
[344] Ioannidis J.P.A. (2005) Why most published research findings are false, PLoS Med, 2(8), e124.
[345] Chan A.W. Hróbjartsson A. Haahr M.T. Gøtzsche P.C. Altman D.G. (2004) Empirical evidence for selective reporting of outcomes in randomized trials: comparison of protocols to published articles, JAMA, 291(20), 2457-2465.
[346] Chan A.W. Altman D.G. (2005) Identifying outcome reporting bias in randomised trials on PubMed: review of publications and survey of authors, BMJ, 330(7494), 753.
[347] Dwan K. Altman D.G. Arnaiz J.A. Bloom J. Chan A.W. Cronin E. Decullier E. Easterbrook P.J. Von Elm E. Gamble C. Ghersi D. Ioannidis J.P. Simes J. Williamson P.R. (2008) Systematic review of the empirical evidence of study publication bias and outcome reporting bias, PLoS One, 3(8), e3081.
[348] Freemantle N. Calvert M. Wood J. Eastaugh J. Griffin C. (2003) Composite outcomes in randomized trials, Greater precision but with greater uncertainty? Journal of the American Medical Association, 289, 2554–2559.

[349] ICH Expert Working Group (1998) ICH harmonised tripartite guideline statistical principles for clinical trials, International Conference On Harmonisation Of Technical Requirements For Registration Of Pharmaceuticals For Human Use, 5 February.

[350] Prenston J. (2005) Composite end-points in clinical trials, Rapid response to: Montori V.M. Permanyer-Miralda G. Ferreira-González I. Busse J.W. Pacheco-Huergo V. Bryant D. Alonso J. Akl E.A. Domingo-Salvany A. Mills E. Wu P. Schünemann H.J. Jaeschke R. Guyatt G.H. (2005) Validity of composite end points in clinical trials, BMJ, 330, 594 doi:10.1136/bmj.330.7491.594.

[351] PLoS Medicine Editors (2005) Minimizing mistakes and embracing uncertainty, PLoS Med, 2(8), e272.

[352] Ioannidis J.P.A. (2008) Why most discovered true associations are inflated, Epidemiology, 19, 640–648.

[353] Ioannidis J.P. (2005) Contradicted and initially stronger effects in highly cited clinical research, JAMA, 294, 218–228.

[354] Hickey S. Roberts H. (2004) Ascorbate: The Science of Vitamin C, Lulu press.

[355] Djulbegovic B. Hozo I. (2007) When should potentially false research findings be considered acceptable? PLoS Med, 4(2), e26.

[356] Djulbegovic B. Hozo I. Schwartz A. McMasters K.M. (1999) Acceptable regret in medical decision making, Med Hypotheses, 53(3), 253-259.

[357] Davies H. (2010) "The Daily Mail list of 'Things that give you cancer'." Facebook, facebook.com/group.php?gid=269512464297; accessed August 16, 2010.

[358] Davies H. "The second Daily Mail list of 'Things that prevent you from cancer'." Facebook, facebook.com/group.php?gid=299519692752; accessed August 16, 2010.

[359] Dobson, R. "Can dogs give you breast cancer? Bizarre medical theories that experts claim may actually be true." Daily Mail Online (October 30, 2007); dailymail.co.uk/health/article-490581/can-dogs-breast-cancer-bizarre-medical-theories-experts-claim-actually-true.html.

[360] Hope J. (2008) Cats and dogs cut their owners' cancer risk by a third, researchers say, Daily Mail, October 8.

[361] Wacholder S. Chanock S. Garcia-Closas M. El ghormli L. Rothman N. (2004) Assessing the probability that a positive report is false: An approach for molecular epidemiology studies, J Natl Cancer Inst. 96. 434–442.

[362] Sterne J.A. Davey Smith G. (2001) Sifting the evidence—what's wrong with significance tests, BMJ, 322, 226–231.

[363] Schena M. (2003) Microarray analysis, Wiley-Liss, New York.

[364] Michiels S. Koscielny S. Hill C. (2005) Prediction of cancer outcome with microarrays: a multiple random validation strategy, The Lancet, 365(9458), 488-492.

[365] Ioannidis J.P.A. (2005) Microarrays and molecular research: noise discovery? The Lancet, 365(9458), 454-455.

[366] Ioannidis J.P.A. Ntzani E.E. Trikalinos T.A. (2001) Replication validity of genetic association studies, Nature Genetics, 29, 306–309.

[367] Colhoun H.M. McKeigue P.M. Davey Smith G. (2003) Problems of reporting genetic associations with complex outcomes, Lancet, 361(9360), 865-872.

[368] Bingel U. Wanigasekera V. Wiech K. Mhuircheartaigh R.N. Lee M.C. Ploner M. Tracey I. (2011) The effect of treatment expectation on drug efficacy: imaging the analgesic benefit of the opioid remifentanil, Sci Transl Med, 3(70), 70, DOI: 10.1126/scitranslmed.3001244.

[369] Hróbjartsson A. Gøtzsche P.C. (2004) Is the placebo powerless? Update of a systematic review with 52 new randomized trials comparing placebo with no treatment, J Intern Med, 256(2), 91-100.

[370] Hróbjartsson A. Gøtzsche P.C. (2001) Is the placebo powerless? An analysis of clinical trials comparing placebo with no treatment, N Engl J Med, 344(21), 1594-602.

371 Bjelakovic G. Nikolova D. Gluud L.L. Simonetti R.G. Gluud C. (2008) Antioxidant supplements for prevention of mortality in healthy participants and patients with various diseases, Cochrane Database of Systematic Reviews, Issue 2. Art. No.: CD007176. DOI: 10.1002/14651858.CD007176.

372 Hickey S. Hancke C. Verkerk R. Schuitemaker G. Hickey A. Roberts H. Noriega L. (2008) Study employed inappropriate statistical analysis, 5 June, in Bjelakovic G. Nikolova D. Gluud L.L. Simonetti R.G. Gluud C. (2008) Antioxidant supplements for prevention of mortality in healthy participants and patients with various diseases, Cochrane Database of Systematic Reviews, Issue 2. Art. No.: CD007176. DOI: 10.1002/14651858.CD007176.

373 Schuitemaker G. Jonsson B. Lawson S. Hickey S. Noriega L. Roberts H. Downing D. (2008) Subjective, selective, and biased, 5 June 2008, in Bjelakovic G. Nikolova D. Gluud L.L. Simonetti R.G. Gluud C. (2008) Antioxidant supplements for prevention of mortality in healthy participants and patients with various diseases, Cochrane Database of Systematic Reviews, Issue 2. Art. No.: CD007176. DOI: 10.1002/14651858.CD007176.

374 Hróbjartsson A, Gøtzsche PC. (2004) Placebo treatment versus no treatment, Cochrane Database Syst Rev, (1):CD003974.

375 Gerss J. Köpcke W. (2009) The questionable association of vitamin e supplementation and mortality—inconsistent results of different meta-analytic approaches, Cell Mol Biol (Noisy-le-grand) 55, Suppl (2009), OL1111–OL1120.

376 WMA (2004) World Medical Association Declaration of Helsinki: Ethical Principles for Medical Research Involving Human Subjects. Ferney-le-Voltaire, France: World Medical Association.

377 WMA (2008) World Medical Association Declaration of Helsinki Ethical Principles for Medical Research Involving Human Subjects, 59th WMA General Assembly, Seoul, October.

378 Rolnick A.J. Weber W.E. (1986) Gresham's law or Gresham's fallacy? Journal of Political Economy, 94 (1), 185–199.

379 Wolinsky H. (2006) The battle of Helsinki: Two troublesome paragraphs in the Declaration of Helsinki are causing a furore over medical research ethics, EMBO reports 7, 7, 670–672.

380 Laffont J. Tirole J. (1991) The politics of government decision-making: a theory of regulatory capture, The Quarterly Journal of Economics, 106(4), 1089-1127.

381 Hanson J. Yosifon D. The situation: an introduction to the situational character, critical realism, power economics, and deep capture, University Of Pennsylvania Law Review, 152, 129-346.

382 Egilman D.S. Presler A.H. Valentin C.S. (2007) Avoiding the Regulatory Capture of the Food and Drug Administration, Arch Intern Med, 167, 732-733.

383 Elliot C. (2004) Six problems with pharma-funded bioethics, Studies in History and Philosophy of Science Part C: Studies in History and Philosophy of Biological and Biomedical Sciences, 35(1), 125-129.

384 FDA (2010) Prescription drug user fee rates for fiscal year 2011, us food and drug administration, Federal Register, 75(149), August 4.

385 Moynihan R. (2002) Alosetron: a case study in regulatory capture, or a victory for patients' rights? BMJ, 325, 592-595.

386 Goldman D.P. Berry S.H. McCabe M.S. Kilgore M.L. Potosky A.L. Schoenbaum M.L. Schonlau M. Weeks J.C. Kaplan R. Escarce J.J. (2003) Incremental treatment costs in national cancer institute-sponsored clinical trials, JAMA, 289(22), 2970-2977.

387 CuttingEdgeInfo (2011) Clinical operations (ph152) benchmarking per-patient trial costs, staffing and adaptive design, cuttingedgeinfo.com, accessed 2011, 10 July.

388 Goldfarb N.M. (2011) Review of: clinical operations: benchmarking per-patient trial costs, staffing and adaptive design, cutting edge information, Journal of Clinical Research Best Practices, 7, 5.

[389] Hoffer A. (2004) Controlled therapeutic trials: disadvantages and advantages, Journal of Orthomolecular Medicine, 19(3), 131.
[390] The Book of Daniel, Chapter 1:1-16, The Bible,
[391] Hemingway P. Brereton N. (2009) What is a systematic review? Bandolier, NPR09/1111.
[392] Consensus Report (2011) Finding what works in health care: standards for systematic reviews, Institute of Medicine, US National Academy of Sciences, March 23.
[393] Juffer F. van IJzendoorn M.H. (2005) Behavior problems and mental health referrals of international adoptees, a meta-analysis, JAMA, 293, 2501-2515.
[394] Porter M. Haslam N. (2005) Predisplacement and postdisplacement factors associated with mental health of refugees and internally displaced persons, a meta-analysis, JAMA, 294, 602-612.
[395] Barone J.E. (2000) Comparing apples and oranges: a randomised prospective study, BMJ, 321(7276), 1569-1570.
[396] Higgins J.P.T. Green S. (2008) Cochrane Handbook for Systematic Reviews of Interventions Version 5.0.0 February, The Cochrane Collaboration.
[397] Kendrick D. Coupland C. Mulvaney C. Simpson J. Smith S.J. Sutton A. Watson M. Woods A. (2007) Home safety education and provision of safety equipment for injury prevention, Cochrane Database of Systematic Reviews, Issue 1, CD005014.
[398] Adams N. Lasserson T.J. Cates C.J. Jones P.W. (2007) Fluticasone versus beclomethasone or budesonide for chronic asthma in adults and children, Cochrane Database of Systematic Reviews, Issue 4, CD002310.
[399] Ferguson T. Wilcken N. Vagg R. Ghersi D. Nowak A.K. (2007) Taxanes for adjuvant treatment of early breast cancer. Cochrane Database of Systematic Reviews, Issue 4, CD004421.
[400] Kaplan A. Wolf C. (1998) The Conduct of Inquiry: Methodology for Behavioral Science, Transaction Publishers, Edison, NJ.
[401] Farris G.F. (1968) The drunkard's search in behavioral science, Prepared for presentation at the Society for Personnel Administration Annual Conference, June 6, Washington DC.
[402] Shamliyan T. Kane R.L. Jansen S. (2010) Quality of systematic reviews of observational nontherapeutic studies, Prev Chronic Dis, 7(6), cdc.gov/pcd/issues/2010/nov/09_0195.htm.
[403] Bailar III J. (1997) The promise and problems of meta analysis, New England Journal of Medicine, 337, 559-561.
[404] Weber W.C. (2011) Why 'Watson' matters to lawyers, The National Law Journal, Feb 14th.
[405] Markoff J. (2011) Smarter than you think, armies of expensive lawyers, replaced by cheaper software, The New York Times, Science, March 4th.
[406] Surowiecki J. (2004) The Wisdom of Crowds, Doubleday.
[407] Levy D.M. Peart S. (2002) Galton's two papers on voting as robust estimation, Public Choice, 113, 357–365.
[408] Beni G. Wang J. (1989) Swarm intelligence in cellular robotic systems, Proceedings. NATO Advanced Workshop on Robots and Biological Systems, Tuscany, Italy, June 26–30.
[409] Hu X. Zhang J. Li Y. (2008) Orthogonal methods based ant colony search for solving continuous optimization problems, Journal of Computer Science and Technology, 23 (1). 2-18.
[410] Feinstein A.R. (1995) Meta-analysis: statistical alchemy for the 21st century, Journal of Clinical Epidemiology, 48(1), 71-79.
[411] Cooper T. Ainsberg A. (2010) Breakthrough: Elizabeth Hughes, the Discovery of Insulin, and the Making of a Medical Miracle, St. Martin's Press.
[412] Willey J. (2011) Wonder cure for diabetes, Daily Express, June 24.
[413] Bosely S. (2011) Low-calorie diet offers hope of cure for type 2 diabetes, The Guardian, June 24.

414 Lim E.L. Hollingsworth K.G. Aribisala B.S. Chen M.J. Mathers J.C. Taylor R. (2011) Reversal of type 2 diabetes: normalisation of beta cell function in association with decreased pancreas and liver triacylglycerol, Diabetologia DOI 10.1007/s00125-011-2204-7.

415 Press office (2011) Diet reverses Type 2 Diabetes, Newcastle University, ncl.ac.uk

416 Cousens G. (2008) There Is a Cure for Diabetes: The Tree of Life 21-Day+ Program, North Atlantic Books.

417 Wilson D.J. (2009) Polio, Biographies of Disease, Greenwood.

418 Klenner F. (1949) JAMA, September 3, 141(1), 1-8. Reported by Landwehr R. in The Origin of the 42-Year Stonewall of Vitamin C, Journal of Orthomolecular Medicine, 6(2), 1991, 99-103.

419 Klenner F. (1949) The treatment of poliomyelitis and other virus diseases with vitamin C", Journal of Southern Medicine and Surgery, 3(7), 211-212.

420 Kneen R. Solomon T. Appleton R. (2002) The role of lumbar puncture in suspected CNS infection-a disappearing skill? Arch Dis Child, 87(3), 181-183.

421 Chezzi C. (1996) Rapid diagnosis of poliovirus infection by PCR amplification, J Clin Microbiol, 34(7), 1722-1725.

422 No authors listed (1997) Case definitions for infectious conditions under public health surveillance, Centers for Disease Control and Prevention, MMWR Recomm Rep, 46(RR-10), 1-55.

423 Hickey S. Roberts H.J. Cathcart R.F. (2005) Dynamic flow, Journal of Orthomolecular Medicine, 20(4), 237-244.

424 Pascuzzi R.M. (1992) Poliomyelitis and the postpolio syndrome, Semin Neurol, 12(3), 193-199.

425 Estrada B. (2007) Poliomyelitis, eMedicine (infectious disease), August 15.

426 CDC (2011) Poliomyelitis, Epidemiology and Prevention of Vaccine-Preventable Diseases, The Pink Book, 12th Edition April.

427 WHO (2008) Poliomyelitis, WHO factsheet, No 114, January.

428 Atkinson W. Hamborsky J. McIntyre L., Wolfe S. (2007) Poliomyelitis, Epidemiology and Prevention of Vaccine-Preventable Diseases, The Pink Book, 10th ed., Public Health Foundation, 101–114.

429 Nathanson N. Martin J.R. (1979) The epidemiology of poliomyelitis: enigmas surrounding its appearance, epidemicity, and disappearance, Am J Epidemiol, 110(6), 672-692.

430 Howard R.S. (2005) Poliomyelitis and the postpolio syndrome, clinical review, BMJ, 330, 1314-1318

431 Watkins A.L. (1949) Progressive disabilities in poliomyelitis, in International Poliomyelitis Congress, Poliomyelitis: papers and discussions presented at the Second International Poliomyelitis Conference, Philadelphia, Lippincott, 142-147.

432 Green W.R. (1949) The management of poliomyelitis: the convalescent state, in Poliomyelitis: papers and discussions presented at the First International Poliomyelitis Conference, Philadelphia, Lippincott, 165-185.

433 Price R.W. Plum F. (1978) Poliomyelitis, in Vinken P.J. Bruyn G.W. Klawans H.L. eds. Handbook of clinical neurology, Vol 34. Infections of the nervous system, part 2,. North-Holland, 93-132.

434 Strebel P.M. Sutter R.W. Cochi S.L. Biellik R.J. Brink E.W. Kew O.M. Pallansch M.A. Orenstein W.A. Hinman A.R. (1992) Epidemiology of poliomyelitis in the United States one decade after the last reported case of indigenous wild virus-associated disease, Clin Infect Dis, 14(2), 568-579.

435 Holland H. (2000) Dr. Henry writes about the Virginia Polio Epidemic of 1950, Lincolnshire Post Polio Network, originally published in the Central Va PPS Support Group (PPSG)'s newsletter, The Deja View, August/September issue.

[436] Walsh F.B. Hoyt W.F. Miller N.R. Newman N.J. Biousse V. Kerrison J.B. (2004) Walsh & Hoyt's Clinical Neuro-Ophthalmology, Lippincott Williams and Wilkins.
[437] Millar A.H. Buck L.S. (1950) Tracheotomy in bulbar poliomyelitis, Calif Med, 72(1), 34-36.
[438] Wackers G. (1994) Constructivist Medicine, PhD thesis, Universitaire Pers Maastricht.
[439] Ariely D. (2008) Predictably Irrational: The Hidden Forces That Shape Our Decisions, Harper Collins.
[440] Landwehr R. (1991) The origin of the 42-year stonewall of vitamin c, Journal of Orthomolecular Medicine, 6(2), 99-103.
[441] 3 News (2010) Living proof: Vitamin C - Miracle Cure? Wed, 18 Aug, 19:30; A family's fight for a dying man, Thu, 19 Aug, 19:00, 3news.co.nz.
[442] Rogers M. (2010) High-dosage vitamin c therapy, ADHB Media Release, September 14.
[443] Coveney P. Highfield R. (1991) The Arrow of Time, Flamingo, London.
[444] Sample I. (2007) The god of small things, The Guardian, Saturday 17 November.
[445] Bell J.S. On the Einstein-Poldolsky-Rosen paradox, Physics, 1, 195-200.
[446] Rifkin E. Bouwer E. (2007) The Illusion of Certainty, Springer.
447 Perlman M.D. Wu L (1999) The emperor's new tests, Statistical Science, 14, 355-381.
[448] Weinstein L. Adam J.A. (2008) Guesstimation: Solving the World's Problems on the Back of a Cocktail Napkin, Princeton University Press.
[449] Fermi E. (1945) Trinity Test, July 16, Eyewitness Accounts, U.S. National Archives, Record Group 227, OSRD-S1 Committee, Box 82 folder 6, "Trinity."
[450] Lagemann R.T. (1977) New light on old rays: N rays, American Journal of Physics, 45(3), 281-284.
[451] Wood R.W. (1904) The N-Rays, Nature 70 (1822), 530–531.
[452] Hippocrates (400 BC) Aphorisms, translated by Francis Adams, classics.mit.edu/Hippocrates/aphorisms.html, accessed 19 Nov 2009.
[453] GreenHalgh T. (1999) Narrative based medicine: Narrative based medicine in an evidence based world, BMJ, 318(7179), 323–325.
[454] Hunter K.M. (1996) Narrative, literature, and the clinical exercise of practical reason, The Journal of Medicine and Philosophy, 21(3), 303-320.
[455] McWhinney I.R. (1978) Medical knowledge and the rise of technology, The Journal of Medicine and Philosophy, 3(4), 293-304.
[456] Tanenbaum SJ. (1993) What physicians know, N Engl J Med, 329(17), 1268-1271.
[457] Pólya G. (1945). How to Solve It, Princeton University Press.
[458] Pólya G. (1992) Mathematics and Plausible Reasoning, Volume 1: Induction and Analogy in Mathematics, Volume 2: Patterns of Plausible Inference (1953), Princeton University Press.
[459] Cioffi J. (1997) Heuristics, servants to intuition, in clinical decision-making, J Adv Nurs, 26(1), 203-208.
[460] Gigerenzer G. (2002) Adaptive Thinking: Rationality in the Real World, Evolution and Cognition Series, Oxford University Press.
[461] Zetterberg H. Hietala M.A. Jonsson M. Andreasen N. Styrud E. Karlsson I. Edman A. Popa C. Rasulzada A. Wahlund L.O. Mehta P.D. Rosengren L. Blennow K. Wallin A. (2006) Neurochemical aftermath of amateur boxing, Arch Neurol, 63(9), 1277-1280.
[462] Kac M. (1985) Enigmas of Chance, Harper and Row.
[463] Czerlinski J. Gigerenzer G. Goldstein D.G. (1999). How good are simple heuristics? In Gigerenzer G. Todd P.M. ABC Research Group, Simple Heuristics That Make Us Smart, Oxford University Press.
[464] Breiman L. Friedman J. Stone C.J. Olshen R.A. (1984) Classification and Regression Trees, Chapman & Hall/CRC.
[465] Strathern P. (2005) A Brief History of Medicine from Hippocrates to Gene therapy, Robinson, London.

466 Klein R. (1989) The politics of the National health service, Longman, London.
467 Jenkins S. (1995) Accountable to none - the Tory nationalization of Britain, Hamish Hamilton, London.
468 Charlton B.G. Miles A. (1998) The rise and fall of EBM, Q J Med, 91, 371–374.
469 Haynes R.B. (2002) What kind of evidence is it that Evidence-Based Medicine advocates want health care providers and consumers to pay attention to? BMC Health Services Research, 2, 3, doi: 10.1186/1472-6963-2-3.
470 Shahar E. (1997) A Popperian perspective of the term 'evidence-based medicine', Journal of Evaluation in Clinical Practice, 3(2), 109-116.
471 Dobbie A.E. Schneider F.D. Anderson A.D. Littlefield J. (2000) What evidence supports teaching evidence-based medicine? Academic Medicine, 75(12), 1184-1185.
472 Couto J.S. (1998) Evidence-based medicine: a Kuhnian perspective of a transvestite non-theory, J Eval Clin Pract, 4(4), 267-275.
473 McDonald C.J.(1996) Medical heuristics: the silent adjudicators of clinical practice, Ann Intern Med, 124(1 Pt 1), 56-62.
474 Hertwig R. Todd P.M. (2003) More Is Not Always Better: The Benefits of Cognitive Limits, In Thinking: Psychological Perspectives on Reasoning, Judgment and Decision Making, ed Hardman D. Macchi L., John Wiley & Son.
475 Siraisi N.G. Medieval and Early Renaissance Medicine: Introduction to Knowledge and Practice, Chicago University Press.
476 Kassel L. (1999) How to read Simon Forman's casebooks: medicine, astrology, and gender in Elizabethan London, Soc Hist Med, 12(1), 3-18.
477 Williams S.J. (2010) Astro-medicine: astrology and medicine, East and West, Bulletin of the History of Medicine, 84(1), 120-121.
478 Schwendimann R. Joos F. De Geest S. Milisen K. (2005) Are patient falls in the hospital associated with lunar cycles? A retrospective observational study, BMC Nurs, 4, 5.
479 Austin P.C. Mamdani M.M. Juurlink D.N. Hux J.E. (2006) Testing multiple statistical hypotheses resulted in spurious associations: a study of astrological signs and health, Journal of Clinical Epidemiology, 59, 964-969.
480 Illich I. (1982) Medical Nemesis, Pantheon.
481 Gossin P. (2002) Encyclopedia of Literature and Science, Greenwood Press, Santa Barbara, CA.

Made in the USA
Columbia, SC
14 February 2020